METHODS IN SOCIAL EPIDEMIOLOGY

J. Michael Oakes
Jay S. Kaufman

Editors

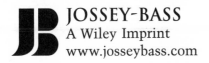

JOSSEY-BASS
A Wiley Imprint
www.josseybass.com

Published by Jossey-Bass
A Wiley Imprint
989 Market Street, San Francisco, CA 94103-1741   www.josseybass.com

Library of Congress Cataloging-in-Publication Data
Methods in social epidemiology / edited by J. Michael Oakes and Jay
  S. Kaufman.
     p. cm.
   Includes bibliographical references and index.
   ISBN-13: 978-0-7879-7989-8 (alk. paper)
   ISBN-10: 0-7879-7989-9 (alk. paper)
   1. Social medicine.   2. Epidemiology—Social aspects.   I. Oakes, J.
Michael, 1967-   .   II. Kaufman, Jay S., 1963-   .
   [DNLM: 1. Epidemiologic Methods.   2. Social Medicine.
WA 950 M59205 2006]
RA418.M48 2006
614.4—dc22   2006008431

Printed in the United States of America
FIRST EDITION
HB Printing 10 9 8 7 6 5 4 3 2 1

TABLE OF CONTENTS

TABLES & FIGURES

Tables

Figures

ABOUT THE EDITORS

J. Michael Oakes, Ph.D., is an Assistant Professor in the Division of Epidemiology and Community Health, University of Minnesota, and is affiliated with the Minnesota Population Center, the University's Metropolitan Design Center, and its Institute for Advanced Study. His research interests include social epidemiology, research methodology, and human research subject protections. Originally trained in sociological methodology and microeconomics at the University of Massachusetts, Dr. Oakes has authored papers exploring neighborhood effects, the measurement of socioeconomic status in health research, and the role of political-economic theory in social epidemiology. His recent work concerns "identification problems," especially in matched propensity score and regression models relying on observational designs. Dr. Oakes teaches graduate-level courses in secondary data analysis (with Stata), SAS programming, and group randomized trials, as well as a doctoral seminar on social epidemiology. He regularly attends National Institutes of Health study sections and consults with a number of not-for-profit community organizations. He established and currently directs the Social Epi Workgroup at the University of Minnesota.

Jay S. Kaufman, Ph.D., is an Associate Professor in the Department of Epidemiology, University of North Carolina at Chapel Hill, a Fellow at the Carolina Population Center, and a Research Fellow at the Sheps Center for Health Services Research. Dr. Kaufman's research interests include social epidemiology, minority health, statistical methodology, and health care. He has published widely on social epidemiology, causal inference, and international health, among other topics, and is an Associate Editor for *Epidemiologic Perspectives and Innovations* and serves on the editorial board of the journal *Epidemiology*. His current research projects include research on social and community factors in the etiology of adverse birth outcomes, social position over the life course in relation to cardiovascular disease, non-parametric methods for covariate control and identification of direct effects for social factors, and racial and ethnic disparities associated with provision of medical care. Dr. Kaufman teaches courses in regression analysis and epidemiologic methods.

ABOUT THE AUTHORS

David Betson, Ph.D., is an Associate Professor and the former Director of the Hesburgh Program in Public Service at the University of Notre Dame. Currently, he is the Chair of the Panel to Evaluate the National Estimates of Participants in the Women, Infant and Children (WIC) Program to Insure Full Funding of the Program. His research has dealt with the impact of tax and transfer programs on the economy and the distribution of income. A particular area of interest is child support policy in which he has written academic papers and consulted with numerous state governments on the development of their child support guidelines.

Tony Blakely, M.B.Ch.B., M.P.H., Ph.D., F.A.F.P.H.M., is an Associate Professor in the Department of Public Health, Wellington School of Medicine and University of Otago. He directs the Health Inequalities Research Programme. Associate Professor Blakely's research interests include socioeconomic and ethnic trends in mortality and cancer incidence, tobacco, neighborhoods and health, the role of health services in social inequalities in health, and longitudinal studies of social factors and health. Dr. Blakely is also interested in epidemiological methods and teaches postgraduate epidemiology and biostatistics and convenes an annual summer school course on "social epidemiology."

Lawrence Blume, Ph.D., is a Fellow of the Econometric Society, Professor at Cornell University, member of the Santa Fe Institute's Economic Program faculty and former Director of the Santa Fe Institute Economic Program and

University of Michigan Associate Professor. Blume's research interests include general equilibrium theory, game theory, decision theory, and social interactions. Topics of recent publications include natural selection in markets, game-theoretic equilibrium concepts, models of social interaction, and the dynamics of statistical discrimination.

Margaret O'Brien Caughy, Sc.D., is Associate Professor of Health Promotion and Behavioral Sciences at the University of Texas School of Public Health, Dallas Regional Campus. Dr. Caughy's research interests include the study of correlates and determinants of poor developmental outcomes among infants and children at risk and the application of this knowledge to the development of intervention strategies. Additionally, Dr. Caughy's research expertise includes measuring communities and neighborhoods, statistical methods, and multilevel modeling. Recent publications have focused on neighborhood poverty and cognitive development, racism and child mental health, social capital and mental health, racial socialization in African American families, and neighborhoods observational assessment.

George Davey Smith, M.D., D.Sc., is Professor of Clinical Epidemiology and Head of the Epidemiology Division at the University of Bristol, Department of Social Medicine. Dr. Davey Smith's research interests include socioeconomic differentials in health; life-course influences on chronic disease in adulthood, and the use of genetic epidemiology in improving understanding of environmental causes of disease.

Steven Durlauf, Ph.D., is the Kenneth J. Arrow Professor in the Department of Economics at the University of Wisconsin, Madison. Dr. Durlauf's research areas include macroeconomics and econometrics. His current research focuses on social interactions, inequality, economic growth, and the applications of decision theory to econometrics. Dr. Durlauf is a Fellow of the Econometric Society, Research Associate of the National Bureau of Economic Research, and currently editing the next edition of the New Palgrave Dictionary of Economics.

Bruna Galobardes, M.D., M.P.H., is a Clinical Research Fellow at the Department of Social Medicine in Bristol University (UK). She studied Medicine and Epidemiology in Barcelona (Spain) before following a Master's Degree in Public Health and a Postdoctoral Fellowship in Epidemiology at the Johns Hopkins School of Public Health (US). She worked at the Division of Clinical Epidemiology in Geneva (Switzerland) before joining Bristol. Her research interests are in the social determinants of health, including measures of socioeconomic position and the life-course epidemiology of individual and population health.

M. Maria Glymour, Sc.D., is currently an Instructor in the Department of Society, Human Development and Health at the Harvard School of Public Health. Her research focuses on how social factors experienced across the life course, such as educational attainment, parents' socioeconomic position, or mid-life work experiences, influence cognitive impairment and other health outcomes in old age. Much of her work explores solutions to methodological problems encountered in analyses of cognitive outcomes in the elderly.

Christopher Hamlin, Ph.D., is a Professor in the History Department at the University of Notre Dame. Dr. Hamlin is trained as an historian of science, although most of his work has dealt with aspects of the history of public health. He is author of *A Science of Impurity* (1990), dealing with the history of concepts of water quality, and *Public Health and Social Justice in the Age of Chadwick* (1998), dealing with the emergence of modern public health. He is currently at work on a book examining the history of ideas about particular natural processes, ranging from population stability to decomposition. Hamlin teaches courses on science and technology studies, the history of medicine, the history of technology, and environmental history.

Peter Hannan, M.Stat., is a Senior Research Fellow in the Division of Epidemiology & Community Health in the School of Public Health at the University of Minnesota. Mr. Hannan's research interests include methodological issues with clustering in community trials, multiple imputation, Bayesian statistical analysis, and correspondence analysis. He has been involved with the Minnesota Heart Health Program, was a statistical consultant to Murray's text "Design and Analysis of Group Randomized Trials," has done the statistical analysis and power calculation sections for many group randomized trials implemented in the Division, and collaborated on a number of methodological papers in his research interest areas. He is widely recognized as a leader in the design and analysis of community trials.

Sam Harper, Ph.D., M.P.H., is a postdoctoral fellow in the Department of Epidemiology and Biostatistics at McGill University in Montreal, Canada. His research interests include conceptual and methodological issues in health inequalities, historical trends in population health and demography, and public health ethics.

Barbara Israel, Dr.P.H., is a Professor of Health Behavior and Health Education at the School of Public Health at the University of Michigan, Ann Arbor. Dr. Israel has published widely in the areas of community-based participatory research (CBPR), social support and stress, social determinants of health, evaluation, and community health education. She has over twenty-five years experience in conducting CBPR in collaboration with partners in diverse ethnic communities and is presently involved in several CBPR projects addressing topics such as environmental triggers of childhood asthma, diabetes management and prevention, and social and physical environmental factors and cardiovascular disease.

Pamela Jo Johnson, M.P.H., Ph.D., trained as a social epidemiologist at the University of Minnesota. She recently completed her dissertation on the effect of neighborhood poverty on American Indian infant death, which was a neighborhood effects study that demonstrated the use of propensity score matching methods as an alternative to multilevel regression modeling for observational inference. Dr. Johnson currently works in the Health Services Research & Policy Division, University of Minnesota, and is affiliated with the Minnesota Population Center. Her interests include applied research methods for social epidemiology, population health, and causal inference. Her research agenda primarily focuses on disparities in health status and access to care, American Indian health, maternal health, and pregnancy outcomes.

Saffron Karlsen, Ph.D., is a Senior Research Fellow within the Department of Epidemiology and Public Health, University College London, London, England. Her work explores the impact of a variety of elements of social disadvantage on the lives of people from different ethnic and religious groups in the United Kingdom and elsewhere, including socioeconomic position, racial and religious discrimination and harassment, ecological effects, and mental and physical health. She also has a number of publications exploring the processes associated with ethnic identification in minority and majority ethnic groups in England.

Paula Lantz, Ph.D., M.S., is Associate Professor and Chair of the Department of Health Management and Policy and Research Associate Professor at the Institute for Social Research at the University of Michigan, Ann Arbor. Dr. Lantz's main areas of research interest are policy issues in women's health and child health, clinical preventive services (such as cancer screening and prenatal care), and social inequalities in health across the life course.

Debbie A. Lawlor, Ph.D., M.Sc., M.P.H., M.F.P.H., M.B.Ch.B., is a Senior Lecturer in Epidemiology and Public Health Medicine at the University of Bristol, Department of Social Medicine. Before starting a career in epidemiology, she worked in clinical practice in Maternal and Child Health in Mozambique and General (Family) Practice in the United Kingdom. Her research interests include life-course epidemiology of coronary heart disease, insulin resistance and diabetes, and women's reproductive health; health inequalities; and the determinants and health effects of physical activity. She has been involved in the management, data collection, and analysis of a number of cohort studies, including the British Women's Heart and Health Study, Aberdeen Children of the 1950s cohort, and European Youth Heart and Health Study.

John Lynch, Ph.D., is a Professor of Epidemiology and Canada Research Chair in Population Health at McGill University in Montreal, Canada. His major research focus is how individual and population life-course processes affect levels and inequalities in population health in richer and poorer countries. Professor Lynch teaches graduate-level courses in population health and social epidemiology.

Peter Marsden, Ph.D., is a Professor of Sociology at Harvard University. Dr. Marsden's research interests center on social organization, especially formal organizations and social networks. He has ongoing interests in social science methodology and developing interests in the sociology of medicine. With James A. Davis and Tom W. Smith, Marsden is a co-Principal Investigator of the General Social Survey, which has tracked attitudes and behaviors of American adults since 1972. He was a lead investigator for three National Organizations Studies conducted between 1991 and 2003. He teaches organizational analysis, social networks, mathematical sociology, quantitative methods, and research methods. He serves as Chair of Harvard's University Benefits Committee and of its Health Plans Subcommittee.

Lynne C. Messer, Ph.D., M.P.H., is a social and reproductive/perinatal epidemiologist whose work explores how social and environmental structure influence women's health and birth outcomes. Her current interests include neighborhood-level sociodemographic deprivation and crime, multilevel modeling methods, and reproductive health. She is currently working on the National Children's Study as an Environmental Protection Agency (EPA)/National Health and Environmental Effects Research Laboratory (NHEERL) postdoctoral fellow through the Department of Environmental Sciences and Engineering at the University of North Carolina School of Public Health. As a member of the Royster Society of Fellows, she earned her Ph.D. from the Department of Epidemiology and her M.P.H. from the Department of Health Behavior and Health Education at the University of North Carolina.

James Nazroo, Ph.D., is a Professor of Medical Sociology and Graduate Tutor of the Department of Epidemiology and Public Health, University College London. He is joint editor of the journal *Ethnicity and Health*. Dr. Nazroo's research interests include ethnic inequalities in health and ethnic differences in health beliefs and behaviors. Central to this is developing an understanding of the links between ethnicity, racism, class, and inequality. Another theme in his current work is social and health inequalities in aging populations. Key publications include the monograph *Ethnicity, Class and Health,* and journal publications related to ethnicity, racial discrimination, social class, and health.

Patricia O'Campo, Ph.D., is Professor in Public Health Sciences at the University of Toronto, Alma and Baxter Richard Endowed Chair in Inner City

Health, and the Director at the Centre for Research on Inner City Health at the St. Michael's Hospital in Toronto. She is Adjunct Professor in the Department of Population and Family Health Sciences at the Johns Hopkins Bloomberg School of Public Health. Dr. O'Campo's research interests include social epidemiology focused on women's and children's health and health policy. Specifically, areas of research include intimate partner violence; welfare reform and women's health; prevention of HIV infection in women; perinatal outcomes with a particular focus on infant mortality and preterm birth prevention; and children's health and development. Recent publication topics include advancing theory and methods of multilevel modeling, social capital and child behavior, racial socialization, and intimate partner violence.

Sean F. Reardon, Ed.D., is Associate Professor of Education and (by courtesy) Sociology at Stanford University. His interests focus on the effects of educational policy on educational and social inequality; the causes, patterns, and consequences of residential and school segregation; the effects of community and neighborhood context on adolescent development and behavior; and applied statistical methods for educational and social policy research. His primary research examines the relative contribution of family, school, and neighborhood environments to racial, ethnic, and socioeconomic achievement disparities. He teaches graduate courses in educational policy research, inequality, and applied statistical methods. He is a recipient of a William T. Grant Foundation Scholar Award and a Carnegie Scholar Award.

Angela G. Reyes, M.P.H., is the founder and Executive Director of the community-based Detroit Hispanic Development Corporation, which was established in May 1997 and has since grown to provide several state-of-the-art programs in the Southwest Detroit community. Ms. Reyes is herself a resident of Southwest Detroit, where she has been active in the community for more than thirty years. She has a Master's Degree in Public Health from the University of Michigan and has been the recipient of several awards for her community work, including the 1992 Michiganian of the Year, Detroit Public Schools Community Service Award, and Hispanic Women Veterans Community Activism Award. Ms. Reyes is a national speaker on issues affecting her community, including youth gangs and violence, substance abuse, community activism, and cultural competency.

Amy Schulz, Ph.D., is a Research Associate Professor in the Department of Health Education and Behavior at the University of Michigan, Ann Arbor and at the Institute for Research on Women and Gender. Dr. Schulz also serves as the Associate Director of the Center for Research on Ethnicity, Culture and Health. Her research focuses on the use of community-based participatory research with a primary focus on understanding social and physical environments and their implications for the health of urban residents.

Mary Shaw, Ph.D., is a Reader in Medical Sociology at the University of Bristol, Department of Social Medicine and the Scientific Director at the South West Public Health Observatory. Dr. Shaw's research interests include social and geographical inequalities in mortality and morbidity, the social and spatial accumulation of health inequalities, poverty and the health of disadvantaged groups (particularly homeless people), health and social policies, and photography in social science.

S.V. Subramanian, Ph.D., is an Assistant Professor of Society, Human Development, and Health in the Department of Society, Human Development, and Health at Harvard University. The main focus of his research is on understanding how different contextual settings influence individual health outcomes and the population disparities in health achievements. Among others, he has specifically investigated the impact of macro contextual factors, such as income inequality and social capital on individual health outcomes. Dr. Subramanian is conducting independent research on the methodological challenges of estimating contextual and neighborhood effects on health. Recent publications include an introductory epidemiology text and journal articles using multilevel modeling.

Jennifer Warlick, Ph.D., is an Associate Professor and Chairperson in the Department of Economics and Policy Studies at the University of Notre Dame. Dr. Warlick's scholarly interests are in the area of poverty policy and the effect of income taxes and transfers on low-income families and the elderly. Dr. Warlick has published in both national and foreign journals and in numerous books regarding income maintenance policy and aging. Her current research focuses on the measurement of poverty and the labor market effects of credentialing low-skill workers. She teaches courses in the economics of poverty, education, and industrial organization.

For
Heather, Maddy, and Henry
&
Lisa, Amelia, and Julian

PREFACE

This text addresses many important methodological issues faced in contemporary social epidemiologic research. The motivation for assembling this material is to increase the potential for social epidemiology to contribute meaningfully to public health knowledge and policy through stronger and clearer methodological foundations. The field is only a few decades old in its current incarnation, and the methodological approaches that characterize work in this sub-discipline are still rapidly evolving. New techniques are continually developed or borrowed from other disciplines. Nonetheless, the bulk of published research in this area is still made up of studies for which the inferential content is modest at best. Some of this ambiguity in interpretation arises from a weak conceptual orientation about the logic underlying many common methods. This is especially true of regression, which is seldom taught with a focus on causal inference.

Without improvements in standard analytic practice, social epidemiology risks being dismissed as naïve or simplistic by policy makers as well as by the wider scientific readership. Popular imagination and scientific credence are extended readily to the rapid developments in molecular biology and genetics, even though their relevance for public health concerns remains largely uncertain. In contrast, the questions posed in social epidemiology have immediate relevance for the most important public health concerns, and yet the results of such studies rarely have the necessary clarity and robustness to alternate explanations (for example, bias, measurement error) that would allow them to enter meaningfully into the public and policy debates. This dilemma will not be solved overnight with the introduction of some exciting new statistical model, but rather slowly, over time, with the training of more careful thinkers and more assiduous analysts.

This volume is intended as a methods text and so is unlike the handful of recent books on social epidemiology and the social determinants of health that focus on substantive findings.

For this reason, little attention is paid to existing knowledge about social epidemiologic relations except by way of motivation or worked examples. It is our intention, however, that this text will compliment these substantive efforts by providing a more thorough investigation of the techniques we use to gather subject matter knowledge in this field and ways in which this research process can be improved.

Is there really a need for a separate text devoted entirely to social epidemiological methods? Why should the interested reader not just rely on the many outstanding methods texts available for epidemiology as a whole? We believe that social epidemiology as a distinct sub-discipline comprises several phenomena that are not very well addressed by traditional epidemiological texts. Foremost among these are human volition, social interaction, and collective action. Because epidemiology is a population science, it is indeed ironic that mainstream epidemiology texts say so little about human interaction, social forces, or social scientific research and understanding more generally. In noting this, we certainly do not intend to minimize the importance of medical or biological knowledge or research; there can be no doubt that these disciplines are also vital to epidemiology. Our point is only that something is missing. A more complete epidemiology includes the social, the biological, and the quantitative, and yet the first of these, which most distinguishes our field from clinical medical investigation, is almost entirely neglected in texts written in the modern period (for example, since the appearance of Kupper, Kleinbaum, and Morgenstern's *Epidemiologic Research* in 1982 and Miettinen's *Theoretical Epidemiology* in 1985). Furthermore, we emphasize that this is obviously not a complete methods text, if such a thing were even conceivable. It is not meant to replace the traditional epidemiology texts, statistical analysis texts, or other foundational works or training. Rather, it augments these works by providing a collection of insights and some original research into the particular challenges facing the study of social relations and institutions on health.

We hope this book serves as a learning guide, a reference tool, and a stepping stone for conceptual advancement. Our target audience is second-year epidemiology doctoral students—those who have some basic training in epidemiologic methods and the capacity and interest to extend these to settings in which the exposures are social phenomena or related to the same. Accordingly, we encouraged contributing authors to write penetrating and cutting-edge chapters that are nonetheless accessible to non-methodologist readers. Because chapter lengths were necessarily limited, we also asked our authors to include abundant citations through which interested readers might continue their study in greater detail.

The text is loosely organized into three parts: Part One, Background; Part Two, Measures and Measurement; and Part Three, Design and Analysis. Part One contains a brief introductory chapter by Oakes and Kaufman that aims to set the stage for the works that follow. The second background chapter is by Hamlin, who considers the intellectual history of methods in social epidemiology. One might well wonder what a history chapter is doing in a methods text. We would argue that it is perilous to ignore past paradigms and conventions, and so we view this chapter as the necessary foundation stone for all that follows.

The second loosely defined part contains seven chapters on measures and measurement. It is difficult to overstate the importance of this work, and there must be no doubt that better measurement is fundamental to any advance. The first chapter is by Galobardes and colleagues, who consider the construct of socioeconomic position and its central role in social epidemiology. Next is an important chapter on the measurement and analysis of race and racial discrimination by Karlsen and Nazroo; much more work is needed in this area and this chapter should move us forward with greater precision and clarity. Betson and Warlick's chapter on measuring poverty comes next. The most enduring finding in all of health research is that poverty is not healthy, and this chapter serves as a much needed reminder that such a seemingly simple idea as poverty is anything but simple to operationalize. Following this, Harper and Lynch contribute an essential chapter in measuring health inequalities. Once again, the deep issues here are difficult and these authors help us to recognize and better appreciate the subjective aspects of these measures. Because residential segregation remains overlooked in much of epidemiology, we wanted to include cutting-edge discussion of the construct and current thinking in this volume. Reardon's chapter not only fills the gap but offers practical insights into how such measurement can and should be done. Finally come two chapters on measuring neighborhood constructs. The first is by O'Campo and Caughy, who carefully consider methods and issues that should move us beyond naïve reliance on census data for community measurement. Community measurement must be more than the tabulation of census data. Nevertheless, census data remain vital to our practice and Messer and Kaufman demonstrate how careful use of such data may be fruitfully employed to answer some difficult questions. Taken together, the chapters in this section would seem to greatly strengthen social epidemiology's foundation by clarifying and extending the measurement tools available to social epidemiologists aiming to understand how social processes interface with health.

The third and final part contains eight chapters on research designs, data analysis, and related issues. The first chapter, by Lantz and colleagues, is special in that it concentrates on community-based participatory research. Such an approach appears to blend well with our view of social epidemiology and merits more attention. Following this is Marsden's thoughtful and informative chapter on understanding, measuring, and analyzing social networks. This chapter should help fill a major gap in the current literature and help strengthen formal approaches to networks. Next comes Blume and Durlauf's penetrating yet accessible review of cutting-edge econometric approaches to modeling social interactions; because it is unlike the bulk of work being done by social epidemiologists, we imagine many will find that this work raises many questions and thus opens many new avenues for fruitful research. Many of the key methodological issues associated with the now common multilevel regression model are carefully addressed by Blakely and Subramanian. Given the near ubiquity of the multilevel model in social epidemiology, this chapter merits repeated study. Perhaps one of this volume's more important chapters is by Hannan, who considers the fundamental statistical aspects of the design and analysis of community trials. It should be clear that we believe more attention to social epidemiological field experiments would be beneficial. Next comes Oakes and Johnson's discussion of how and why propensity score matching methods may benefit social epidemiologic inquiry. The last two chapters are by Glymour, who explains and demonstrates, in a remarkably lucid fashion, both the use of instrumental variables technique and directed acyclic graphs. Both methods seem to hold great promise for improving social epidemiological analyses and understandings. All told, because these eight analysis chapters are infused with aspects of social interaction and causal inference, this part represents an important resource for those aiming to advance social epidemiology.

No preface is complete without acknowledgments. As in the assembly of all such works, we find ourselves in the debt of many—in fact, too many to mention, but a few merit extra special thanks from both of us. First, we gratefully acknowledge the remarkable group of contributing authors; their hard work and positive attitudes nearly made this project fun. Second, we extend extra special thanks to Mary Hearst, a doctoral candidate at the University of Minnesota, who labored tirelessly to coordinate people, paper, and content. This book would not have been completed without her. Finally, we both thank our publisher Andy Pasternack and his colleagues at Jossey-Bass. Andy encouraged us to undertake this project long before we were ready to, and he remained remarkably patient as we missed several self-imposed deadlines.

Additionally, JMO offers special thanks to his teachers, including Doug Anderton, Pete Rossi, Sam Bowles, and the late but still great Andy Anderson. He also thanks Ichiro Kawachi for years of support and encouragement, his irreverent students, and members of the Social Epi Workgroup at the University of Minnesota for asking such tough questions. JSK gratefully acknowledges the patient and generous mentoring of Sherman James and Richard Cooper in his formative intellectual development as a social epidemiologist and the encouragement, prodding, and occasional needling of several influential colleagues, including Irva Hertz-Picciotto, George Kaplan, Jim Koopman, John Lynch, Dan McGee, Carles Muntaner, Charlie Poole, Ken Rothman, and David Savitz.

JMO – Minneapolis, MN
JSK – Chapel Hill, NC
September 2005

PART ONE

BACKGROUND

CHAPTER ONE

INTRODUCTION: ADVANCING METHODS IN SOCIAL EPIDEMIOLOGY

J. Michael Oakes and Jay S. Kaufman

The aim of this brief introductory chapter is to highlight some of the fundamental methodological issues facing social epidemiology. In many cases, these
are the background issues that this volume's contributing authors have weaved
into each of the chapters that follow.

It is necessary to first define social epidemiology and social epidemiologic
methodology, as these definitions underlie all of the discussion that follows. Subsequently, we discuss three fundamental issues that typically arise in the application of social epidemiologic methodology. We conclude by offering a short and
speculative discussion on methods not included in this text that may help advance
the field beyond its present limitations.

What Is Social Epidemiology?

Epidemiology is the study of the distribution and determinants of states of health
in populations. We define *social* epidemiology as the branch of epidemiology that
considers how social interactions and collective human activities affect health. In
other words, social epidemiology is about how a society's innumerable social
arrangements, past and present, yield differential exposures and thus differences
in health outcomes among the persons who comprise the population. Defining
social epidemiology in this broad way permits the analysis of not only how social

factors serve as exposures that affect health outcomes but also how such factors/exposures emerge and are maintained in a distinctive distribution.

Social epidemiology is thus concerned with more than the identification of new disease-specific risk factors (for example, a deficit of social capital); it also considers how well-established exposures, such as cigarette smoking, lead paint, and lack of health insurance, emerge and are distributed by the social system. With such a focus, social epidemiology must consider the dynamic social relationships and human activities that ultimately locate toxic dumps in one neighborhood instead of another, make fresh produce available to some and not others, and permit some to enjoy resources such that they can purchase salubrious environments and competent health care. In short, social epidemiology is about social allocation mechanisms (that is, economic and social forces) that produce differential exposures that often yield health disparities, whether deemed good or bad.

Social epidemiology is different from the bulk of traditional epidemiologic practice, which tends to operate with a model based on the fictitious Robinson Crusoe. Recall that this character is someone in an environment devoid of social context, whose health depends only on biological relationships and the vicissitudes of island weather. Social interaction and thus political and economic power play no role in Robinson's health, although the same is perhaps not so true for his "friend" Friday. Such interactions are central to social epidemiology, however. Without any attention to social arrangements and institutions, epidemiologic research on humans is almost indistinguishable from an application to, say, livestock.

It is the incorporation of purposive human interaction and agency (that is, social coordination and conflict) that links social epidemiology to the social sciences and raises enormous methodological obstacles to inference—obstacles that leading social scientists have long sought to overcome. But social epidemiology is not a social science, at least as traditionally conceived. Although the methods and models of, say, a social epidemiologist and medical sociologist might be identical, the distinction between social epidemiology and social science lies in the focus, outcome variable, or more formally the "explanandum" of each discipline. The goal of social science—including sociology, economics, political science, and anthropology—is to understand and explain the social system. In other words, social science's outcome variable (that is, explanandum) is society, social forces, or the like. A social scientific study that considers/models health outcomes does so to learn about society. By contrast, the outcome variable for social epidemiology is health. Whereas social epidemiologists may borrow theory, methods, and constructs from social science, they do so in an effort to understand health rather than social forces or related phenomena. This means that social epidemiology, although related to the social sciences, firmly remains a branch of epidemiology. Accordingly, social epidemiology should not discount the potential impact of genes, microbes, or other factors frequently found in other subfields within epidemiology. The inevitable decline in the importance of (sub)disciplinary boundaries is a necessary step for the integration of these diverse considerations, as it frequently requires multidisciplinary teams to properly address the important research questions in their true complexity.

Although each day seems to bring more interest and activity in social epidemiology, it is important to appreciate that the questions we consider are anything but new. Not only did the ancient Greeks wonder about the relationship between social conditions and health but John Snow's famous cholera investigations, which many say mark the dawn of epidemiology and germ theory more generally, were infused with the same paradigm. Furthermore, what is too often overlooked is that questions concerning the relationship between social institutions (for example, government or societal norms) and human welfare date back to at least Hobbes and many great, more contemporary, political thinkers such as Keynes, Hayek, Freedman, and Sen, who continue to contribute to insights into the fundamental normative question: *How must we organize . . . to improve health*?

What Is Social Epidemiologic Methodology?

Methods are rules or procedures employed by those trying to accomplish a task. Sometimes such rules or procedures are written down. For example, cookbooks provide methods for baking better cookies or cakes. In much the same way, research methods are rules and procedures that researchers working within a disciplinary framework employ to improve the validity of their inferences. At risk of taking the analogy too far, researchers who abide by good research methods may more reliably produce valid inferences in much the same way that bakers who abide by excellent recipes tend to produce tasty cookies and cakes. There are always exceptions, but the point seems to hold generally.

Social epidemiologic methodology is naturally the study of methods in and for social epidemiology. To reiterate a point raised in the Preface, social epidemiologic methodology includes not only the broad collection of study design, measurement, and analytic considerations that has evolved over the previous century in mainstream epidemiology but also methods needed to address social epidemiology's special or unique questions and data. This latter group of methods arises more clearly from the social sciences, although a long tradition of considering these points in relation to communicable disease is also discernable in the history of epidemiology (Eyler 1979; Hamlin 1998; Ross 1916).

Methodological research is largely concerned with studying the logic of and improving techniques for scientific inference. The broad objective is to learn what conclusions can and cannot be drawn given specified combinations of assumptions and data (Manski 1993). Because methodologists strive to determine what conclusions may be legitimately drawn given a set of assumptions, it is natural that this group of researchers often views existing practice more skeptically. Many methodologists might readily propose that a fundamental problem in applied research is that substantive investigators frequently fail to face up to the difficulty of their enterprise. We would venture to guess that many of the contributors to this volume would themselves articulate a similar position, that much published research is naïve with respect to assumptions being relied upon and to the many alternate explanations being ignored. The solution to this problem is rarely the use of more elaborate statistical methodology, however, as such solutions tend to be more assumption-laden rather than less so. Rather, the solution is for methodological training that stresses the fundamental logical principles behind study design and quantitative analysis of data and for greater rigor in the criticism of such models. Disciplines that become overly fascinated with the technique of analysis can easily become distracted from more elemental issues in the logic of inference, a nagging concern in economics, sociology, and other social sciences (Leamer 1983; Lieberson and Lynn 2002).

Three Fundamental Issues

In this section we briefly comment on three issues fundamental to social epidemiologic methodology: causal inference, measurement, and multilevel methodology.

Causal Inference

Perhaps the most fundamental and yet intractable problem of all research, especially observational research, is that of causal inference. The centrality of this concern rests with the need to have science be successfully predictive of the future and thus serve as a guide for how human activity may manipulate conditions for preferred outcomes. Because social epidemiology seeks to identify the effects of social variables, we must necessarily adopt a model of human agency that posits various actions taken or not taken and their consequences (Pearl 2000). Because a causal effect is *defined* on the basis of contrasts between various of these (potentially counterfactual) actions, many authors argue that we must immediately exclude non-manipulable factors, such as individual race or ethnicity and gender, from consideration as causes in this sense (Kaufman and Cooper 1999). The modifiable exposures that are typically of interest to social epidemiologists include factors such as income, education, and occupation, which are potentially influenced through social policies or by various specific educational or social interventions. For example, the existence of a governmental income supplementation program changes income distributions in the population, allowing some families to live above the poverty line that would have lived beneath it in the absence of this policy (Basilevsky and Hum 1984; Orr et al. 1971). The contrast of these two policy regimes or between many specific variations of this intervention is the basis for the definition of a causal effect of interest in etiologic observational research.

For simplicity of exposition, consider a binary outcome ($Y = 1$ if disease occurs during the period of observation, $Y = 0$ otherwise), although extension to other outcome distributions is straightforward. For example, suppose that $Y = 1$ represents a subject in the defined population dying before the end of follow-up, whereas $Y = 0$ indicates that the subject is alive at end of follow-up. Consider social exposure $X = 1$ as the policy that provides income supplementation up to the poverty line and $X = 0$ as the absence of such a policy. As a notational convention to represent intervention, many sources in the statistical and epidemiologic literature make use of a subscript on the outcome variable ($Y_{X = x}$) to indicate the variable conditioned on forcing the target population to exposure level x (for example, Holland 1986). Pearl has employed several notional conventions (Pearl 2000, p. 70), including the "SET" notation, which expresses intervention as $SET[X = x]$. Using this notation, the outcome distribution under the various interventions is readily expressed as $Pr(Y = y \mid SET[X = x])$, which may be translated as the probability of an outcome Y being the value y given the value of intervention X is set at x. These distributions of Y enable computation of outcome contrasts between all possible values of x taken by X. For example, for the causal effect of income supplementation on mortality, common contrasts would include the difference or ratio between the risk of death in the target population during the specified time period if the income supplementation policy were in effect versus if it were not in effect.

Although the hypothesis of a causal relation between income supplementation and mortality seems plausible, it is also entirely possible that states or counties with such programs have lower age-specific mortality risks than states or counties without such programs for extraneous reasons. If this were true, it would suggest that some part of the empirical association observed between income supplementation and mortality may arise not from the causal link between them but rather owing to their mutual response to other conditions, such as the level of the state cigarette tax, which affects both revenues available for income supplementation and the death rate through its affects on smoking behavior.

The task is to contrast the proportion of the target population who would die if subjected to a policy of income supplementation to the proportion who would die if there was no policy in place for income supplementation: $\Pr(Y = 1 \mid \mathrm{SET}[X = 1])$ versus $\Pr(Y = 1 \mid \mathrm{SET}[X = 0])$. The problem in observational data is that nothing is actually SET, and so we must manipulate the observed quantities in some way to more validly estimate the causal effect. Clearly the crude contrast of observed mortality proportions, $\Pr(Y = 1 \mid X = 1)$ versus $\Pr(Y = 1 \mid X = 0)$, is not adequate, as these conditional probabilities may differ not only because of the causal effect of X but also because of the correlated perturbation in X and Y by their common cause.

The usual epidemiologic solution is to condition in some way on measured covariates that represent the common causes of X and Y. The logic behind this strategy is that within the categorizations of the covariates, there can be no confounding by these quantities (Greenland and Morgenstern 2001). Formally, this adjustment provides a statistically unbiased estimate of the true causal effect for X on Y when, within each stratum of covariate Z, observed exposure X is statistically independent of the potential response $(Y \mid \mathrm{SET}[X = x])$ for each imposed value x (Rosenbaum and Rubin 1983). To the extent that one can enumerate and accurately measure all of the important common ancestors of exposure and outcome, this conventional epidemiologic solution is entirely adequate for the specification of the desired causal effect from observational data in point-exposure studies with no interference between units. For exposures related to human behavior, however, the task of identifying and measuring these common antecedents is often daunting.

Even in randomized experiments, but especially in observational studies, causal inference requires a strong theoretical foundation to justify assumptions of causal order, of no bias due to omitted covariates, and of effect homogeneity. This level of theoretical justification is often lacking in epidemiology, and is especially uncommon in social epidemiology (Oakes 2004). Regression modeling is particularly insidious in this regard, as the method has become so routine as to seem facile, when, in fact, the statistical and the extra-statistical assumptions required are often heroic (see Berk 2004; McKim and Turner 1997). Some authors are assiduously cautious with their language, yet many others imply causal relationships when they employ euphemisms such as "effect," "impact," "influence," "dependent variable," or "outcome" (Oakes 2004). The motivations are laudable, but in the end such "findings" may do more harm than good. Surely there are opportunity costs and risks to the public's trust and understanding (Caplan 1988; Greenlund et al. 2003; Hogbin and Hess 1999).

Basic descriptive and predictive models devoid of causal import can be quite useful (Berk 2004). But at some point policymakers will want to use the results of social epidemiologic investigation to improve health, and causal understanding is desirable in this case. While prediction and causality are related, they are almost always distinct because the latter is tied to action rather than observation. Too see this, recall that a rooster's crow does not raise the sun, but it predicts it with regularity. Such an alarm clock may be quite helpful to the sleepy farmer. But this model is merely predictive, because no matter how many times the sleepy farmer might get his rooster to crow later, the sun will rise in accordance with a completely different causal mechanism.

The subfield of social epidemiology is now suitably mature and sophisticated that we must state our analytic goals more clearly: does an author seek a causal, predictive, or perhaps "merely" descriptive model? Unlike fields such as climatology, social epidemiologists are often interested in actually enacting policies or interventions in order to improve the public's health. We therefore need to privilege causal explanations and to *aim* to build causal models. The yardstick is not perfection but usefulness, but it does not seem that multiple-regression procedures are getting us very far in this regard (Berk 2004).

Measurement of Social Phenomena

It was the poet Yeats (1938) who grasped the essential idea with the words "measurement began our might." Yet, although there can be no doubt that measurement of biological phenomena is quite advanced and that the field of psychometrics has aided progress on individual-level measures, such as IQ and depression (Nunally and Bernstein 1994), measures of social phenomena and other aggregate constructs remain remarkably primitive (Duncan 1984; Lazarsfeld and Menzel 1961). For example, several authors have revealed a striking lack of attention to the measurement of the central construct of socioeconomic status (SES) in health research (Oakes and Rossi 2003). The situation appears even worse when it comes to measures of ecological settings such as neighborhoods, schools, and workplaces. The fact is that the methodology needed to evaluate these measure remains in its infancy (Sampson 2003).

It is unclear why so little progress has been made on the measurement of constructs fundamental to social epidemiologic inquiry, especially in light of a consensus agreement on the basic consequences of measurement error: it has been known for over 100 years that measurement error generally biases (attenuates or accentuates) effects (Gustafson 2004; Jurek et al. 2005; Nunally and Bernstein 1994; Yatchew and Griliches 1984). Surely one reason for the slow pace of progress is that the task is difficult. Unlike counting red blood cells or calculating a subject's body mass index, relevant constructs in social epidemiology are always between persons and are often group-level phenomena. This means that such measures reflect complex functions of individual action, interactions, and largely unknown feedback systems: this greatly complicates things. Other reasons for the slow progress probably include the fact that there is little practical incentive for work on social measurement within epidemiology. For better or worse, it is clear that conventional epidemiology has not devoted much attention to the social sciences (Oakes 2005), which means that whereas health outcome assessments may be thoroughly scrutinized by reviewers and editors, social exposure assessment may be accomplished crudely or reflexively without drawing much negative attention (Jones and Cameron 1984). As Berk (2004, p. 238) laments, "Many investigators appear to proceed as if fancy statistical procedures can compensate for failures to invest in proper data collection." Progress in conceptualization and measurement is key to advancement of social epidemiology, and more attention should be devoted to it.

Multilevel Methods

Much has been published in recent years within social epidemiology about multilevel theory and multilevel models (Diez-Roux 2000; Kaplan 2004). This is clearly a salutary development for the field because the point of such discussions—that context matters—is timely and important. Yet, whereas several scholars have ably considered some of the statistical issues of the multilevel regression model (see Chapter Thirteen), few have fully discussed the fundamental methodological issues inherent in a true multilevel methodology, namely, an approach that incorporates the critical and dynamic tension between individuals and groups. At some point several slippery questions must be considered, including whether a group is an entity independent of its constituents. Asked differently, is there a group without the specific individuals who comprise it? Another question is how groups or aggregate phenomena change over time; what are the mechanisms? These issues rest at the core of multilevel theory and models, and more attention needs to be devoted to them. To be sure, such issues are difficult, and we can offer no facile recipe or simple conclusion. Obviously, a full treatment is far beyond our scope here.

To better understand multilevel theory, we turn to the work of Coleman, who in 1990 tried to present the key issues by discussing Weber's 1905 classic explanation of the rise of capitalism in the Protestant West (Coleman 1990; Weber [1905] 1958). According to Coleman, Weber was trying to explain how society evolved from pre-capitalistic to capitalistic by describing changes that occurred among individuals within the societies under investigation. Weber's research question was how and why some societies changed so dramatically over a relatively brief period of time. For purposes here, the important point is that Weber's explanation of social change rested on the changes within and among the individuals who made up the societies. According to Weber, it was the adoption and

FIGURE 1.1. CONCEPTUAL FRAMEWORK
FOR MULTILEVEL THINKING

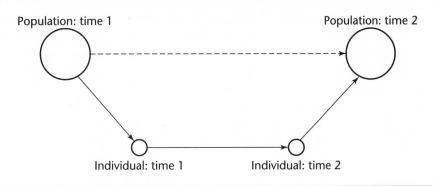

(Adapted from Coleman 1990, fig. 1.3)

internalization of the Calvinist religious ethic by individuals that eventually led to the growth and dominance of capitalism at the societal level.

Coleman tried to better formalize the issues by drawing a trapezoidal figure (which we affectionately call the "Coleman bathtub"). We adopt this pedagogical device and present a similar figure (Figure 1.1). Although simple on its face, this figure contains a great deal of useful information for advancing multilevel methods in social epidemiology.

The larger circle to the left represents the population or society at time one or *before* any change. The larger circle to the right represents the population at time two or *after* some change. Alone, these two larger circles represent a change in a population/society over time. That is, the two larger circles and the dotted-line arrow linking them represent our central question: how did society change? In concrete terms, one might observe a change in the rate of cigarette smoking over time. A social epidemiologist observing this might ask how and why this change occurred. Her goal might be to try to explain this change so that better interventions to reduce the smoking rate could be developed and tested. How then might we understand the social or epidemiologic change?

A methodological individualist, Coleman insists that such social change comes about only through changes in individual people and their interactions. Societal or group-level change does not just happen mysteriously without the involvement of actual persons; social change must be grounded in the activity of constituent individuals. It follows that the change in smoking rates can only be explained by understanding what happened to the smokers and non-smokers, and their relationships, under investigation.

Individual change is diagrammed in Figure 1.1. The smaller circle to the left represents a given person living in the society at time one. The smaller circle to the right represents the same person at time two, after some change. The arrow linking this person at time one to himself or herself at time two represents personal growth or change, a psychological (or perhaps medical) phenomena. Note well that, however interesting, this change is not our focus here; indeed, for social epidemiology, personal change is only important to the extent it reflects or implies change at the societal or population level.

Most important here are the (near) vertical arrows to the left and to the right. The downward pointing arrow to the left, from the larger circle to the smaller, represents the impact or influence of society on an individual. This is the *macro-to-micro* transition. The arrow to the right, from the smaller to the larger circle, represents the impact of the individual on society. This is the *micro-to-macro* transition. Together, these "micro-macro" transitions represent the most important but most difficult methodological challenge for a multilevel social epidemiology. The fundamental questions are how and why society "gets into" individuals and how and why do individuals interact to produce complex social organizations and related outcomes.

Macro-to-micro transitions may come as resource constraints, social norms, laws, and all other such forces that affect individual behavior. Especially important are the concepts of socialization and endogenous preferences. Although difficult to study, the former idea appears easily understood: socialization is the process of learning and internalizing the rules of proper behavior and the consequences of behaving improperly. Parents and teachers socialize offspring and students. What then of the related notion of endogenous preferences? The term *endogenous preference*s implies that what we like and dislike is at least partly learned from others and the constraints faced (Bowles 1998). Simply put, our circumstances affect our preferences if not our entire world view. These notions of socialization and endogenous preferences may be interpreted as implying that our own likes and dislikes are all social constructs, which is a slippery and controversial conclusion because it seems to cast suspicion on the very existence of free will and individual volition (Sunstein 1986).

Moving in the other direction, micro-to-macro transitions may come as efforts of individuals to change laws, lower-prices, or promote collective actions, such as anti-smoking demonstrations. To keep this discussion accessible and brief, we shall greatly oversimplify and assert that all micro-to-macro transitions may be viewed as collective actions where individuals somehow act together for seemingly common goals. Collective action problems are ubiquitous in society and well studied in the social sciences. The key point is that there are fundamental interdependencies and interactions among persons engaged in a social goal, which means that simple aggregations of presumed individual behavior fails to explain or predict outcomes (Olson 1971). Consider two notable examples of collective action problems: voting, and protection of a field for grazing sheep. First, the issue of voting in an election is at once simple and complex. Simply understood, persons vote to express their preference for one candidate or object to another. But a paradox arises, because as the probability that anyone's vote will be decisive approaches zero, an individual has no incentive to waste even a moment in order to vote. So why do so many people do it? More generally, why does any voluntary group effort occur when individuals typically have no incentive to participate? The second example of collective-action phenomena may be found in the so-called "commons problem." In short, the classic commons problem occurs when individual sheep farmers have incentive to graze more sheep (Hardin 1968). The trouble is that when all shepherds do so the common land is overgrazed, the sheep starve, and each farmer loses his fortune. This is a collective action problem that illustrates how individuals seeking their own self-interest can yield collective outcomes that no individual would want; in other words, private rationality can lead to collective irrationality.

Both micro-macro transitions highlight the crucial role of interdependencies in social phenomena that affect social (that is, population-level) change. For the most part, social epidemiology has not addressed these fundamental issues in theory, measurement, or analysis, leaving much work still to be done. Coleman and others have suggested that the best way through this thicket is to conceptualize the micro-macro transitions not with respect to particular persons or even any persons but rather as a system of socio-structural positions that tend to emerge from the characteristics of the micro-macro transitions. Accordingly, the transitions can be conceived of as the "rules of the game" that transmit the consequences of an individual's action to other individuals and yield macro-level phenomena (Coleman 1990). New and insightful work in multilevel theory includes Durlauf's 2002 article on social capital, Durlauf and Young's 2001 edited volume on dynamic social interactions, and Bowles' 2004 novel microeconomics text.

Advancing Further Still

Although it seems appropriate to briefly comment on some potential steps beyond this volume that would appear to enhance the practice and import of social epidemiology, we do so with some trepidation. It is simply difficult to know how our subfield will evolve or co-evolve with more mainstream epidemiology. Nevertheless, some speculation on three approaches may be useful for discussion, debate, and further study.

First, success might be enhanced if social epidemiologists considered and conducted more randomized experimental studies. While Hannan and Glymour discuss many aspects of community trials and natural experiments in Chapters Fourteen and Seventeen, respectively, it is worth pointing out that there have been other applications of experimental methods that seem potentially useful to social epidemiology. The first type includes efforts to manipulate constructs important to social epidemiology through laboratory-like factorial experiments. For example, McKinlay et al. (2002) used videotape vignettes in an experiment aimed to determine: (1) whether patient attributes (specifically a patient's age, gender, race, and socioeconomic status) independently influence clinical decision-making; and (2) whether physician characteristics alone (such as gender, age, race, and medical specialty) or in combination with patient attributes influence medical decision-making (see also Feldman et al. 1997). If nothing else, such efforts are useful because they clearly require sharply formed *a priori* hypotheses and offer some control over confounding.

Somewhat relatedly, there may be benefit in resurrecting the seemingly overlooked method of factorial surveys, which aim to experimentally examine judgments and preferences by combing factorial experiments with survey methods (Rossi and Nock 1982). Classic examples include the work of Nock and Rossi (1979), who used the method to understand the *independent* effects of factors considered when judging a household's socioeconomic status. More recently, Schwappach and Koeck (2004) employed the method to better understand judgments about medical errors. Furthermore, though rarely used in this fashion, the method would seem to hold some promise for understanding variation in social norms (Rossi and Berk 1987). Finally, there is the growing and recent work of evolutionary economists and their like-minded kin who use simple experiments to better understand social interactions and outcomes (Henrich et al. 2005; Sunstein 2000). Paying greater attention to such work and extending it would seem to hold great promise for social epidemiology.

Second, it seems prudent to devote greater attention to cross-validation—a procedure where predicted values from, for example, a regression model are compared with actual observations. Cross-validation is one of the true tests of a (statistical) model because until tested, parameter estimates are shielded from scrutiny and perhaps public view because true values are not known—sampling variability offers enormous protection (Kennedy 1988). Box (1994) draws an analogy to a criminal investigation: no matter how good it might be, detective work (that is, model building) without prosecution and adjudication (validation) is worthless if not irresponsible.

Ironically, the medical and public health literatures, especially as related to obesity, are replete with cross-validation studies focused on validating instruments or biological relationships (for example, Beekley et al. 2004; Craig et al. 2003;

Finan et al. 1997; Goran and Khaled 1995; Thomsen et al. 2002; Vander Weg et al. 2004). Indeed, diagnostic medicine has not tolerated non- or poorly validated instruments since the publication of Ransohoff and Feinstein's landmark paper (see also Zhou et al. 2002). Yet as far as we know, no social epidemiologic models have been formally validated or tested in this way. The reason, it would seem, is that researchers rarely have access to a second independent sample from their target population. Presuming awareness of validation methods, the fact is that second samples are expensive. It is possible to validate a model with the same data used to estimate it (Hastie et al. 2001). But building and validating a model with the same data, even subsets of it, can be very misleading; the model is likely to appear better than it really is. This is because it is too easy to capitalize on chance or a particular realization of the stochastic process (Browne 2000; Zucchini 2000). Once again, Berk (2004, p. 130) captures the point:

> model selection can lead to the problem of "overfitting." If a goal of data analysis is to make inferences from a sample to a population or to natural processes that generated the data (or to forecast), testing lots of different regression models can lead to a final model that reflects far too many idiosyncrasies in the sample . . . the final fit is then an overfit. . . .

Although a general problem for all observational science, overfitting may be particularly rampant in social epidemiology, and such mistakes may serve to impede scientific progress and improvements to the public health.

Finally, we note that the most widely applied method for evaluating the impact of social exposures on health is one that is not covered to any extent in this volume or used in most social epidemiologic research, despite its importance and arguable advantages in relation to other methods. This is the qualitative or narrative historical approach. In broad outline, the basic idea is to tell the story of the exposures and outcomes in the specific socio-historical context in which they actually occurred rather than in an abstract and idealized context defined by statistical models. The strength of this approach is clearly that it does not presume to state some set of universal rules that exist for all vaguely similar situations at all times but rather is the explanatory narrative of one unique configuration of events. The weakness of this approach is exactly the same: if we only know how exposure and outcome were related in one particular instance in the past, of what practical use is this information to us for the future? Furthermore, if no generalization to other settings is formally justified, then the explanatory mechanism proposed by the author is not prospectively testable and therefore not refutable, because those exact circumstances will never be replicated. Instead, critique can only come in the form of counterarguments and alternative explanations, and therefore the evaluation of competing explanations remains necessarily subjective. This is the fundamental tension between the idiographic and nomothetic scientific paradigms.

Narrative historical depictions can certainly be highly quantitative, in the sense that they involve numerical summaries of the events that occurred. These depictions may also be characterized by specific causal explanations in the form of counterfactuals (that is, arguing that events are the results of specific precipitating conditions that, had these conditions not pertained earlier, would have come out differently). For example, from 1991 through 1994, there was an epidemic of neuropathy in Cuba in which more than 50,000 people experienced vision loss. The causal explanation appears to be an acute nutritional deficiency subsequent to the collapse of the Soviet Union (which had subsidized the Cuban economy) and concomitant tightening of the U.S. economic embargo (Ordunez-Garcia et al. 1996). This explanation is causal because it implies that, had the Soviet subsidies continued, the epidemic would have been reduced or avoided entirely. But it differs in numerous ways from the inferences gleaned from statistical models. For example, although the factual conditions may be represented with great precision, the outcome distribution under the counterfactual condition is not generally identified quantitatively in the narrative approach. Indeed, an important strength of this analytic approach is that it successfully avoids the seductive generality of statistical models, the results of which are described in universal terms, without reference to the specific circumstances in which the data-generating mechanism operated. And by representing the counterfactual outcome distribution qualitatively as opposed to quantitatively, this also avoids the illusion of numerical precision for contrasts that fall outside the realm of the observed data (King and Zeng 2003).

Important social epidemiologic works that adopt this analytic strategy include Randall Packard's *White Plague, Black Labor* (Packard 1989) and Eric Klinenberg's *Heat Wave: A Social Autopsy of Disaster in Chicago* (2002). Unfortunately, however, this approach lends itself more naturally to book-length treatment or, at very least, to the longer article lengths typical of the humanities and social sciences. The restrictive length and structuring requirements of many biomedical journals make it almost impossible to engage in these kinds of arguments in our mainstream epidemiology journals. One notable exception is the "Public Health Then and Now" column in *The American Journal of Public Health*. By contrast, several social sciences recognize that the narrative historical approach is an essential tool for investigating and characterizing the complex relations between social arrangements and their consequences (King et al. 1994).

The bulk of the current volume is organized around the paradigm of the experimental trial as the standard for scientific inference. But for social epidemiology to thrive in the decades to come, we must also become comfortable with the realization that some scientific questions will not be answered best by treating observational data as though they arose from controlled experiments. For some highly complex systems, such as human social structures, the costs of generality in terms of oversimplification and unjustified assumptions may easily be too great to warrant the fantasies of regression equations and exogenous errors and the like. If the statistical models must become so baroque that they obscure rather than facilitate understanding and insight, then it is time to consider alternate approaches that more readily acknowledge subtlety, uniqueness, and peculiarity.

References

Basilevsky, A., & Hum, D. (1984). *Experimental social programs and analytic methods.* New York: Academic Press.

Beekley M. D., Brechue W. F., deHoyos D. V., Garzarella L., Werber-Zion G., Pollock M. L. (2004). Cross-validation of the YMCA Submaximal Cycle Ergometer Test to Predict VO2max. *Research Quarterly for Exercise and Sport, 75,* 337–342.

Berk, Richard. (2004). *Regression analysis. A constructive critique.* Thousand Oaks, CA: Sage Publications.

Bowles, Samuel. (1998). Endogenous preferences: The cultural consequences of markets and other economic institutions. *Journal of Economic Literature, 36,* 75–111.

Bowles, Samuel. (2004). *Microeconomics: Behavior, institutions, and evolution.* Princeton, NJ: Princeton University Press.

Box, George. (1994). Statistics and quality improvement. *Journal of the Royal Statistical Society, Series A 157,* 209–229.

Browne, M. W. (2000). Cross-validation methods. *Journal of Mathematical Psychology, 44,* 108–132.

Caplan, A. L. (1988). Professional arrogance and public misunderstanding. *Hastings Center Report, 18,* 34–37.

Coleman, James S. (1990). *The foundations of social theory.* Cambridge: Belknap.

Craig, C. L., Marshall, A. L., Sjostrom, M., Bauman, A. E., Booth, M. L., Ainsworth, B. E., et al. (2003). International physical activity questionnaire: 12-country reliability and validity. *Medicine and Science in Sports and Exercise, 35,* 1381–1395.

Diez-Roux, A. V. (2000). Multilevel analysis in public health research. *Annual Review of Public Health, 21,* 171–192.

Duncan, O. D. (1984). *Notes on social measurement: Historical & critical.* New York: Russell Sage.

Durlauf, S. N. (2002). On the empirics of social capital. *Economics Journal, 112,* 459–479.

Durlauf, S. N., & Young, H. P. (2001). *Social dynamics.* Washington, DC: Brookings Institution Press.

Eyler, J. M. (1979). *Victorian social medicine: The ideas and methods of William Farr.* Baltimore: Johns Hopkins University Press.

Feldman, H. A., McKinlay, J. B., Potter, D. A., Freund, K. M., Burns, R. B., Moskowitz, M. A., et al. (1997). Nonmedical influences on medical decision making: An experimental technique using videotapes, factorial design, and survey sampling. *Health Serv Res, 32,* 343–366.

Finan, K., Larson, D. E., & Goran, M. I. (1997). Cross-validation of prediction equations for resting energy expenditure in young, healthy children. *Journal of the American Dietetic Association, 97,* 140–145.

Goran, M. I., & Khaled, M. A. (1995). Cross-validation of fat-free mass estimated from body density against bioelectrical resistance: Effects of obesity and gender. *Obesity Research, 3,* 531–539.

Greenland, S., & Morgenstern, H. (2001). Confounding in health research. *Annual Review of Public Health, 22,* 189–212.

Greenlund, K. J., Neff, L. J., Zheng, Z. J., Keenan, N. L., Giles, W. H., Ayala, C. A., et al. (2003). Low public recognition of major stroke symptoms. *American Journal of Preventative Medicine, 25,* 315–319.

Gustafson, P. (2004). *Measurement error and misclassification in statistics and epidemiology.* Boca Raton, FL: Chapman & Hall/CRC.

Hamlin, C. (1998). *Public health and social justice in the age of Chadwick: Britain, 1800–1854.* New York: Cambridge.

Hardin, G. (1968). Tragedy of the commons. *Science, 162,* 1243–1248.

Hastie, T., Tibshirani, R., & Friedman J. (2001). *The elements of statistical learning: Data mining, inference and prediction.* New York: Springer-Verlag New York, Inc.

Henrich, J., Boyd, R., Bowles, S., Camerer, C., Fehr, E., & Gintis H. (2005). *Foundations of human sociality: Economic experiments and ethnographic evidence from fifteen small societies.* New York: Oxford University Press.

Hogbin, M. B., & Hess, M. A. (1999). Public confusion over food portions and servings. *Journal of the American Dietetic Association, 99,* 1209–1211.

Holland, P. W. (1986). Statistics and causal inference. *Journal of the American Statistical Association, 81,* 945–960.

Jones, I. G., & Cameron, D. (1984). Social class analysis—An embarrassment to epidemiology. *Community Medicine, 6,* 37–46.

Jurek, A. M., Greenland, S., Maldonado, G., & Church, T. R. (2005). Proper interpretation of non-differential misclassification effects: Expectations vs. observations. *American Journal of Epidemiology, 34,* 680.

Kaplan, G. A. (2004). What's wrong with social epidemiology, and how can we make it better? *Epidemiologic Reviews, 26,* 124–135.

Kaufman, J., & Cooper, R. (1999). Seeking causal explanations in social epidemiology. *American Journal of Epidemiology, 150,* 113–119.

Kennedy, P. (1988). *A guide to econometrics* (4th ed.) Cambridge, MA: MIT Press.

King, G., Keohane, R. O., & Verba, S. (1994). *Designing social inquiry: Scientific inference in qualitative research.* Princeton, NJ: Princeton University Press.

King, G., & Zeng, L. (2003). *When can history be our guide? The pitfalls of counterfactual inference.* (vol.) Retrieved December 12, 2005, from http://gking.harvard.edu/preprints.shtml: Harvard University.

Klinenberg, E. (2002). *A social autopsy of disaster in Chicago.* Chicago: University of Chicago Press.

Lazarsfeld, P. F., & Menzel, H. (1961). On the relation between individual and collective properties. In A. Etzioni (Ed.), *Complex organizations: A sociological reader.* New York: Holt, Rinehart, and Winston.

Leamer, E. (1983). Let's take the con out of econometrics. *American Economic Review, 73,* 32–43.

Lieberson, S., & Lynn, F. B. (2002). Barking up the wrong branch: Scientific alternatives to the current model of sociological science. *Annual Review of Sociology, 28,* 1–19.

Manski, C. F. (1993). Identification problems in the social sciences. In P. V. Marsden (Ed.), *Sociological Methodology 1993* (Vol. 23, pp. 1–56). Washington, DC: Blackwell Publishers, for the American Sociological Association.

McKim, V. R., & Turner, S. P. (1997). *Causality in crisis? Statistical methods and the search for causal knowledge in the social sciences*. Notre Dame, IN: Notre Dame University Press.

McKinlay, J. B., Lin, T., Freund, K., & Moskowitz, M. (2002). The unexpected influence of physician attributes on clinical decisions: Results of an experiment. *Journal of Health and Social Behavior, 43*, 92–106.

Nock, S. L., & Rossi, P. H. (1979). Household types and social standing. *Social Forces, 57*, 1325–1345.

Nunally, J. C., & Bernstein, I. (1994). *Psychometric theory*. New York: McGraw Hill.

Oakes, J. M. (2004). The (mis)estimation of neighborhood effects: Causal inference for a practicable social epidemiology. *Social Science & Medicine, 58*, 1929–1952.

Oakes, J. M. (2005). An analysis of AJE citations with special reference to statistics and social science. *American Journal of Epidemiology, 161*, 494–500.

Oakes, J. M., & Rossi, P. H. (2003). The measurement of SES in health research: Current practice and steps toward a new approach. *Social Science & Medicine, 56*, 769–784.

Olson, M. (1971). *The logic of collective action: Public goods and the theory of groups*. Cambridge, MA: Harvard University Press.

Ordunez-Garcia, P. O., Nieto, F. J., Espinosa-Brito, A. D., & Caballero, B. (1996). Cuban epidemic neuropathy, 1991 to 1994: History repeats itself a century after the "amblyopia of the blockade." *American Journal of Public Health, 86*, 738–743.

Orr, L. L., Hollister, R. G., & Lefcowitz, M. J. (1971). *Income maintenance: Interdisciplinary approaches to research*. Madison, WI: Institute for Research on Poverty.

Packard, R. M. (1989). *White plague, black labor: The political economy of health and diseases in South Africa*. Berkeley: University of California Press.

Pearl, J. (2000). *Causality: Models, reasoning, and inference*. New York: Cambridge University Press.

Ransohoff, D. F., & Feinstein, A. R. (1978). Problems of spectrum and bias in evaluating the efficacy of diagnostic tests. *New England Journal of Medicine, 299*, 926–930.

Rosenbaum, P. R., & Rubin, D. B. (1983). The Central Role of the Propensity Score in Observational Studies for Causal Effects. *Biometrika, 70*, 41–55.

Ross, R. (1916). An application of the theory of probabilities to the study of a priori pathometry. Part I. *Proceedings of the Royal Society of Medicine, Series A, 92*, 204–240.

Rossi, P. H., & Berk, R. A. (1987). Varieties of normative concensus. *American Sociological Review, 50*, 333–347.

Rossi, P. H., & Nock, S. L. (1982). *Measuring social judgements: The factorial survey approach*. Beverly Hills, CA: Sage.

Sampson, R. J. (2003). Neighborhood-level context and health: Lessons from sociology. In I. Kawachi & L. F. Berkman (Eds.), *Neighborhoods and health* (pp. 132–146). New York: Oxford.

Schwappach, D. L., & Koeck, C. M. (2004). What makes an error unacceptable? A factorial survey on the disclosure of medical errors. *International Journal for Quality in Health Care, 16*, 317–326.

Sunstein, C. R. (1986). Legal interference with private preferences. *The University of Chicago Law Review, 53*, 1129–1174.

Sunstein, C. R. (2000). *Behavioral law & economics*. New York: Cambridge University Press.

Thomsen, T. F., McGee, D., Davidsen, M., & Jorgensen, T. (2002). A cross-validation of risk-scores for coronary heart disease mortality based on data from the Glostrup Population Studies and Framingham Heart Study. *International Journal of Epidemiology, 31,* 817–822.

Vander Weg, M. W., Watson, J. M., Klesges, R. C., Eck Clemens, L. H., Slawson, D. L., & McClanahan, B. S. (2004). Development and cross-validation of a prediction equation for estimating resting energy expenditure in healthy African-American and European-American women. *European Journal of Clinical Nutrition, 58,* 474–480.

Weber, M. (1958). *The Protestant ethic and the spirit of capitalism.* New York: Scribners. (Original work published 1905).

Yatchew, A., & Griliches, Z. (1984). Specification error in probit models. *Review of Economics and Statistics, 67,* 134–139.

Yeats, W. B. (1938). Under Ben Bulben. In *Last Poems and Two Plays.* Shannon: Irish University Press.

Zhou, X.-H., Obuchowski, N. A., & McClish, D. K. (2002). *Stastistical methods in diagnostic medicine.* New York: Wiley.

Zucchini, W. (2000). An introduction to model selection. *Journal of Mathematical Psychology, 44,* 41–61.

CHAPTER TWO

THE HISTORY OF METHODS OF SOCIAL EPIDEMIOLOGY TO 1965

Christopher S. Hamlin

Although social epidemiology is a recently emergent sub-discipline of public health, its issues and approaches are not new. In this chapter, social epidemiology is treated conceptually, as a *fundamental component* of medical inquiry with a long history, if only recently with a distinct identity. This historical introduction is intended as an aid to thinking: we are able to practice our professions more creatively, critically, and responsibly if we can see them evolve over a long time span; see how they vary under different social, cultural, political conditions; identify the determinants of their trajectories; and distinguish what is essential from what is incidental or contingent.

That *fundamental component* is best defined as the understanding of disease incidence and disease causation[1] as well as health experience more broadly, in terms of factors usually designated as social. These factors include economic position (that is, income, wealth, and economic security relative to others), family and

---

[1]It is appropriate to recognize both causation and incidence, as causation is conceived so variously. Some are comfortable with multiple levels and kinds of causation; others want to focus on a necessary or even a necessary and sufficient cause. In fact, as MacMahon and Pugh observe, cause is often dictated by disciplinary conventions or perceived possibilities for remediation. The widely used *risk factor* conflates levels and kinds of causal efficacy with circumstances. A social epidemiologist may or may not be concerned with cause, depending on how she or he interprets the term (MacMahon and Pugh 1970).

community structure, class, culture, and legal and political system. Ethnicity and race may be relevant as constructs that tie many of these together. Elements of the "social" also overlap significantly with other areas of medicine and approaches to epidemiology where, in terms of a common but troublesome dichotomy, "social" meets "biological." Thus, focus on environment and occupation may be concerned with the presence of microbes or toxins as well as with less specific influences on health and circumstances that govern production of these agents and exposure to them. Likewise, focus on lifestyle components like diet and exercise may be concerned not only with calories and cardiovascular condition but also cultures of eating and access to means of exercise and the value attached to it. And finally, although disease states may often be linked to sex, age, or genotype, a social epidemiology might integrate these with exploration of the influence of age and gender roles within cultural or ethnic contexts (with regard to expectations of sexual behavior or of dress, for example).

As "epidemiology," social epidemiology is concerned with the peculiar health and disease experiences of populations, but this concern is mainly methodological: the effects of social circumstances on the health of individuals *can only be discerned* by comparison of groups similar in some respects and different in others. Yet, as we shall see, a population orientation is not essential to an interest in the health effects of the social; such a focus has long been an element of clinical medicine both in the West and beyond.

As a medical science, social epidemiology has been important for four reasons. The first is as a way to elucidate the complexity of causation in diseases that are not accounted for by single agents or simple processes (for example, heart disease). Second, even where pathogenic agents and processes are well recognized, it may be a means of identifying other elements in a network of determinants that together constitute sufficient cause, particularly elements for which intervention may be most practicable. Thus, factors governing shoe-wearing are important in hookworm control. Third, it may guide interventions that improve health generally, not simply by lowering rates of specific diseases. Finally, social epidemiology may be a key to a non-reductive pathology, which recognizes the important interactions between milieu, a sense of self, and somatic state.

A final introductory point is the relation of social epidemiology to social medicine. To the eminent historian of medicine George Rosen, author of the classic 1947 review, *What is Social Medicine?*, a social medicine was neither more nor less than medicine itself, properly conceived (Rosen 1947). It would include an investigative arm, a *social epidemiology*. For Rosen and others of his generation, exploration of the social distribution of health and disease would have been tightly tied to exploration of the distribution of medical care and preventive action and, in turn, to the coordinated transformation of society to secure better health

(Porter 1997, 1999). Although one might argue that the findings of modern social epidemiology imply transformations—of medical institutions, social structures, or both—the continued vulnerability of socialized medicine along with the unreliability of health as an imperative for public action have combined to isolate social epidemiology: it flourishes, but not as part of the comprehensive social medicine that seemed so obvious to Rosen and others.[2]

It may seem that modern social epidemiology is but a product of maturation of statistical techniques, which now allow us to discover causes of disease hitherto invisible. It is better seen as standing on three legs: on paradigms of etiology that make room for social causation, on conceptions of social structure and dynamics, and on means of measuring social determinants. These arose relatively independently. These are treated separately and then as a union.

Can the "Social" Cause Disease?

In the history of the West, for much of the last two millennia, issues of "social" causes of disease would have been discussed within a heritage dominated by the Hippocratic authors of the early fourth century B.C. and by the Roman philosopher-physician Claudius Galen, c. 130–200. They would have been discussed in terms of a science of hygiene, concerned more with causes of health than of disease.

Although medical authors of later centuries would sometimes pit the empiricist and geographic tradition of the Hippocratics against theory-laden Galenic pathology, with its focus on individual temperament, the traditions in fact complemented one another and produced a medical paradigm clearly distinct from that of modern medical science. Remarkably, both traditions were prominent in medical training well into the middle of the nineteenth century. True, few would then have identified themselves as Galenists; the details of Galenic anatomical and clinical science had long been superseded, but fundamental categories, questions, and modes of medical explanation persisted (King 1982; Temkin 1973, p. 179). For social epidemiology, the most important persistent elements were the Hippocratic tradition of medical topography and two concepts from Galen: the six things non-natural and the philosophy of cause.

In early modern Europe, particularly in the eighteenth century, the most important of the Hippocratic texts (with the exception of the famous oath) was the text on *Airs, Waters, and Places*. Its author was simply recognizing a geographical

---

[2]Thus, Rosen begins his article by pointing out the truism that the biological, the realm of disease, invariably is mediated by the social.

distinctiveness of health experience (Brockliss and Jones 1997; Glacken 1969; Riley 1987). Sometimes this could plausibly be attributed to soil, water, or wind, or what one could guardedly call heredity; sometimes it was an inexplicable feature of place. Although the ancient writer is not much concerned with what we would call the "social," eighteenth-century revivers of the tradition were more attuned to the integration of nature and culture, particularly in towns. Authors were interested in how people made their livings, not simply in terms of exposure to dangerous materials but also in terms of psychosocial determinants of health: overexcitement and exhaustion, anxiety and insecurity, and opportunity for exercise. They were also interested sometimes in the stability and adequacy of food supply, in the adequacy of the family as a health-securing institution, in movements of population and their causes, and in the capacity of local governments to regulate the urban environment and meet needs for the necessities of life as well as for medical care.

Unlike the original Hippocratic texts, which alert the traveler and the physician, many of these later texts were concerned with the problem of effective government, both with regard to the potential medical catastrophes of epidemic or siege and to the health of the newly important bourgeoisie, to whose welfare that of the state was increasingly closely tied (Coleman 1974). The theoretical basis for this concern was the Galenic concept of the six things non-natural. Following Aristotle, Galen had equated *healthy* with *natural*. An organism that grew according to its natural *telos* or path was healthy. Whatever interfered or distorted—poisons, for example, or physical injuries—was thus anti-natural. But Galen recognized a third set of influences. These were neither intrinsically health-producing nor health-destroying: their effect depended on the circumstances, including quantity and temporality, of the body's engagement with them. They were air (including eudiometric quality, temperature, humidity, and throughput), sleep, exercise, diet, excretions, and the passions of the mind. In the many centuries before there was much knowledge of specific disease agents, monitoring and adjusting the six non-naturals was the main art of the physician. Traveling for a change of air, moderating one's diet, accelerating replacement of bodily fluids, or diverting one's mind from worry might improve the health of the wealthy client.

So long as that client could readily gain health by changing his or her way of living—and those treated by physicians usually were thus free—there was little incentive to regard these influences as *social* determinants of disease. As a medicine for the elite came to be applied to classes more constrained in their options, however—first to the middle class, then to workers, and even to a desperate underclass—the many ways in which society impeded health became inescapable.

Galen also provided a philosophy of causation that directed attention to multiple levels and kinds of cause, avoiding the problem of mutual exclusivity that would characterize discussion in the aftermath of the germ theory. Here too, his treatment drew on Aristotle, though it better anticipates John Stuart Mill, the source for the modern epidemiologists MacMahon and Pugh (1970, p. 12). Mill writes: "The cause, then, philosophically speaking, is the sum total of the conditions, positive and negative taken together; the whole of the contingencies of every description, which being realized, the consequent invariably follows."[3]

Mill asks a different causal question than do many medical scientists. He is interested in necessity, not in necessary cause, not in "what x must be present for y to follow" but "what are the full determinants of y?" The approach was hardly unproblematic. To view cause as the totality of determinants by itself offered no way to discriminate the potency of particular causes and left most events vastly overdetermined (Carter 2003). Yet, as MacMahon and Pugh suggest, such a network outlook does generate broader options for intervention.

But Galen also organized causes into classes. Although Galen-inspired schemes of classification sometimes became bewilderingly complex, their key distinctions were between proximate and remote causes and, among the latter, between exciting and predisposing causes. "Proximate" cause referred to the changes that comprised the disease itself that warranted the diagnosis. All other causes were remote, but "predisposing" causes referred to a matrix of background conditions, whereas an "exciting cause" was usually a sudden exogenous element that transformed a hitherto stable situation into a case of disease. As infectious epidemic diseases became increasingly paradigmatic in medical philosophy, "exciting cause" would become increasingly predominant. Usually it would mean "infectious agent," yet that was not always appropriate, as an infection might lie latent, as in the case of tuberculosis.

Prior to 1850, most medical texts would have carried a chapter on etiology in general. William Osler's landmark 1892 textbook was the first major nineteenth-century English text to forego one. It was not that the approach had been refuted or because Osler was preoccupied with infectious disease; the enormous accumulation of clinical knowledge of specific diseases had simply overwhelmed general considerations. Discarded by germ theorists on the one hand and by eugenicists on the other, the Galenic approach would nevertheless reappear in simplified form in twentieth-century epidemiology in old metaphors of multiple causation: seed and soil or spark and fuel (Greenwood 1935; Paul 1958).

---

[3]A decade later, evidently independently, the eminent pathologist-philosopher Lester King used the same quotation from Mill (King 1982, p. 206–7) in discussing the continuing relevance of a Galenic approach to causation.

To most pre-1850 medical writers, the domain of predisposing causes included the "social."[4] A single example will suffice: the March 1839 essay of the Scottish physician Somerville Scott Alison (no relation to the more famous William) on "the Propagation of Contagious Poisons, by the Atmosphere . . . ," a work that predates the great sanitary revolution (Alison 1839). Although he does not exclude contagia or miasmata, Alison finds them largely "superfluous" in accounting for disease, and he is better labeled a "predispositionist."[5] Scant and bad food, bad weather, poor clothing, and depression are sufficient as causes of disease. Each of these will have prior causes; thus poor diet will be due to high prices, and in turn to "arbitrary regulations of rulers, or . . . scarcity." To Alison, "cause" means chains and networks: "one cause of disease produces another, and so on, till the tendencies to, and the excitants of, pestilence, are so strong and so numerous, that whole communities are affected." He recognizes a role for an exciting cause, (for example, vitiated air) that will "act as a spark amid fuel." He acknowledges a reciprocal reinforcement of physical and psychological causes within a particular social environment. With hunger will come depression and inability to effect the environmental changes needed to maintain health: "a mother so situated will, in her misery, amid her actual sufferings, and with the dark yet immediate prospect of further hardships, forget the necessity, . . . of removing impurities . . . of retaining the persons and clothes of her family clean—and of washing the furniture, the walls, and the floor of her pestilence-haunted cabin." Those in such conditions, Alison declares, "can scarcely, for any length of time, escape disease." Along with public and private cleanliness, prevention will require "an active and cheerful state of mind, sufficient clothing, and wholesome diet." For Alison, as later for Marx, cause is a matter of vital energy: disease occurs when debilitating forces overwhelm resistance (Alison, 1839, pp. 62, 140–143, 153–155, 206).

This Galenic outlook is pertinent to modern social epidemiology for three reasons. The first is that, at least philosophically, no single class of remote causes trumped the others in accounting for disease. Causes that undercut resistance or that brought a victim into contact with harmful agents or the harmful agents themselves all warranted attention, although they might be differentially preventable. Second, practitioners viewed health as more than absence of disease. Whether or

[4]It would also have included hereditary or constitutional factors, but because there was no strong conceptual reason to force an ontological distinction between nature and nurture, these factors too might come under the "social."

[5]Alison was also the author of one of the best socio-medical treatises of the period, a study of the Scottish coal-mining town of Tranent done in connection with Edwin Chadwick's famous inquiry on the health of the laboring classes. Alison explicitly distinguishes "vitiated air" from "marsh miasma."

not they were philosophical vitalists (most were), their emphasis on predisposition led to a focus on a qualitative state of constitution, which was a product of social location. Although modern immunology would emerge from biochemistry and cell biology and would focus on the body's abilities to respond to generic or particular invading agents, what we would now regard as overall immunological status resembles the "constitution" of these medical thinkers. The third reason is the inclusion of states of mind as causal factors. Depression in Alison's text is less a psychological or a biochemical state than a social condition with psychological and biochemical manifestations. The Galenic causal paradigm is overlooked, yet much of what contemporary epidemiologists seek in a way beyond the "black box" of the risk-factor was addressed in the Galenic outlook (Susser and Susser 1996a, 1996b).

What Is the "Social" and How Does It Work?

Conditions might affect health; to call them social required a theory to understand what society was and how it worked. Such theorizing is a product of the eighteenth century. Prior to that time, it would have been appropriate to think in terms of a *social order*, but hard to conceive of *society* as a dynamic system of interaction. For most writers, the social order was composed of ranks or estates. Largest and lowest was the peasantry, who might be free as yeomen or enslaved as serfs. There would also have been an artisanal or commercial class and a class of nobility and royalty. Some would distinguish miners or mariners or the church and the military. Within ranks, there would be a sexual order too. Although power clearly lay at the top, such models were usually presented more in terms of mutual dependencies than as trophic systems.[6]

Such models did not recognize social mobility; effectively, rank was species. Differing health experiences were part of what distinguished ranks. Thus, peasants were expected to be fecund and robust but subject to famine. Aristocrats overindulged and were nervy. The commercial classes were too sedentary; artisans suffered from trade-specific diseases and hazards. To find that mortality (or morbidity or fertility) differed among these groups was hardly surprising, but nor was it problematic. Thus Bernardino Ramazzini's (1633–1714) much-noticed treatise, *On the Diseases of Workers* (1700), was a major contribution to occupational epidemiology but not to occupational public health. Such knowledge might

---

[6]Indeed, the famous botanist Linnaeus described an ecosystem in terms of the stations of society: thus, the peasantry were mosses, the yeomen grasses, the gentry herbs, and the higher nobility trees (Linnaeus 1977, 136).

(or might not) prove useful in treatment or in advising persons with particular constitutions what trade to follow, but that knowledge brought no imperative to prevention. Rather, early death was simply a component of the life that one elected (or that God chose for one) and that was recompensed in one's years of living.

The question arose, however, of what in the *ancien* biological regime of wars, famines, and epidemics kept the social ranks stable (Braudel 1985)? In his 1742 work, *Die göttliche Ordnung . . . (The Divine Ordering of the Human Condition with Regard to Birth, Death, and Propagation)*, a Prussian army chaplain, Johann Peter Süssmilch (1707–1777), answered the question: God's providence. Süssmilch was struck that slightly more males than females were born (the ratio was 21:20) but that the sexes were equal at the time of marriage. He noted, with apparent approbation, that mortality rates over the life course produced a reverse bell curve: high for the very young and very old, low for young adults. He confirmed that towns were deadlier (one death per 25–32 persons) than the countryside (one per 40–45), a fact that would provide the index of preventable death that would underwrite nineteenth-century urban hygiene.

But during Süssmilch's lifetime, the question was shifting. An emphasis on a permanent social order was giving way to a concept in which society was less "plan," more "system." No longer was the central problem that of explaining stability; rather, it was to determine the operation of a universe of social forces, modeled on the Newtonian physical universe. The new view did not privilege stasis; an understanding of the workings of these forces permitted (and, some would say, necessitated) human progress, which, according to enthusiasts like the English radical William Godwin and the French statesman-mathematician Condorcet, would lead eventually to blissful immortality.

The units in these social systems were not ranks or stations but individuals. Collectively, their self-interested behavior in a condition of freedom constituted society and was to be the motor of progress. But accompanying this new representation was a recognition that many human beings were not free: biologically, politically, or spiritually. Progress could occur only when they were. The several humanitarian and evangelical movements and the cultivation of sentiment of the late eighteenth century reflect this concern. In the second (1761) edition of his work, Süssmilch himself had moved from celebrating godly stasis to calling for improved morality (in order to lower urban death rates), the liberation of the peasantry, and land reform and reclamation schemes to improve their welfare (Meitzen 1891, pp. 34–35). In his reflective *English Sanitary Institutions* (1890), the English public health reformer John Simon would include campaigns against slavery and cruel and unusual punishment and for civil liberties as early forms of sanitary reform.

But how to measure social progress? In a broad and sometimes also in a narrower sense, the integrative measure of progress would be health in much the sense that the World Health Organization understands it: "a state of complete physical, mental and social well being and not merely the absence of disease or infirmity" (World Health Organization 1968). Liberty and an appropriate spiritual state would manifest themselves in a condition in which most human beings possessed the means to a "competence," a sense of personal and political responsibility, and sufficient education to act effectively in one's own interests. The many mappers of social condition, beginning after the Napoleonic wars, at first in France and later in England, classified populations and commented on whether the people looked well-fed, happy, and healthy; whether their work or living conditions were debilitating; whether they had resources to carry them through periods of scarcity; and whether sex, drink, political activity, or sheer fecklessness were putting them at risk. Overall mortality rates might be taken into account as well as the effects of high mortality in generating large numbers of dependent spouses or children. *Demoralization*, a term much used by English investigators of the period, referred not so much to immoral behavior but to an apathy that was destructive spiritually, socially, and physically.

There was, then, by the early nineteenth century, a climate for thinking hard about how modes of social organization acted reciprocally with social forces to create conditions in which human beings flourished. While one might measure conditions, there was great disagreement about dynamics and about which was cause and which was effect. Most fundamental was the conditions–character debate, which is still with us. In its starkest form, the question was whether character—a prior mental-spiritual state—led to certain social conditions with particular health consequences or whether prior social and health conditions determined character. During the 1830s and 1840s, followers of the social, industrial, and educational reformer Robert Owen (who held the latter view) toured English cities debating churchmen from a variety of denominations (Harrison 1969). In fact, usually discussions were less polarized: the question was, "Which kinds of conditions interact with states of mind to produce which kinds of social and health progress?" Or, put differently, "What are the social determinants of human flourishing and health?"

Three perspectives were particularly important in answering that question: those of Jeremy Bentham, of T. R. Malthus, and of a group of Scottish moral philosophers of whom the best known is Adam Smith.

Working within a framework of utilitarianism drawn in turn from the materialistic psychology of John Locke and David Hartley, the independently wealthy Jeremy Bentham (1748–1832) spent much his career deducing, by means of a "felicific calculus," details of legal and institutional devices that would direct the human atoms inserted into them along paths of virtue and progress. The utilitarian ethic Bentham espoused was expressed as happiness and measured (and theorized) biomedically: pleasure, like pain, was a state of the nervous system; health was the integral of pleasure. Bentham's influence was powerful but multivalent: it led both to intrusive total institutions (for example, prisons, poor houses, and schools) that sought to regulate all aspects of life and to heavy reliance on nature to provide incentives for humans to protect their health (Foucault 1979).[7] But underlying the seemingly divergent deductions was agreement that a good society was the product of good government, which in turn rested upon a science of social dynamics rather than on tradition or claims of right.

The followers of Bentham and, in France, of an independent utilitarian tradition were generally optimistic.[8] Not so the followers of T. R. Malthus (1766–1834). Reacting to his father's admiration of Condorcet, the young Anglican clergyman Robert Malthus began examining the assumptions underlying the predictions of human progress by Condorcet and Godwin. The result was the first, relatively short edition of his *Essay on Population* (1798), in which Malthus reduced social physics to two forces: the sexual drive and the need to eat. Together, they produced an eternal oscillation between overpopulation and starvation. The condition of human health was not high and could not significantly improve. Health was ultimately predicated on food; extension of health to the many (perhaps through the new technology of vaccination) meant extension of population and, consequently, hunger leading to excess death until population once more equilibrated with food. Like Süssmilch, Malthus thought he had found God's demographic order, but where Süssmilch had simply touted providential stability, Malthus exposed its mechanisms. By resisting sexual desire and working exceptionally hard to expand their means to support the children they would beget, individual (men) might improve their physical (and spiritual) condition. Yet this would not improve health generally; it would merely insulate them and their dependents from the margins where the "terrible corrective" occurred.

Whereas Malthus addressed himself to men, later theorists of a demographic transition would see the condition of women as a more powerful determinant of health. Food supply would turn out to be significantly more elastic than Malthus had appreciated, yet the framework he began persists in many questions of social epidemiology. How do social settings figure in reproductive decisions that in turn affect, at a variety of levels and by a variety of means, health conditions and the ability to improve community health (Szreter 1993)?

Neither Bentham nor Malthus had much room in their systems for human vulnerability. Both assumed a fully healthy human agent capable of making choices

---

[7]In most cases, "nature" meant nature plus existing property rights.
[8]The French tradition, also rooted in Locke, runs through Diderot, Condillac, St. Simon, Fourier, and Comte.

and acting upon them. For Malthus, reproductively irresponsible persons were weak, stupid, or temporarily insulated from the consequences of their actions by poorly thought-out social structures, such as public relief programs. From the 1740s until the 1830s, however, Scottish moral philosophers of the so-called "common sense" school were developing a more complicated model of human behavior. In contrast to the sensualist utilitarianism of Locke and Bentham, they saw the mind as composed of a number of innate faculties, which accounted for important elements of social and moral behavior as well as aspects of cognition. Allowing us to feel the pain of others—the faculty of sympathy, for example, famously explicated by Adam Smith (1723–1790)—helped produce sociability.

In part because the medical paradigm in which they worked highlighted the nervous system, Scottish medical professors shared the philosophers' interest in the workings of the mind, but they were confronted more often with failures of the faculties than with their successes. They attributed these chiefly to elements of the environment. They thus developed a perspective that underlies the third type of social epidemiology referred to earlier, of psychosocial–somatic reciprocity. States of the mind affected and were affected by states of the body and of social and physical environment; environment was affected by human agency and capacity that in turn depended on states of mind and body. Hence, human beings overwhelmed by what Galen had called the passions of the mind—fear, anger, desperation—might not respond to the incentives Bentham or Malthus would impose. Malthus had argued that the hardness of life would prod one to improve one's health; yet perhaps desperation, rather than heightening self-reliance, led only to a descending spiral of self-destructive behavior. The ability of one's so-called character to act to improve one's health itself depended on a preexisting condition of health that made accurate judgment and sustained action possible.

The Scottish philosophers not only supplied theory; they developed comparative historical-political-moral-sociological study to a remarkable degree. Societies past and present could be analyzed in terms of the workings of the faculties, dependent upon the reciprocal relations among the natural resources and modes of production and distribution, forms of government, the moral status of the citizenry, and their degree of prosperity and well being.

By the mid-nineteenth century, a few had begun to suggest the inadequacy of this view of society as the composite of individual actions. Rather, society was an emergent entity with laws of its own. The most important exponent of such a view was the Belgian physicist Adolphe Quetelet (1796–1874). Like Süssmilch, Quetelet was struck that many human phenomena that could not be explained by the equilibration of interests seemed inexplicably to cling to an average state. They seemed to represent laws of random distribution around a mean. So much was this the case that Quetelet and the English astronomer-philosopher John Herschel wondered if human free will was moot: what one did, another would undo. Later in the century the pioneering sociologist Emile Durkheim would go further to suggest that the social domain could produce forms of behavior that individuals not only would not have chosen but might have summarily rejected. It would follow that remediation must address not only the interests of individuals but their dependence on this emergent social domain.

At the time that Durkheim was positing an important role for this domain, others, frustrated with the failure of market or welfarist policies to improve social conditions, were beginning to understand these failures in hereditarian terms. Problems were intractable because the hierarchical social order reflected a natural order. They might even be worsening, because welfare programs counteracted the natural selection of the human population that would normally occur. Society would be improved only by wiser breeding. This eugenics movement began in England but spread rapidly throughout the world (Kevles 1995). It also diversified. Some would associate hereditary inferiority with race; others would not. Although it is infamous as the foundation of sterilization and genocide, by no means did eugenists uniformly ignore the social. Many argued, for example, that a comprehensive understanding of social hygiene must be the basis of a comprehensive program of social prophylaxis, which could serve as a corrective of widespread hereditary inadequacy. In fact, eugenist and sociological perspectives would often be tied closely together during the first half of the twentieth century.

The ferment of liberal social physics of the late eighteenth and early nineteenth century is rightly seen as the birthplace of modern public health. But although it led both to the development of data on population health and to hypotheses about social causation, it did not lead to adequate means for testing those hypotheses. Appeals to what people would or should do under different circumstances overshadowed convincing empirical demonstrations of what they were doing.

How Can We Demonstrate the Effects of the "Social"?

Although now viewed as a branch of applied mathematics applicable to a wide range of problems in natural and social science, until 1900 statistics was distinguished by its subject—the state—and not by its methods, which were not even distinctly mathematical (Griffen 1913). In part, a mathematics of relation depended on having the variables to relate; the qualitative dominated because the quantitative was unavailable. The denominator of most medical statistical determinations, population, was highly problematic. How did one get a stable number from flux?

Could a flawed and partial enumeration still perhaps be good enough? Perhaps when multiplied by some appropriate constant? But what constant? For much of the eighteenth century it was not even clear whether human numbers were rising or falling (Glass 1973).

The statistical accounts that German academics began to offer their princes in the late seventeenth century were to be useful digests of information on the condition of the state. This was Süssmilch's tradition, although he was more concerned than many with numerical regularities (John 1884). This so-called *kameralwissenschaft* had a medical branch that would evolve into the medical police movement of the eighteenth century. This focused on such matters as regulating marriage, controlling prostitution, the quality and availability of medical care, and urban hygiene but also sometimes on relieving poverty (Frank 1941; Rosen 1974). Generally, however, statisticians were more concerned with economic, technological, and moral issues (health might be relevant as a determinant of military power or of moral and, in turn, political stability). A similar science of government, developed in France by J. B. Colbert in the late seventeenth century, lapsed but would be revived after 1750. In Scotland it would be taken up by the state Church, in England in the 1830s by local statistical societies of concerned amateurs, and in America by state governments and occasionally by the national government.

Statisticians had recognized early that amassed data, however rigorously collected, meant nothing. Secrets could be revealed only by manipulation. This might mean arithmetic techniques (reduction to a mean, for example), but it usually meant creative juxtapositions of information through tables that allowed one to trace the course of variables across time or space, sometimes in relation to other variables. Tables then were no mere means of representing; in conjunction with the workings of the mind, they constituted a scientific instrument that gave access to an aggregate domain hitherto invisible. Table construction slowly evolved into graphical representation. So basic a technique as plotting data on a two dimensional grid, although conceptualized abstractly in the middle ages, did not become widespread until late in the nineteenth century, entering medicine as part of clinical science. Meitzen, writing in 1885, would present such "chronograms" as a novel means of analysis (1891, p. 196).

Limitations of technique did not preclude causal claims. Almost always, the claims have a large degree of arbitrariness—a statistician chances on a striking difference or selects numerical facts to defend a cherished position. Whereas demographic databases were gaining in completeness and comparability throughout the nineteenth century, the quality of statistical argumentation remained variable. Dubious comparisons for patently ideological reasons are so plentiful that modern commentators have sometimes wondered how their makers could overlook their obvious weaknesses (Cullen 1975). In part, the rhetorical character of statistics reflects the absence of accepted means of settling many of the most fundamental statistical questions, such as which of several variables was most closely correlated with a condition of interest. Meitzen would answer such a question by plotting the variable in question (which might well be an average, representing an unknown distribution) and then plotting beneath it, in order of likelihood, the possible determinants. One did this until one found the single variable that most closely matched the curve, which was something one saw rather than calculated (Meitzen 1891, p. 141).

Although there were improvements in mathematical medical statistics prior to the late nineteenth century (notably by William Farr, statistical assistant to the Registrar General of England and Wales, who standardized age structures of populations [Eyler 1979]), most historians recognize a scientific revolution in the development of techniques by a loosely knit (and often combative) group of English biometricians of whom the best known were Francis Galton and Karl Pearson. In a relatively short period, from roughly 1890 to 1920, they developed most of the major mathematical techniques for determining the strength of relation of variables as well as for handling error and for managing variability within data sets. Their revolution involved the gradual arithmetization of graphical techniques, but also the creative use of existing arithmetic practices—thus in Pearson's hands, the least-squares method, developed for correcting error in astronomical observations—became a way to measure departure from a regression line (Magnello 2002; McKenzie 1981).

In explaining their relatively late arrival, historians of these methods have noted that the Galton-Pearson project differed from those of earlier demographers. Galton, a founder of the eugenics movement (Pearson was a later convert), was interested in individuals rather than populations. He required mathematics to distinguish that component of a succeeding generation's phenotype ascribable to heredity. That meant a means to both handle variability and compare the strength of various determinants. As a positivist uneasy with such metaphysical concepts as "cause," Pearson would be more interested in developing the mathematics of correlation. In 1897, Pearson's colleague George Yule began deploying these methods on a question of social medicine, the causes of pauperism, a work that required techniques of multiple regression (Desrosières 1998). Pearson also took an interest in medical applications, and by 1911 a group interested in medical statistics had gathered around him. In 1922, one of his students, Major Greenwood, was appointed Reader in Medical Statistics at the University of London (Magnello 2002). In the United States, Raymond Pearl, newly appointed professor of Biometry and Vital Statistics at Johns Hopkins, was deploying the same methods (Marks 1997; Pearl 1923). Pearsonian methods begin to appear regularly in the

American Journal of Hygiene (forerunner of the *American Journal of Epidemiology*) from the mid-1920s.

Toward a Social Epidemiology

A theory of disease causation, a conception of a dynamic society, and a set of methods of inference were preconditions for the emergence of social epidemiology, but the three legs did not converge automatically. Rather, beginning in the early nineteenth century, small groups of medical practitioners sought to explore social causation, and, more rarely, social prophylaxis, linking the first two legs.

For much of the nineteenth and the twentieth century, however, they were working against a strong tide: interest in social causation was declining in the face of growing faith in the accessibility of single, necessary causes of infectious diseases. This was the revolution associated with Ignaz Semmelweis, William Budd, and John Snow. It would be the foundation of a disciplinary identity in epidemiology (the Epidemiological Society began in 1861). Later in the century, that orientation would be reinforced by bacteriologists and the first generation of immunologists. The interventions that epidemiology sometimes allowed were so dramatic that interest in the full range of component causes (including social determinants) came to seem an archaic and perverse philosophical crotchet. Indulging it could not aid the sick, and it hopelessly entangled public medicine into moral and political matters where it lacked standing and was in any case clueless as to how to proceed. The so-called "new public health" that emerged in American cities in the 1880s severed links with hygiene and welfare more broadly (Cassedy 1962). It would attack disease by attacking microbe haunts and (sometimes literally) ill persons; prevention would be a matter of isolation and disinfection. The social seemed somehow an impediment to knowledge.

Yet on the margins of the germ theory, social approaches survived. In the first place, notwithstanding new knowledge and powerful interventions, death rates as well as other forms of misery remained high. Phenomena such as infant diarrhea (and infant mortality, more broadly), malnutrition, venereal disease, occupational diseases, as well as the incidence of many endemic infectious diseases, seemed more amenable to structural and political changes and to what are rightly called modes of social control, such as health education. Thus a more macroscopic perspective, integrating the incidence of several diseases into a site- or class-specific mortality, might be more useful than seeking out individual causal agents and studying their transmission.

Second, even in cases where diseases could be shown to have a single necessary cause, it was becoming clear that many factors other than its presence affected disease incidence and course. In Galenic terms, the necessary cause was not always the exciting cause. The paradigmatic social disease was tuberculosis, the leading cause of death in the late nineteenth century (Barnes 1995). In some cities nearly everyone tested was infected. The variability of effects might stem from variations in the virulence of the microbe (or, put differently, from the adequacy of techniques for distinguishing it). Or it might be due to what was emerging as the concept of an immune status. Yet the further this got from serological reactions, the less it was explanation and the more it was simply a proxy for multiple and complicated factors—in effect, all those that Galenists would have labeled as predisposing causes. (A third form, an inquiry into the epidemiology of chronic and noninfectious diseases would not flourish until the mid-twentieth century.)

Those interested in questions of social causation worked within distinct national traditions. The most important were in France from 1790 to 1850, in Scotland from 1820 to 1850, in England from the 1840s, in Germany beginning in 1848, and in Sweden beginning in the 1920s.

The French hygienic movement which peaked in the 1830s, following the founding in 1829 of the *Journal d'Hygiene Physique et de Medicine Légale,* was an outgrowth of the Hippocratic medical topographies carried out toward the end of the old regime but, more importantly, of an aggressive revolutionary empiricism, captured in Xavier Bichat's dictum that medical students should "Read little, say little, observe a lot." To Bichat and his colleagues, the classical medical philosophy of cause was so much verbiage: better to stick to what one could see and measure. Within the body, this meant lesions on tissues discovered on autopsy; outside the body, it meant populations living in certain conditions and dying at certain rates. The most important exponents of this *hygiene publique* were Alexander Parent-Duchâtelet and Louis-Rene Villerme. Their exhaustive investigations made a strong case for social causation. Place a person in an environment and they would take on the biological and moral features characteristic of it. Yet the approach was subject to a general critique that had been directed at the use of this "numerical method" in hospital medicine. Health was the property of individuals; the situation of each individual in an aggregate was more or less different from the average situation; thus how could knowledge of the average dictate medical action (Desrosières 1998)? And were the units of aggregation even the most useful ones? For the hygienists, knowledge of social distribution of disease did not clearly warrant action, partly, it has been argued, because the hygienists were philosophical liberals distrusting public intervention in natural social processes (Coleman 1982; LaBerge 1992).

Scottish medicine, a generation earlier the world's best, kept abreast of developments in France, but the Scots' approach was theoretical and dynamic, the antithesis of French empiricism and positivism. William Pulteney Alison (1790–1858), for most of his career professor of either the theory or the practice of medicine at Edinburgh, was a contagionist and champion of the approach of Semmelweis and Budd. Yet it did not follow that knowledge of contagia could prevent fever. Fever incidence and mortality, he argued, was a product of poverty, acting through mechanisms that facilitated transmission (that is, overcrowded housing, high mobility in search of work or food) or undermined resistance (undernourishment, anxiety, and lack of shelter, heat, and adequate clothing). In urban Scotland, fever broke out among famine refugees from Ireland or the Scottish highlands. Alison framed the question of cause in the context of Scottish moral philosophy. How had the faculties of the mind interacted with existing political and economic institutions to generate a population that regularly became indigent? His answer addressed the issues of demographic transition. Possibility for upward social mobility would lead to reproductive prudence, hence to a population which would not readily succumb to fever; changed modes of land tenure would facilitate that (Hamlin, forthcoming).

In England, the key issue would be what levels of social explanation (and social change) to entertain. There, as in Scotland, an individualistic political economy was ascendant in the first half of the nineteenth century, but English social policy was on an opposite trajectory from Scottish (and Irish). In the Celtic nations, the poor, including the sick poor, had had no entitlement to relief. England had long recognized such a right. There the concern was that it was being abused by those who preferred to depend on the public purse rather than the labor market. The Benthamite Edwin Chadwick, architect and administrator of a reformed poor law in 1834, faced the problem of how to steer claimants on the public weal back into the labor force without driving them into disease and death. His answer was to identify a domain of social provision—labeled "physical causes of disease"—in which the state could act effectively to prevent disease without interfering in markets for food and work. This would be sanitation: good water, water closets, and effective waste removal (Hamlin 1998).

Chadwick justified the approach with a semi-social disease theory, a version of a miasmatic theory developed chiefly for tropical fevers (those which would later prove to be insect-transmitted) but used much more widely (Pelling 1978; Pickstone 1992). A focus on these quasi-specific aerial poisons generated in various sorts of decomposing matter allowed Chadwick to focus on social and governmental structures that allowed those materials to accumulate. In this way he opened a vast arena for health progress both by raising standards of environmental health and establishing a role for medical expertise in local government.[9] His

[9]This was not novel, there having been municipal health officers in Islamic and medieval European cities from an early period. English medical officers were, however, more epidemiologically oriented than had been customary.

successors were not so fixated on sanitation, yet it would continue to dominate public medical intervention and, especially with regard to enteric diseases, would be largely compatible with the emerging microbial view of disease. In effect, for roughly a half century, a focus on infrastructural reform walled off English public health from consideration of other social causes of ill health. An enormous epidemiological effort was directed toward proving that the healthy society was the clean one. Although the health consequences of increasingly vivid class stratification continued to be dealt with haphazardly by medical institutions, there was resistance to seeing them as distinct sociomedical problems.

What dissent existed rarely rose to the level of controversy (Hamlin 1995). The statistician William Farr, the medical reformer Henry Rumsey, and the nursing reformer Florence Nightingale pointed out from time to time that health statistics presented a more complicated picture than sanitary reform could address. In her *Notes on Nursing* (1859), Nightingale focused on the constituents of health (which were remarkably similar to the Galenic non-naturals). Good air was very important but so too was good food, quiet, and a solicitous interest in one's well being. Perhaps these might be provided to the hospital patient or the middle-class invalid, but could these determinants of health prevail universally? During the 1880s, adequate housing came to seem the key integrating determinant of health. Whereas Chadwick had initially included poor housing among physical causes, it had gained only a minimal presence on the public health agenda. Housing belonged to the domain of the market. Thus the first generation of local public health officers found themselves in the absurd position of chasing poor persons from one overcrowded dwelling to another. And those who tried to put into effect slum clearance legislation often found the market to be more interested in converting slum areas to commercial use than in providing affordable housing to the many.

To the German philosopher Karl Marx, for whom industrializing England was the field site for studying the grand clash of labor and capital, none of this was surprising. It was the essence of capital, Marx argued in the work of that title, to extract ever greater surpluses, which could have been translated into health, from the worker. Such mining of health would stop only when the working classes became biologically unable to reproduce the labor force (Marx 1939). Much of Marx's empirical case came from medicine, yet he failed to appreciate the potential of treating exploitation in terms of differential health.

A fuller recognition of social impacts on health would develop in England in the half-century after 1880. It would come through thorough social surveys—of Charles Booth, B. Seebohm Rowntree, Beatrice Webb, Clementina Black, and others (Himmelfarb 1991). Local public health officers had been reporting much of the same information for fifty years, but the surveys garnered attention because they came from a nonmedical elite and also perhaps because they coincided with the increasingly strident demands of a newly enfranchised working class. The surveys did make room for public health administrators such as Arthur Newsholme and George Newman to take up more socially oriented studies in the 1910s and '20s, on infant mortality, for example, studies which would increasingly reflect the biometric techniques of the Pearson school (Eyler 1997). They also gave rise to what may be called a golden age of academic social medicine, from the 1930s through the 1950s, associated with Richard Titmuss and John Ryle and later with Thomas McKeown, Gerry Morris, and A. Bradford Hill. Although their heritage includes important demographic generalizations and contributions to the methodology of epidemiological inference, the movement was not mainly methodological. Rather, it reflected a conviction that the level of community and society, and not of the individual, was the level at which health experience was determined and should therefore be the focus of medical inquiry and intervention—a return to the outlook of William Pulteney Alison (Porter 1997, 1999).

It was in Germany that the union of medicine and social reform was most politicized. The young Rudolph Virchow, who in 1847 attributed typhus in Silesia to a poverty induced by serfdom, was one of a group of radical medical scientists active in the liberal revolutions of that year. Virchow's later career as a socialist parliamentarian meant that social medicine would have a political identity that it lacked elsewhere; it would also acquire an academic identity. Yet German medical politics was more complicated. Among the many instances of rivalry between north and south (Prussia and Bavaria) in the newly unified Germany was that between the schools of Robert Koch and Max von Pettenkofer. Against Koch's tendency to focus on isolation of necessary agents of infectious diseases, Pettenkofer asserted a soil-seed-climate model. Disease (cholera) required a specific agent, activated by certain environmental conditions (changes in groundwater levels in Pettenkofer's view), and a susceptible constitution (that is, a state of predisposition) that would include social and political determinants. Although Pettenkofer's model included the social and Koch's largely ignored it, it would be wrong to see the latter as somehow reactionary. In the wake of the Hamburg cholera outbreaks in 1891–92, Koch urged improvement of the water. Opponents of this much-needed expenditure prevailed on Pettenkofer to argue that cholera causation was too complicated a process to succumb to a simple technical fix (Evans 1990).[10] Whether a focus on social causes of disease will improve health will depend on how much those factors are subject to change.

[10]Curiously, followers of Pettenkofer would pay much more attention to the meteorological than the social component of the theory: It would be known as the "groundwater" theory.

By contrast, a medical picture of society arose in a remarkably apolitical fashion in early twentieth-century Sweden. Sweden escaped much of the ideological turmoil of the nineteenth century. Although social conditions were hardly ideal, its social structure and paternalist central state were not seriously challenged. During the century, concerns about underpopulation gave way to concerns about overpopulation and eventually to eugenic concerns about national degeneration. More than in most other nations, government attention focused on chronic problems: tuberculosis, alcoholism, venereal disease, and a general malaise that rendered otherwise healthy persons (chiefly women) unproductive members in a modernizing society. In the view of the Swedish state, these were symptomatic of pervasive social problems and the diagnosis and solution to these problems properly belonged to the domain of medicine. For roughly the first third of the twentieth century, many of the policies were those of benevolent despotism. Public good required constraint of individuals; thereafter, interventions were increasingly seen as liberating, as establishing the social-biological foundations for both health and freedom (Johannisson 1994).

The growing concern with chronic forms of ill health, so conspicuous in Sweden, was also present in other nations. An epidemiologic transition was occurring. As infectious diseases came under control in the middle third of the twentieth century (before acquired immune deficiency syndrome [AIDS], Ebola, severe acute respiratory syndrome [SARS], and new forms of flu made clear that the control was only temporary), chronic and degenerative diseases (and, for some demographics, accidents and violence) began to dominate mortality tables (Fox 1993). Mental illnesses as well as cancer and heart diseases, all growing rapidly, seemed to warrant an epidemiology that recognized a multiplicity of partial causes. The latter would be the subject of the pioneering Framingham Study begun in the late 1940s, which would follow a large population to discover determinants of heart disease (Susser 1985).

But as the medical gaze broadened to include ever more of the social, troublesome issues arose concerning which social factors to focus on and of how to translate social diagnoses into social prophylaxis. Some of these could be attributed to the statistical problem of confounding; but such issues were most striking in politically charged situations, often involving race and class. The famous research in the U.S. South, by Joseph Goldberger and later Edgar Sydenstricker during the 1920s and 1930s, established pellagra as a deficiency rather than a parasitic disease. That research identified social causes of malnutrition but ignored the degree to which class was a proxy for race (Marks 2003). The Roosevelt coalition depended on southern Democrats. To attribute health problems to social causes was politically acceptable, to blame them on racialist institutions was not.

Multivariate analysis became widespread after 1970, employing newly available computational capability and bringing hope that egregious oversights could be eliminated. It also brought with it the language of "risk factors." The term could be seen to endorse the positivist Pearsonian vision in avoiding the messy term "cause." We did not need to know cause, in the sense of mechanism, to see where precautions might be taken (and, of course, such knowledge would help to guide study of mechanisms). Yet in black-boxing the problem of how a particular victim came to have a particular disease (precisely what Galen's complicated philosophy had addressed), risk-factor thinking ironically raised again that embarrassing philosophical problem of cause. Complaining of the "mindless abuse" of powerful statistics packages, Susser concluded that conducting such studies in ignorance of what was known about cause would be "as likely to obscure as to reveal reality." (Susser 1985, p. 156). Such critical reflections did, however, re-accustom epidemiologists to thinking in multicausal terms. They made clear, for example, that there were levels of remoteness of cause and that interventions for improving health outcomes were not restricted to a single level. They suggested the value of integrating incidence of several diseases as products of a single social determinant (Galenists had often argued that predisposing causes were usually general and could culminate in a variety of diseases).

Thus, whereas Austin Bradford Hill in 1965 offered a set of guidelines to explain why he and many colleagues could rationally infer that cigarette-smoking caused lung cancer (Hill 1965), still others were moving backward to look into the causes of cigarette smoking or into the social setting of a host of unhealthy practices of which smoking was only one. Generally, such hypothesizing would be guided not only by considerations of the viability of intervention but also by hypotheses about mechanisms and sometimes about interactions that were at once physical, psychological, and social. The most conspicuous of these would be the relative deprivation hypothesis of Richard Wilkinson (the flagship of modern social epidemiology) (Kawachi et al. 1999). But it would employ pathological processes that Galen had reflected on, invoke a Durkheimian sense of the power of society, utilize Pearsonian techniques of measurement, and in many respects mark the resurgence of the social medicine of William Pulteney Alison and Rudolph Virchow. Yet it is still the case that a social epidemiology tied to a social medicine will be guided by assumptions about which parts of society are fixed and which can be seen as appropriate targets for intervention.

Although this chapter has reviewed the three legs of social epidemiology—concepts of causation, concepts of society, and mathematical means of linking the two—and explored their union in several national contexts in the late nineteenth and early twentieth centuries, it has stopped short of bringing that heritage up to the present. On the one hand, there are excellent treatments for much of this period (Susser 1985); on the other, it will become familiar to students as they read the classic works in the field and acquire their own disciplinary identity. That will be important, but it will be equally important to think about the field from outside it and before it, which has been our concern here.

References

Alison, S. S. (1839). *An inquiry into the propagation of contagious poisons, by the atmosphere; as also into the nature and effects of vitiated air, its forms and sources, and other cause of pestilence; with directions for avoiding the action of contagion, and observations on some means for promoting the public health.* Edinburgh: Maclachlan, Stewart.

Barnes, D. (1995). *The making of a social disease: Tuberculosis in nineteenth-century France.* Berkeley: University of California Press.

Braudel, F. (1985). *The structures of everyday life.* Vol. I. *The limits of the possible* (S. Phillips, Trans.). New York: Harper and Row.

Brockliss, L., & Jones, C. (1997). *The medical world of early modern France.* Oxford: Clarendon.

Carter, K. C. (2003). *The rise of causal concepts of disease: Case histories.* Aldershot, UK: Ashgate.

Cassedy, J. (1962). *Charles V. Chapin & the public health movement.* Cambridge, MA: Harvard University Press.

Coleman, W. (1974). Health and hygiene in the encyclopedia: A medical doctrine for the bourgeoisie. *Journal of the History of Medicine 29,* 399-421.

Coleman, W. (1982). Death is a social disease: Public health and political economy in early industrial France. Madison: University of Wisconsin Press.

Cullen, M. J. (1975). *The statistical movement in early Victorian Britain: The foundations of empirical social research.* New York: Barnes and Noble/Harvester.

Desrosières, A. (1998). *The politics of large numbers: A history of statistical reasoning* (C. Naish, Trans.). Cambridge, MA: Harvard University Press.

Englander, D., & O'Day, R., (1995). *Retrieved riches: Social investigation in Britain, 1840–1914.* Aldershot, UK: Scolar Press.

Evans, R. J. (1990). *Death in Hamburg: Society and politics in the cholera years, 1830–1910.* London: Penguin Books.

Eyler, J. (1997). *Sir Arthur Newsholme and state medicine, 1885–1935.* Cambridge: Cambridge University Press.

Eyler, J. M. (1979). *Victorian social medicine: The ideas and methods of William Farr.* Baltimore, MD: Johns Hopkins University Press.

Figlio, K. (1984). Was social medicine revolutionary? Rudolph Virchow and the revolution of 1848. *Bull. Society for the Social History of Medicine, 34,* 10–12.

Foucault, M. (1979). *Discipline and punish: The birth of the prison.* New York: Random House.

Fox, D. (1993). *Power and illness: the failure and future of American health policy.* Berkeley: University of California Press.

Frank, J. P. (1941). Academic address on the people's misery. *Bulletin of the History of Medicine 9,* 88–100.

Glacken, C. (1969). *Traces on the Rhodian shore: Nature and culture in western thought from ancient times to the end of the eighteenth century.* Berkeley: University of California Press.

Glass, D. V. (1973). *Numbering the people: The eighteenth-century population controversy and the development of census and vital statistics in Britain.* Farnborough, UK: Saxon House.

Greenwood, M. (1935). *Epidemics and crowd diseases.* New York: Macmillan.

Griffen, R. (1913). *Statistics* (ed. with an introduction by Henry Higgs, with the assistance of George Udny Yule.) London: Macmillan.

Hamlin, C. (1992). Predisposing causes and public health in the early nineteenth-century public health movement. *Social History of Medicine 5,* 43–70.

Hamlin, C. (1995). Could you starve to death in England in 1839? The Chadwick-Farr controversy and the loss of the 'social' in public health. *American Journal of Public Health 85*(6), 856–66.

Hamlin, C. (1998). *Public health and social justice in the age of Chadwick: Britain 1800–1854.* Cambridge, UK: Cambridge University Press.

Hamlin, C. (forthcoming). William Pulteney Alison, the Scottish philosophy, and the making of a political medicine. *Journal of the History of Medicine.*

Harrison, J.F.C. (1969). *Quest for the new moral world: Robert Owen and the Owenites in Britain and America.* New York: Scribner.

Hill, B. (1965). The environment and disease: Association or causation. *Proceedings of the Royal Society of Medicine 58,* 295–300.

Himmelfarb, G. (1991). *Poverty and compassion: The moral imagination of the late Victorians.* New York: Knopf.

Johannisson, K. (1994). The people's health: Public health policies in Sweden. In D. Porter (Ed.), *The history of public health and the modern state.* (pp. 165–182). Amsterdam: Rodopi.

John, V. (1884). *Geshicte der Statistik. Erster Teil. Von dem Ursprung der Statistik bis auf Quetetet (1835).* Stuttgart: Ferdinand Enke.

Kawachi, I., Kennedy, B. P., & Wilkinson, R. (1999). *The society and population health reader,* (Vol 1: Income Inequality and Health.) New York: New Press.

Kay-Shuttleworth, J. P. (1970). *The moral and physical condition of the working classes employed in the cotton manufacture in Manchester.* (2nd ed.). London: Frank Cass.

Kevles, D. (1995). *In the name of eugenics: Genetics and the uses of human heredity.* Cambridge, MA: Harvard University Press.

King, L. (1982). *Medical thinking: A historical preface.* Princeton, NJ: Princeton University Press.

La Berge, A. (1992). *Mission and method: The early-nineteenth-century French public health movement.* Cambridge: Cambridge University Press.

Linnaeus, C von. (1977). *Select dissertations from the Amoenitates academicae.* New York: Arno.

MacMahon, B., & Pugh, T. (1970). *Epidemiology: Principles and methods.* Boston: Little, Brown.

Magnello, E. (2002). The Introduction of Mathematical Statistics into Medical Research: The Roles of Karl Pearson, Major Greenwood, and Austin Bradford Hill. In E. Magnello, & A. Hardy (Eds.), *The road to medical statistics* (pp. 95–123). Amsterdam: Rodopi.

Marks, H. (1997). *The progress of experiment: Science and therapeutic reform in the United States, 1900–1990.* Cambridge: Cambridge University Press.

Marks, H. (2003). Epidemiologists explain pellagra: Gender, race, and political economy in the work of Edgar Sydenstricker. *Journal of the History of Medicine and Allied Sciences, 58,* 34–55.

Marx, K. (1939). *Capital: A critical analysis of capitalist production,* (S. Moore & E. Aveling, Trans. from the 3rd German edition). New York: International Publishing.

McKenzie, D. (1981). *Statistics in Britain 1865–1930*. Edinburgh: Edinburgh University Press.

Meitzen, A. (1891). *History, theory, and technique of statistics. Part first: History of statistics* (R. Falkner, Trans.). Philadelphia, PA: American Academy of Political and Social Science.

Mikkeli, H. (1999). *Hygiene in the early modern medical tradition*. Helsinki: Academia Scientiarum Fennica.

Paul, J. L. (1958). *Clinical epidemiology*. Chicago: University of Chicago Press.

Pearl, R. (1923). *Introduction to biometry and statistics*. Philadelphia: W. B. Saunders.

Pelling, M. (1978). *Cholera, fever, and English medicine, 1825–1865*. Oxford: Oxford University Press.

Pettenkofer, M. (1941). *The value of health to a city* (H. E. Sigerist, Trans. with an introduction). Baltimore, MD: Johns Hopkins University Press.

Pickstone, J. V. (1992). Dearth, dirt, and fever epidemics: Rewriting the history of British 'public health', 1780–1850. In T. Ranger & P. Slack (Eds.), *Epidemics and ideas: Essays on the historical perception of pestilence.* (125–148). Cambridge: Cambridge University Press.

Porter, D. (1997). The decline of social medicine in Britain in the 1960s. In D. Porter (Ed.), *Social medicine and medical sociology in the twentieth century* (Wellcome Institute Series in the History of Medicine, *Clio Medica* 43, pp. 97–119). Amsterdam and Atlanta: Rudolpi.

Porter, D. (1999). *Health, civilization and the state: A history of public health from ancient to modern times.* London: Routledge.

Riley, J. C. (1987). *The eighteenth-century campaign to avoid disease*. London: MacMillan.

Rosen, G. (1947). What is social medicine?: A genetic analysis of the concept. *Bulletin of the History of Medicine 21*, 674–733.

Rosen, G. (1974). Cameralism and the concept of medical police. In G. Rosen (Ed.), *Medical police to social medicine: Essays on the history of health care* (pp. 120–141). New York: Science History.

Rusnock, A. (2002). *Vital accounts: Quantifying health and population in eighteenth-century England and France.* Cambridge: Cambridge University Press.

Susser, M. (1985). Epidemiology in the United States after World War II: The evolution of technique. *Epidemiologic Reviews, 7*, 147–177.

Susser, M., & Susser, E. (1996a). Choosing a future for epidemiology: I. Eras and paradigms. *American Journal of Public Health 86* (5), 668–673.

Susser, M., & Susser, E. (1996b). Choosing a Future for Epidemiology: II. From Black Box to Chinese Boxes and Eco-Epidemiology. *American Journal of Public Health 86* (5), 674–677.

Szreter, S. (1993). The idea of demographic transition and the study of fertility change: A critical intellectual history. *Population and Development Review 19* (4), 659–701.

Temkin, O. (1973). *The rise and fall of a medical philosophy*. Ithaca, NY: Cornell University Press.

Weindling, P. (1984). Was social medicine revolutionary? Rudolph Virchow and the revolution of 1848. *Bull. Society for the Social History of Medicine, 34*, 13–18.

Winslow, C.E.A. (1980). *The conquest of epidemic disease: A chapter in the history of ideas (1943)*. Madison: University of Wisconsin Press.

World Health Organization (1968). *Constitution of the World Health Organization in WHO Basic Documents, 19th ed.* Geneva: WHO.

PART TWO

MEASURES AND
MEASUREMENT

CHAPTER THREE

INDICATORS OF SOCIOECONOMIC POSITION

Bruna Galobardes, Mary Shaw, Debbie A. Lawlor, George Davey Smith, and John Lynch

Societies are stratified in multiple ways that lead to degrees of economic, political, social, and cultural advantage. These multiple systems of social stratification are important mechanisms through which societal resources and goods are distributed to and accumulated over time by different groups in the population. In this chapter, we consider one dimension of social stratification—that related to socioeconomic position (SEP). We use SEP as a generic term that refers to the social and economic factors that influence which positions individuals or groups will hold within the structure of a society (Krieger et al. 1997; Lynch and Kaplan 2000; Galobardes et al. 2006a, 2006b). It thus encompasses a variety of other terms, such as social class and social or socioeconomic status that are often used interchangeably in epidemiology despite having different theoretical bases.

There is a huge literature showing that better health is generally more closely associated with social advantage than with social disadvantage. Trying to document and understand how different aspects of social stratification are linked to different health states has been a major focus of social epidemiology in many countries for more than 150 years (Engels 1958; Sydenstricker 1933; Villerme 1830; Virchow 1848). There is variation, however, in the magnitude of this association with specific diseases (Davey Smith et al. 1996a, 1996b), and there is a much smaller but equally important literature showing that social advantage is not always associated with better health (Davey Smith 2000; Lawlor et al. 2005; Vagero and Leinsalu 2005). These variations and exceptions are crucially important to understanding how aspects of social stratification are differentially linked to health across place and time (Davey Smith 2003).

Different SEP indicators can establish groups with differential exposures and identify specific as well as generic mechanisms relating SEP to health (Naess et al. 2005). There is no single best indicator. On one hand, each indicator will emphasize a particular aspect of social stratification, which may be more or less relevant to different health outcomes at different stages in the life course. On the other hand, most SEP indicators are, to different degrees, correlated with each other, because they all measure aspects of underlying socioeconomic stratification.

In this chapter, we present a very brief theoretical background that illustrates the conceptual origins of most indicators of SEP, followed by a comprehensive list of these indicators. They are presented in an order best suited to the narrative of the chapter. We purposely abandoned the tradition of presenting education first, followed by occupation and income, to avoid assigning an established use or importance to the indicators. Most of these indicators characterize SEP in industrialized societies, reflecting the fact that most work on SEP measures has been developed in these countries and has generated measures appropriate to this context. Nevertheless, it is increasingly important to establish such measures for industrially developing countries. The two following sections include considerations for specific subgroups of the population and area-level measures of SEP. We then comment on life course measurement of SEP and conclude with some recommendations.

For a detailed account of the theoretical and historical background of measures of social stratification, the reader should refer to other sources (Goldthorpe 1980; Marshall et al. 1989; Wright 1997). These concepts have also been elaborated for health researchers elsewhere (Bartley 2004; Oakes and Rossi 2003). We present here an introduction to illustrate the different origins of some of the indicators described later in the chapter.

The work of two social theorists, Karl Marx and Max Weber, informs most of the concepts underlying the use of SEP in social epidemiology. Marxian-based social stratification refers to structural relations between groups defined by their relationship to the means of production and how owning classes exploit the nonowning classes in society. Class relations are characterized by the inherent conflict between exploited workers and the exploiting capitalists or those who control the means of production and power. For Marx, this was a purely structural relation that was exogenous to any individual. It was "hard-wired" into the capitalist system of exploiting the surplus production of workers. Current adaptations of social class classifications based on Marx's ideology of social class exist in the work of Erik Olin Wright in the United States (Wright 1985) and Lombardi et al. (1988) in Brazil.

In contrast to Marx, Weber suggested that society is hierarchically stratified along many dimensions, creating groups whose members share a common position leading to shared "life chances." These life chances are created by individuals from their ability to beneficially trade their education, skills, and attributes in the marketplace; Weber originated the use of education, occupation, and income as measures of these dimensions. Thus Weber places more emphasis on human agency in creating life chances than does Marx's more structural approach.

Occupation-Based and Work-Related Indicators

Indicators based on occupation are widely used, particularly in the United Kingdom where social stratification has traditionally been conceptualized in terms of occupation and is recorded systematically on all death certificates. Although these occupation-based indicators share the same variable, they have different theoretical bases, categorize occupations differently, and therefore offer a variety of interpretations. In addition to measuring SEP, occupation can also be used as a proxy indicator for occupational exposures. This different use overlaps with SEP because most occupational exposures carrying a risk for health tend to occur among groups of lower SEP.

Most occupational classification schemes, with some important exceptions, have not been recently updated and probably cannot account for today's occupational structure. The decrease in manual occupations with concomitant increase in low-level service occupations has altered the stratification that occupation generates in terms of SEP, and so classifications such as manual and non-manual worker may lose some of their meaning in economies which include a large number of low-paid, non-manual service jobs. This will result in cohort effects (that is, effects specific to groups born at the same time but that differ between groups born at different times) that should be taken into account to correctly interpret these associations. In addition, women moved into the labor force in increasing numbers in the last decades in industrialized societies and their job stratification may not be well-characterized with schemes based on men's job distribution. Unemployed people are often excluded in occupation-based classifications, resulting in underestimation of socioeconomic differentials (Martikainen and Valkonen 1999). Other groups commonly excluded are retired individuals, people whose work is inside the home (mainly affecting women), students, and people working in unpaid, informal, or illegal jobs. Although previous occupation can be assigned to those who are retired and to some unemployed people, and husband's occupation is often used to assign women's SEP, this may inadequately index current social circumstances.

Occupational measures are in some sense transferable: measures from one individual or combinations of several individuals can be used to characterize the SEP of others connected to them. For example, the occupation of the "head of the household" or "the highest status occupation in the household" can be used as an indicator of the SEP of dependents (for example, children) or the household as a unit.

Although occupational classifications measure particular aspects of SEP, they also share some more generic mechanisms that may explain the association between occupation and health-related outcomes. For example, occupation (parental or own adult) is strongly related to income and therefore any association between occupation-based SEP and health may indicate a direct relationship between material resources and health. Occupations reflect social standing or status and may be related to health outcomes because of certain privileges—such as easier access to and better quality of health care, access to education and more salubrious residential facilities—that are more easily achieved for those of higher standing. Finally, occupation-based SEP may reflect social networks and psychosocial processes and may also be a proxy for occupational exposures.

British Occupational-Based Social Class (Prior to 1990 Known as the Registrar General's Social Classes)

This scale is based on the prestige or social status that a given occupation has in society. Britain has classified the population according to occupation and industry since 1851. In 1911, the Registrar General's Annual Report presented a summary of occupations representing "social grades" in relation to fertility and mortality; there is evidence suggesting that adjustments to the classification were constructed "in the light of knowledge of mortality rates" (Rose 1995). After revisions in 1990 this measure was more explicitly related to the skills needed to perform a particular occupation.

In this scheme, occupations are categorized into six levels or classes, ranked from higher to lower prestige (Table 3.1). A seventh category includes all individuals in the armed forces irrespective of their rank therein, which is generally excluded in health studies. A common use of this classification reduces the six levels into two broad categories of manual and non-manual occupations. Adaptations of the British Registrar General's Social Class have been extensively used in other countries, making comparability between studies easier.

It could be argued that the relationship of this classification—as (theoretically) a measure of prestige or social standing—to health should be interpreted as due to the advantages given by elevated social standing and increased prestige. In practice it is often interpreted as a generic indicator and thus generic interpretations are attached to it. Based on criticisms over its lack of theoretical basis, the Office

TABLE 3.1. OCCUPATIONAL GROUPS DEFINED WITH THE REGISTRAR GENERAL SOCIAL CLASSES.

I	Professional	Non-manual
II	Intermediate	
III-N	Skilled non-manual	
III-M	Skilled manual	Manual
IV	Partly skilled	
V	Unskilled	
VI	Armed forces	

for National Statistics in the United Kingdom has since 2000 used the new UK National Statistics Socio-Economic Classification as its official occupation classification (described in this section).

Erikson and Goldthorpe Class Schema (Also Known as the "Goldthorpe Schema")

This classification uses specific characteristics of employment relations to classify occupations. It covers a wide spectrum of employment relations that ranges from an employment based on high levels of trust and independent working practices with delegated authority to occupations that are based on a labor contract with very little job control (Chandola 1998; Erikson and Goldthorpe 1992). Occupations are classified into eleven groups (Table 3.2). An important characteristic that differentiates this scheme from other occupational based classifications is the lack of an implicit hierarchical rank. Therefore it may not capture a gradient in health across its groups.

The clearly defined theoretical basis of this indicator offers an explicit interpretation for its association with health outcomes. Under this scheme, differences in health outcomes between groups are mainly attributed to differences in working relations and work autonomy, different contract and reward systems and terms of remuneration, and different job promotion prospects (Chandola 1998). The scheme also inherently reflects material resources, as aspects of employment relations such as decision latitude and job autonomy are usually co-terminus with material rewards accorded to different types of jobs (Davey Smith and Harding 1997).

This indicator was conceived for international comparisons and has been used in this context in European studies (Kunst et al. 1998; Mackenbach et al. 1997, 2003). In addition, several studies have assessed its construct and criterion validity. Working relations are likely to change over time, however, and therefore this scheme will also require continuous updating (Rose and O'Reilly 1998).

TABLE 3.2.   OCCUPATIONAL GROUPS DEFINED WITH THE ERIKSON AND GOLDTHORPE SCHEMA.

I	Higher-grade professionals, administrators and officials; managers in large industrial establishments; large proprietors
II	Lower-grade professionals, administrators and officials; higher-grade technicians; managers in small industrial establishments; supervisors of non-manual employees
IIIa	Routine non-manual: higher
IIIb	Routine non-manual: lower
IVa	Small proprietors with employees
IVb	Self-employed without employees
IVc	Farmers/smallholders
V	Foremen and technicians
VI	Skilled manual
VIIa	Semi- and unskilled manual
VIIb	Agricultural workers

Note: This classification is not a hierarchy despite the numbering that is used to refer to each group.

UK National Statistics Socio-Economic Classification

From 2000, the Office of National Statistics in the United Kingdom created the National Statistics Socio-Economic Classification (NS-SEC), replacing the Registrar General's scheme in all official statistics and surveys in the United Kingdom. The NS-SEC is explicitly based on differences between employment conditions and relations, similar to the Erikson and Goldthorpe class schema (Chandola and Jenkinson 1999). People are placed in groups according to occupations with different employment relations and conditions, such as whether they have a wage rather than a salary, their prospects for promotion, and levels of autonomy (Table 3.3). Only the grouping that collapses into three categories can be considered hierarchical.

Marxist-Based Social Class Classifications

In the United States, Wright has developed an adaptation of Marx's theory of social classes, constructing an indicator that categorizes individuals as to whether they are exploited workers or those who own the means of production. Strictly speaking, this is the only correct interpretation of *social class* as defined by Marx. Lombardi et al., in Brazil, have developed a Marxist-based indicator similar to Wright's (Horta et al. 1997; Lombardi et al. 1988).

Wright's scheme classifies individuals according to their positions in three forms of exploitation related to the ownership and control of assets: (1) ownership

TABLE 3.3. OCCUPATIONAL GROUPS DEFINED WITH THE NS-SEC SCHEME.

8 classes		5 classes		3 classes	
1	Higher managerial and professional occupations	1	Managerial and professional occupations	1	Managerial and professional occupations
1.1	Large employers and higher managerial occupations				
1.2	Higher professional occupations				
2	Lower managerial and professional occupations				
3	Intermediate occupations	2	Intermediate occupations	2	Intermediate occupations
4	Employers in small organizations and own account workers	3	Employers in small organizations and own account workers		
5	Lower supervisory and technical occupations	4	Lower supervisory and technical occupations	3	Routine and manual occupations
6	Semi-routine occupations	5	Semi-routine and routine occupations		
7	Routine occupations				
8	Never worked and long-term unemployed		Never worked and long-term unemployed		Never worked and long-term unemployed

of capital assets, (2) control of organizational assets, and (3) possession of skills or credential assets. This defines twelve locations where cells one and two represent the capitalist class, cell three the petty bourgeoisie or self-employed, cells four to ten include contradictory class locations, and cells eleven and twelve the working class (Table 3.4). Individuals in the contradictory class locations belong simultaneously to the capitalist *and* the working class (capitalist in terms of controlling skills and credentials and exploiting workers; workers because they do not own capital assets and are controlled by capitalists) (Krieger et al. 1999; Wright 1985). Wright has developed variations of this classification (Wright 1997).

Differential health outcomes across groups according to this scheme are explained in terms of exploitation between classes and the conflict generated by

TABLE 3.4. OCCUPATIONAL GROUPS DEFINED WITH WRIGHT'S SCHEME.

	Relation to means of production				
	Owners	**Non-owners**			
Own sufficient capital to hire workers and does not work	1 Bourgeoisie	4 Expert managers	7 Semi-credentialed managers	10 Uncredentialled managers	+
Own sufficient capital to hire workers but must work	2 Small employers	5 Expert supervisors	8 Semi-credentialed supervisors	11 Uncredentialled supervisors	Relation to organization/ > 0 management
Own sufficient capital to work for self but cannot hire workers	3 Petty bourgeoisie	6 Expert non-managers	9 Semi-credentialed workers	12 Proletarians	−
		+	>0	−	
		Relation to skills/credentials			

contradictory locations within this class system (Muntaner et al. 2003). Although relatively underused in social epidemiology, this scheme has been used in several studies. In the United States, Muntaner et al. (1994; 1998), Schwalbe and Staples (1986), and Krieger et al. (1999) have used Wright's classification in epidemiological research. Wright's social class scheme has also been used in studies conducted in Spain (Muntaner et al. 2003) and Israel (Wohlfarth 1997; Wohlfarth and van den Brink 1998). In the United Kingdom, Macleod et al. (2005) have applied Wright's notion of contradictory class location to investigate the role of material circumstances versus perceived social status on health.

Other Occupation-Based Indicators

There are numerous country-specific occupation-based classifications, which mainly use the educational requirements and income returns of occupations to obtain an SEP scheme. In the United States in 1917, Edwards created a hierarchy of occupations based on his intuition of whether an occupation required

TABLE 3.5. OCCUPATIONAL GROUPS DEFINED WITH THE U.S. CENSUS OCCUPATIONAL SCALE.

I	Managerial and professional
II	Technical, sales, and administrative support
III	Service occupations
IV	Farming, forestry, fishing
V	Precision production, craft, repair
VI	Operators, fabricators, laborers

intellectual or manual work (Liberatos et al. 1988). Generally, it was correlated with the educational and income level required for each occupation, which later became the basis for this scheme and it is used to classify occupations in the U.S. census. It classifies occupations into occupational subgroups that are collapsed into a smaller number of major socioeconomic groups (Table 3.5) (Diez-Roux et al. 1995; Sorlie et al. 1995).

Other occupation-based classifications used in the United States are the **Nam-Powers' Occupational Status Score,** which assigns to each occupation a score derived from the cumulative percentile of all occupations that had been ordered on the basis of average education and income, and the **Duncan Socioeconomic Index (SEI),** which initially combined occupational prestige obtained through public opinion (1947 National Opinion Research Center prestige study) and a weighted measure of education and income for the occupations not available through the initial source. See Liberatos et al. (1988) and Oakes and Rossi (2003) for more details on these and other occupation-based indicators developed in the United States.

The **Cambridge Social Interaction and Stratification scale (CAMSIS),** mainly used in the United Kingdom, is different from other occupation-based classifications. It uses patterns of social interaction in relation to occupational groups to determine the nature of the social structure and an individual's position within it, providing a hierarchical measure of social distance. For example, people working in pairs of occupations that rarely cited each other as friends are considered to have greater social distance, whereas those pairs of occupations that frequently cited each other were considered of close social distance. This provides a numerical indication of how similar (socially close) or dissimilar (socially distant) any two occupations are (Chandola and Jenkinson 2000; Prandy 1999). The Cambridge scale is a continuous measure, although it is often categorized into groups. Results with this scheme are interpreted as corresponding to (dis)similarities in lifestyles and health behaviors but also reflect general and material advantage (Chandola 1998; Prandy 1999).

Work-Related Indicators

Although individuals who do not hold an occupation are difficult to classify in most occupation-based schemes, working life and conditions in themselves have been used as indicators of SEP. For example, **unemployment** can be used as an indicator based on exclusion from the workforce. Other work-related indicators that can be used to measure socioeconomic circumstances are **job insecurity** and **type of employment** (temporary, wage, salary, commission, and so forth) (Benavides et al. 2000). These conditions are associated with worse health through a variety of mechanisms: lack of material resources for those who are unemployed, social isolation, loss of self-esteem, and the stress of potential job loss in conditions of job insecurity.

Education

Education is frequently used as a generic indicator of SEP in epidemiological studies. It is based in the "status domain of Weberian theory" (Liberatos et al. 1988). Despite this generic use of education as an SEP indicator, there are specific interpretations that can be argued for associations with health outcomes (Blane 2003; Fuchs 1979; Liberatos et al. 1988; Yen and Moss 1999). Most commonly, education is thought to capture the knowledge-related assets of an individual (Lynch and Kaplan 2000). The knowledge and skills attained through education may affect an individual's cognitive functioning, make them more receptive to health education messages and more able to communicate with and access appropriate health services, or provide the cognitive resources that affect "time preferences" (living in the here and now versus investing in the future) for modifying risk behaviors. A recent attempt to measure knowledge in terms of "cultural literacy" and assess its role in the association between education and health highlighted the great difficulty in trying to unpack some of the specific ways in which education and knowledge may affect health (Kaufman 2002; Kelleher 2002).

Within the life course framework (see Life Course Socioeconomic Position discussed on p. 67), education is increasingly seen as partly reflecting one's early life circumstances (Beebe-Dimmer et al. 2004; Davey Smith et al. 1998). Education captures the transition from parents' to adulthood SEP and also strongly determines future employment and income (Lynch and Kaplan 2000; Davey Smith et al. 1998; Blane et al. 1999). As an exposure, it reflects material, intellectual, and other resources of the family of origin, begins at an early age, is influenced by access to and performance in primary and secondary school, and reaches final attainment in young adulthood for most people. Therefore, it captures some of the long-term influences of both early life circumstances on adult health as well as the influence of adult resources (for example, through employment status) (Morris et al. 1996; Davey Smith et al. 1998; White et al. 1999). Reverse causality could partly explain some of the associations, however, because ill health in childhood may limit educational attendance or attainment and predisposition to adult disease, generating "health selection" (Davey Smith et al. 1994).

Education is measured as either a continuous or categorical variable. When using education as a continuous measure, with number of years of completed education, the assumption is that a greater amount of time spent in education confers health protection. In this model, every additional year of education contributes similarly to health outcomes. In contrast, using education as a categorical variable with pre-specified categories representing milestones in the educational process assumes that completion of specific achievements is important in determining SEP (Liberatos et al. 1988). Choice of measure should reflect the underlying mechanism that may relate education with the specific health outcome.

It is important to note that the meaning and attainment of educational level varies for different birth cohorts and in different countries. The proportion of the population reaching higher levels of education has dramatically increased in many countries. This is particularly so among women or minorities who have experienced marked changes in educational opportunities. As a result, the absolute number of years of education does not always correspond to the relative amount of education the person achieved within their birth cohort. Older cohorts, in studies that combine several birth cohorts, will be over-represented among the lower-educated groups (Hadden 1996). Few studies have taken birth cohort into account when using educational levels. In a study of cardiovascular disease mortality among women, the authors classified participants into low, medium, or high levels of education, these categories being defined with specific relevance to their birth cohort (Beebe-Dimmer et al. 2004). Stratification of the analysis by age group may also be required (for example, examining health inequalities by educational attainment within five-year age groups) (Sihvonen et al. 1998). A further limitation of educational levels exists, particularly among minorities, for individuals that have obtained their education outside the country of residence, in a different educational regime in which indicators of education may have very different implications than within the host country.

Despite the potential mechanisms that are used to explain the association between education and health, neither number of years of education nor levels of attainment provide any information about the quality of the educational experience. For health outcomes where knowledge, cognitive skills, and analytical abilities were relevant, the variables currently used in social epidemiology would fail to capture this aspect of the educational exposure.

Finally, the widespread use of education as an indicator of SEP reflects that it is relatively easy to measure in self-administered questionnaires, and response rates to educational questions tend to be high compared with other more difficult-to-assess measurements such as income. Importantly, it can be obtained from everybody who has completed their full-time education independently of working circumstances (Liberatos et al. 1988).

Income

Income and wealth are the SEP indicators that most directly measure material circumstances (Liberatos et al. 1988; Lynch and Kaplan 2000). The mere possession of money is unlikely to have a direct effect on health unless the possession of money per se increases a sense of control and perceptions of social advantage. Although such a psychosocial comparison mechanism may operate, its effects would differ across outcomes. It seems more plausible that more of the effect of income on health can be understood by the way in which money and assets are converted via expenditure into providing health enhancing environments (work, residential) and consumption of health enhancing commodities (food, exercise) and services (health care). Despite widespread use in economics, measures of consumption are rarely used in epidemiological studies. Nevertheless, most epidemiological studies of income and health assume it is the consumption mechanism that operates even though the exposure is assessed as income. Thus, income is interpreted as primarily influencing health through a direct effect on material resources that affect more proximal factors in the causal chain such as behaviors. For example, income allows access to better quality material resources such as food and shelter and better, easier, or faster access to services, some of which have a direct (health services, leisure activities) or indirect (education) effect on health. Higher income can also provide social standing and self-esteem and facilitate participation in society. Finally, the association between income and health outcomes can be due to reverse causality, where people with poor health suffer a loss of income. This reverse causality can be more prominent in certain outcomes such as mental health (Dohrenwend et al. 1992). Income is the SEP indicator that can change most on a short-term basis, although this dynamic aspect is rarely taken into account in epidemiological studies (Duncan et al. 2002) and its effect on health may accumulate over the life course (Lynch et al. 1997). In a U.S. study, persistent low income and income instability in the middle income group were both predictive of a higher mortality risk (McDonough et al. 1997).

Most often household rather than individual income is measured. Although individual income will capture individual material characteristics, household income may be a useful indicator for women in particular who may not be the main earners in the household. Using household income information to apply to all the individuals in the household assumes an even distribution of income according to needs within the household, which may or may not be true. For income to be comparable across households, additional information on family size or the number of people dependent on the reported income should be collected (Krieger et al. 1997). This can be then transformed into "equivalized income" (Ecob and Davey Smith 1999; McClements 1977) that adjusts for family size and reduced associated costs of living (Liberatos et al. 1988). Not all available income is equally shared within the household, however, as mothers from poor and working families tend to use available money to cover the needs of their children and partner before their own (Krieger et al. 1997).

Individuals can be asked to either report their absolute income or to place themselves within pre-defined categories; the latter seems to increase response to this question. Ideally we want to be able to collect information on disposable income, as this reflects what individuals or households can actually spend, but often we collect gross incomes or incomes that do not take account of in-kind transfers that function as hypothecated income (such as food stamps in the United States). Questions about income should include money received from jobs, social security, retirement annuities, unemployment benefits, public assistance, interest dividends, income from rental properties, child support, and informal income. Information on some of these may be difficult to obtain, and study participants may not want to disclose all information.

There is evidence that personal income is a sensitive issue and people may be reluctant to provide such information (Turrell 2000), although this may have been overstated (Dorling 1999). In different settings (including different countries, different birth cohorts, different genders) income may be a more or less "sensitive" indicator (with respect to participants' willingness to disclose this information accurately) relative to educational attainment and occupation. There are, however, more sophisticated methods for eliciting accurate income information (especially for in-person interviews; Galobardes and Demarest 2003; Pleck and Sonenstein 1998), but these will increase the cost and time to collect these data.

The meaning of current income for different age groups may also vary and be most sensitive during the prime earning years. Income for young and older adults may be a less reliable indicator of true SEP, because income typically follows a curvilinear trajectory with age. Income generally rises on entry into the labor market until the peak earning years in middle-age, where it stabilizes and then declines after retirement. Although highly desirable as a measure of life course income, calculating such lifetime income trajectories is difficult in practice and may best be done using population registries of the type that exist in Nordic countries.

Finally, income can be measured as a relative indicator establishing levels of *poverty* (for example, percentage above or below the official poverty level in a given year; Lynch et al. 1997).

Wealth

Wealth includes financial and physical assets such as the value of housing, cars, investments, inheritance, pension rights (Muntaner et al. 1998), and accumulated income. In terms of health, it is assumed that combining all these resources is a better measure of SEP and consequently a better predictor of health than income alone. The relative importance of wealth versus income, however, is likely to change over the life course (wealth being more important in older age owing to the accumulation of assets over time and the impact of retirement on income; Lynch 2001) or in population subgroups (for example, for a given level of income, black and Hispanic households have less wealth than white households; Smith 1995).

Whereas income captures the resources that are available for periods of time, wealth incorporates the accumulation of these resources. Wealth provides stable and long term security and acts as a reserve that can increase the ability of a household to go through periods of economic instability without suffering major changes in other social and socioeconomic circumstances (Berkman and Macintyre 1997). In addition, wealth needs to be interpreted in a specific context. For example, for a similar level of wealth, a person from a northern European country would be more likely to obtain resources through the social welfare system than a person in the United States and will therefore have a different ability to cope with socioeconomic difficulties (Berkman and Macintyre 1997). As with income, the main effects of wealth on health are likely to be indirect through its conversion into consumption.

Housing Characteristics and Housing Amenities

Housing conditions are used as an SEP indicator, particularly in the United Kingdom. They are used in industrialized and non-industrialized countries, although the characteristics assessed will differ in the two settings. Indeed, housing indicators can be very specific to the population or area where they are developed. For example, the number of rooms or even specific types of rooms (bedrooms and bathrooms) may be relevant as an SEP indicator in an industrialized country whereas the type of flooring (mud, concrete) or walls (tin, mud, concrete) are more meaningful in a non-industrialized country. Housing characteristics are mainly markers of material circumstances. Housing is generally the key component of most people's wealth and accounts for a large proportion of the outgoings from income.

Housing and its context is an important, multifaceted indicator of SEP. In addition to measuring overall SEP, housing characteristics may be direct exposures or markers of exposures for specific diseases and can be associated with health outcomes through these specific mechanisms. For example, the association of the number of windows with tuberculosis infection and death, in historical studies, (Shaun and Egger 2002), may have indicated both a general and a specific mechanism linking this indicator of SEP to this particular outcome. Because tuberculosis is an airborne pathogen, having access to a larger number of windows, and thus fresh air, may have reduced exposure to the infection. Indeed, there continues to be great interest in the built environment and its direct effect on health (Howden-Chapman 2004).

The most commonly used characteristic is **housing tenure**—whether housing is owner-occupied (owned outright or being bought with a mortgage) or rented from a private or social landlord. In rural populations, ownership of a farm and farm size may better define housing characteristics (Shaw 2004). **Household amenities,** such as access to hot and cold water in the house, having central heating and carpets, sole use of bathrooms and toilets, toilet in or outside the home, having a refrigerator, washing machine, telephone, and so forth, are also frequently used. These household amenities are markers of material circumstances and may also be associated with specific mechanisms of disease. For example, lack of running water and a household toilet may be associated with increased risk of infection (Dedman et al. 2001; Shaw 2004). The meaning of these amenities will vary by context and cohort. Very few people in contemporary industrial society will live in a house without running hot water, an indoor toilet, or bathroom facilities and therefore some of these measures are not able to differentiate individuals in these populations. These indicators will have relevance, however, in developing country populations and as indicators of childhood SEP in older adults in contemporary developed country populations (Claussen et al. 2003; Lawlor et al. 2003, 2004). One amenity that has proved to be a useful SEP indicator in the United Kingdom but that has been used less in other populations is **car access** (Abramson et al. 1982; Davey Smith et al. 1990; Macintyre et al. 1998). In rural areas of industrialized countries, car ownership may not be a useful indicator of SEP as even the poorest households often own cars out of sheer necessity (Asthana et al. 2002). In addition, car access in the United States is less likely to provide socioeconomic information given that in this country most households are likely to have access to at least one car. In non-industrialized countries, other assets that have been used as indicators of SEP in health-related research include number of livestock and owning a bicycle, refrigerator, radio, sewing machine, TV, or clock (Cortinovis et al. 1993; Filmer and Pritchett 2001; Montgomery et al. 2000). Asset indicators have also been created through combinations of these (Subramanian et al. 2004).

In addition to household amenities, **household conditions,** such as dampness, type of building materials used, and number of rooms in the dwelling, among others, have been assessed. The latter is used to assess **overcrowding,** which reflects material circumstances in industrialized and non-industrialized countries (Banguero 1984; Kuate-Defo 1994; Lenz 1988; Marsella et al. 1975). Crowding is calculated as the number of persons living in the household per number of rooms available in the house (excluding kitchen and bathrooms). Overcrowding is then defined as being above a specific threshold (for example, two or more persons per room). Overcrowding can plausibly affect health outcomes through a number of different mechanisms: overcrowded households are often households with few economic resources and there may also be a direct effect on health through facilitation of the spread of infectious diseases. Burstrom et al. (1999) have shown how crowding was related to increased risk of death from measles but not other causes of childhood mortality. Because measles is spread by human contact, the measure of crowding suggests a specific mechanism (greater person-to-person contact) associated with this marker of socioeconomic disadvantage.

More recent indicators have been developed that use different housing conditions. In the United States, a **"broken windows" index** included housing quality, abandoned cars, graffiti, trash, and public school deterioration at the census block level (Cohen et al. 2000). This indicator was more useful in explaining the variance in gonorrhea rates than a poverty index that included income, unemployment, and low education. In Switzerland, the **"social standing of the habitat"** combined characteristics of the building, its immediate surroundings, and the local neighborhood of residential buildings to assign SEP (Galobardes and Morabia 2003). Concordance of this measure with education or occupation was good for people of either high or low SEP but not for those with medium education or occupation, showing the greater heterogeneity of socioeconomic circumstances among people labeled as "middle class."

Housing characteristics and amenities are extensively used as measures of SEP. They are relatively easy to collect and may also provide some indications of specific mechanisms linking SEP to particular health outcomes. Results from studies that use housing indicators, however, are difficult to compare when the context varies.

Composite Indicators

A number of composite measures have been used to assess SEP at the individual level. There are also composite indicators that measure SEP at the area level (see Area-Level Measures of SEP on p. 63). Composite indicators have been especially prominent in the United States where Weberian notions of SEP have been much more prominent than a Marxist approach; however, increasing interest in determining specific mechanisms for—rather than merely describing—socioeconomic inequalities in health has lead to these measures being less frequently used (Geronimus and Bound 1998; Liberatos et al. 1988). Nevertheless, composite indicators may be efficient when SEP is measured as a confounding factor rather than as the main exposure of interest, as these composite measures incorporate and therefore adjust for different aspects of SEP. This is not theoretically unlike developing "confounder scores" as efficient summary measures of confounding.

Individual studies have designed and used specific composite indices, often dependent on the data available to that particular study. There are also some standard composite indicators that were frequently used: **Hollingshead Index of Social Position** (Hollingshead and Redlick 1958), **Duncan Index, Nam-Powers Socioeconomic Status, Warner's Index of Status Characteristics** (Liberatos et al. 1988). These are based variously on education and occupation data but have not been updated with current changes in the occupational structure and so are rarely used nowadays. For more detailed explanations of these indicators we refer the reader to Liberatos et al. (1988).

Recently, Oakes and Rossi (2003) have proposed a new composite indicator of SEP. They define socioeconomic status as "differential access (realized or potential) to desired resources." Based on this conceptualization, their indicator incorporates three domains: material capital, human capital, and social capital. In a pilot study, they found that this indicator, compared with more traditional measures, captured more of the social complexities involved in SEP.

Proxy Indicators

It is important to stress that the indicators included in this section are not measures of SEP per se but proxies for SEP and usually only used when direct indicators are not available. They are markers of SEP because of their strong correlation with more direct indicators of SEP and thus they may provide valuable information when direct measures are not available.

The **number of siblings** has been used as a proxy SEP indicator because, in some contemporary industrialized societies, larger numbers of children are associated with poorer SEP (Hart and Davey Smith 2003; Wamala et al. 2001). This is not necessarily the case in other populations or societies. Number of siblings may have a direct effect on health outcomes, as it may increase the risk of early-life infection. Indeed, number of siblings is most strongly associated with stomach cancer mortality, an outcome of H. pylori infection in early life (Hart and Davey Smith 2003). Number of siblings, however, may also reflect other mechanisms through which family size can affect health outcomes in individuals and family members. For example, the positive association between parity and coronary heart disease among women may in part reflect family lifestyle resulting in obesity in all family members and in part reflect pathophysiological processes related to large numbers of pregnancies (Lawlor et al. 2003).

Infant and maternal mortality rates have been used as ecological measures of an area or country SEP (Forsdahl 1977). Other characteristics such as **maternal marital status, having a single mother** or **being an orphan, illegitimacy, broken family,** and **death of father or mother at an early age** are circumstances that often result in low SEP (for example, economic hardship and unemployment due to the inability of obtaining a flexible job can be associated with single motherhood). Several studies report worse health in these subgroups (Lundberg 1993; Modin 2003; Osler et al. 2003; O'Leary et al. 1996), although adverse health outcomes could also be caused by other factors associated with these circumstances but unrelated to SEP. For example, infant and maternal mortality may reflect climatic factors leading to infectious diseases (such as malaria infection) in addition to reflecting SEP; broken family or death of mother or father at an early age could lead to ill health due to depression. So, when using SEP proxies, it is clearly important to consider alternative explanations of their association with health outcomes.

SEP Indicators in Specific Populational Groups

In this section, we briefly present some additional aspects to consider when measuring SEP in specific populational subgroups.

Women

Traditionally, married women were assigned their husband's occupational SEP, and in earlier studies, an unmarried woman's position was indexed with her father's SEP. Societal changes occurring in the last century in industrialized societies suggest that other approaches might be necessary to validly measure women's SEP in these populations. Nevertheless, partner's SEP may still be relevant or modify a women's SEP, particularly among older women (Krieger et al. 1999). Thus, accounting for birth cohort effects is particularly relevant with occupation-based indicators and education when defining SEP in women across different age groups. Occupation-based indicators that were defined with men's workforce distribution exclusively might not be appropriate to capture women's occupational positions, which are more highly concentrated in some sectors of the workforce. New classifications, such as the NS-SEC, and classifications based on clearly defined working relations (for example, the Goldthorpe Schema and Wright's social class stratification) might index a woman's SEP better. Household-based occupation can be traditionally defined (men's SEP determines the household's SEP) or the highest level can be assigned (independently of who in the household holds the higher occupational level).

Individual income can only be used for women working outside the house. In a given occupation or similar educational level, however, women's income is generally lower than men's, thus, household income might be more relevant in determining women's health and access to health services. Yet, traditionally women have used available income to cover children and partner's needs, thus the household income, particularly in poor households, might not reflect the actual income that is available for women's health needs.

Elderly

Morbidity and mortality are higher among groups of lower SEP, thus we could expect elderly people with lower SEP to be a more selected group in terms of health (those who have survived despite their lower SEP), which would result in the narrowing of health inequalities in the elderly. Health inequalities at old and very old age are reported, however, suggesting that the effect of SEP on health persists into old age (Arber and Ginn 1993; Ebrahim et al. 2004; Grundy and Holt 2001).

Considering life course SEP is particularly relevant among the elderly. In terms of occupation-based indicators, the last, longest, or average occupation is often used, although this approach assumes continuity in the person's SEP and the ability to maintain similar SEP from working into retirement life. Whereas this might be possible in middle to high socioeconomic groups, it is less likely for those in lower manual occupations. It may also not be appropriate for cohorts that have gone through periods of job insecurity and high unemployment. Arguably, this may not affect the SEP that is measured through status or prestige of the last occupation and therefore the prestige that the person carries on into retirement. It will, however, have important financial consequences that may determine an important shift in income level and therefore in SEP measured through material circumstances. A loss in material assets due to lost income may be balanced by wealth and pensions acquired during the working years. This is unlikely among those who held occupations with the lowest incomes, who are more likely to become unemployed and may not have been able to accumulate wealth.

Financial assets are particularly important in determining worse health in the elderly (Arber and Ginn 1993). Income and housing tenure are related to self-reported chronic diseases, functional ability, and oral health (Avlund et al. 2003). Material circumstances among the elderly will be strongly related to the occupational class the person held during working life, as this will be the main determinant of income and the pension the person will receive during retirement (Arber and Ginn 1993). Indeed, studies have shown that occupational position is still important and predicts subjective health and disability in men and women after retirement (Arber and Ginn 1993; Breeze et al. 2001). Moreover, previous occupational position was more important in determining disability than current material circumstances in the elderly (Lauderdale and Cagney 1999), suggesting an important role for status and other factors not related to current material circumstances.

Car ownership, a relevant indicator in the UK context, should be interpreted with caution in the elderly, as health-related problems may preclude car use. Health selection as a mechanism for health inequalities needs to be particularly explored in the elderly. Health problems developed throughout the life course may influence occupation and the possibility of acquiring wealth.

Children

Children's SEP is usually classified by their parents SEP. Most often this information will be obtained directly from the parents, particularly for small children. Asking older children and adolescents about their parent's education, occupation, or income may result in non-trivial levels of missing data and greater measurement error (Wardle et al. 2002). Some studies report good levels of agreement between parent's occupation reported by children and adolescents and the parents (West et al. 2001); however, these discrepancies most likely reflect methodological differences, and having someone to help and motivate children and adolescents to complete the questionnaire is likely to be important. Indicators based on household characteristics seem to be less problematic. For example, number of telephones in the home, car ownership, and bedroom-sharing as a proxy for overcrowding were used to derive a family affluence scale (FAS) in a World Health Organization survey in Scotland (Currie et al. 1997). Each item separately and the FAS had a progressive relation with father's occupation among those children that provided accurate information (Currie et al. 1997). A similar scale was constructed in England that included ownership of a computer and option of free school meals but did not include ownership of a telephone (Wardle et al. 2002). This scale showed good agreement with parental social class, although there was a bias toward lower FAS values among adolescents that did not provide information on parental occupation or education. An additional measure for a children's SEP is their own income, measured with earned money and money given by parents that they are free to spend (Currie et al. 1997). Father's occupational class and FAS showed similar associations with adolescent health behaviors with the exception of smoking and beer drinking, which were not associated with FAS but showed strong inverse associations with father's occupation (Currie et al. 1997). Interestingly, in this same study a higher level of own income was associated with unhealthy behaviors, such as smoking, beer drinking, eating chips, watching TV but also with exercising, suggesting that adolescents increased behaviors that required disposable income, whether these behaviors were healthy (exercise) or unhealthy (smoking) (Currie et al. 1997).

Ethnic Groups

The origin and processes of social stratification may vary in different ethnic groups; therefore the same indicator of SEP may not capture equally the socioeconomic distribution in different ethnic groups. Accordingly, the choice of SEP indicator within a particular group should reflect the stratification that best describes socioeconomic inequalities in health for this group. More often, the socioeconomic circumstances between different ethnic groups are compared and used to explain health inequalities in health outcomes; however, in this case, the same SEP indicator may have different meanings for different ethnic groups. For example, for a specific educational, occupational, or income level, blacks in the United States have less wealth and worse housing conditions compared with whites; for a given educational level, blacks receive lower income than whites (Davey Smith 2000). Characteristically, racist societies have a nearly non-overlapping distribution of SEP indicators among ethnic groups or races. In this situation, trying to establish direct or indirect effects (for example, through SEP) of ethnicity or race cannot produce valid inferences (Kaufman and Cooper 2001).

Area-Level Measures of SEP

Area-level indicators of SEP are mainly used in two ways: first, to determine the effect that area socioeconomic circumstances have on a health outcome beyond individual SEP; second, area-level measures of SEP are used as proxies for individual-level SEP when individual measures are not available. It is important to keep these distinctions in mind, because in the first case, the area-level SEP indicator is an object of study in itself as a contextual exposure. In the second case, the area-level SEP indicator is only a proxy for an individual-level measure. Similar indicators are used in both cases but the interpretation and the methodological issues involved in each situation differ.

Area-level indicators of SEP are obtained by aggregating individual-level measures of SEP to the area level of interest. These can be aggregates of the single individual-level indicators already described, such as proportion of unemployed, proportion in blue-collar or manual occupations, proportion with higher education, average income, and so forth, aggregated to the appropriate area level (for example, census tract, county, constituencies, census ward). Composite indicators using aggregates of several individual-level indicators have been widely used in the United Kingdom, where these area measures are referred to as **indices of deprivation** that serve to characterize areas on a continuum from deprived to affluent. Generally, the individual-level indicators are obtained from routine data, census, or other administrative databases that were collected for other purposes. In the United Kingdom, the geographical variations in deprivation obtained with these indicators have important policy implications, as they serve to allocate public resources to areas. They are also used in health-related research and have been applied in the United States as well (Krieger et al. 2002, 2003).

The most well-known indices of deprivation in the United Kingdom are the following. The **Townsend Deprivation Index** measures multiple deprivation with four variables from the British census: the proportion of unemployment (proportion of economically active residents ages 16–64 who are unemployed), the proportion of households with no car, the proportion of households that are not owner occupied, and the proportion of households with overcrowding (> one person per room) (Townsend et al. 1988). The Townsend Score for each area is a summation of the standardized scores (z scores) for each variable; a greater score indicates higher levels of material deprivation. Other similar indices are the **Carstairs deprivation index** (Carstairs and Morris 1989) and the **Jarman or Underprivileged Area** score (Jarman 1983). The **Breadline Britain Index** has different conceptual origins (Gordon and Pantazis 1997). This is a consensual measure of poverty, combining survey data with census data and using weights to account for the different probability that sub-groups in the population have of suffering from a particular type of deprivation (Gordon 1995). The Breadline Britain index is based on the proportions of: unemployment, people with no car, households non-owner occupied, lone-parent households, households with persons with long-term illness, and unskilled and semi-skilled manual occupations (social class IV and V) in an area. A version of the index without the health component can be derived and might be preferable for health-related research. This modified version has been found to have a close relationship with the geography of mortality in Britain (Shaw et al. 1999).

When area-level measures of SEP are used as proxies for individual-level indicators, the estimate of the association with SEP and the health outcomes is likely to be an underestimate of the true individual level effect (Davey Smith et al. 1998), but associations could be biased in either direction by the ecological fallacy. In general, the larger the area, the greater the underestimate is likely to be. Moreover, the variability in SEP picked up by the area-level indicators will always be smaller than that of the individual-level indicator. For example, if we use average income in a given area as a proxy for individual-level income, the lowest value in area income will always be higher than the lowest individual income, and the other way around for the highest income (Davey Smith et al. 1999). If the area socioeconomic characteristics have an effect on health outcomes independent of the individual SEP, however, the association of individual SEP will be overestimated when area-level indicators are used to predict individual level effects, because the area effect will be interpreted as individual-level effect. Whether underestimation (or overestimation) and its magnitude affect a given study will depend on the specific health outcomes, the area measures, and area size (Davey Smith et al. 1998; Geronimus and Bound 1998). In addition, using area measures for individuals relies on the area indicators measuring the same construct as the individual-level variable, which may not be the case (Schwartz 1994).

Area-level measures of SEP are needed when the goal is to investigate whether socioeconomic aspects of the place where a person lives, over and above individual characteristics, affect that person's health. "Where" a person lives can be a neighborhood, city, or higher administrative area (for example, health authority in the United Kingdom, region, county, or country level) (Diez-Roux 2002; Tunstall et al. 2004). There have been numerous studies of such "area effects," mainly in the United States but also elsewhere, with most studies finding a relatively small, in comparison with individual-level variables, independent neighborhood effect on various health outcomes and health behaviors (Pickett and Pearl 2001). Several of these studies, however, adjusted for only one measure of individual SEP, whereas when life course individual SEP was accounted for, area SEP was no longer associated with mortality (Davey Smith et al. 1997). By contrast, in a study of British women, 60–79 years of age, area-level SEP and individual life course SEP both contributed to CHD prevalence (Lawlor et al. 2005).

There are some methodological issues to consider in estimating area-level associations with health outcomes. It is unclear whether the associations between area-level measures of SEP and health outcomes are related to the socioeconomic characteristics of the area independently of the (lifetime) characteristics of the people living in these areas (Naess, Claussen et al. 2005; Diez-Roux 2002; Macintyre et al. 2002; Pickett and Pearl 2001; Reijneveld et al. 2001). This is a conceptual and an empirical problem, particularly within a life course framework (see Life Course Socioeconomic Position, on page 67), as historical SEP information on both areas and individuals is required if we are to understand how area-level processes affect health over time independently of individual SEP. It is unlikely that adjustment for one or two adult indicators of SEP, as used in most research conducted up until now, is sufficient for capturing the full extent of individual SEP effects (Davey Smith et al. 1997). A more generic question is whether area SEP can even be conceptualized independently of the SEP of individuals living in the area (Oakes 2004). For example, changing the proportion of poor individuals living in an area would automatically change the area SEP defined in terms of income. This lack of independence between individual and area in terms of socioeconomic circumstances is additionally illustrated by the fact that it is difficult to find examples of measures of SEP conceptually defined at the area level that are not simple aggregates of individual-level SEP. One potential exception in this regard is distributional indicators of SEP, such as the extent of income or educational inequality. Here, it is not the average income in an area that is the supposed contextual exposure but rather the unequal distribution of income among the individuals living in the area. More unequal income distribution can only be defined at an area level because it represents the relation of one individual's income to others in the same area and so has no meaning at the individual level. There have been several examples of this type of research in social epidemiology (Lynch et al. 2004a, 2004b; Subramanian and Kawachi 2004). Nevertheless, income inequality is not independent of individual income, as it will change according to changes in individuals' incomes. It has also been argued that area SEP acts as a proxy for other environmental exposures (Diez-Roux 2004a). For example, areas of different SEP have different levels of retail investment that results in the type and quality of foods being unequally available across different areas.

Additional limitations occur with studies that do not explicitly state the mechanisms through which a determined area-level exposure can influence a health outcome. Most data, including the area-level boundaries themselves, are obtained from administrative databases limiting the available information to what had been collected, often for other than health purposes. For example, the relevant area boundary for the outcome of interest may not be available, as is the case for neighborhood effects that are being explored by such surrogates as census blocks or tracks (Diez-Roux 2004b). Discussion of these and other methodological and conceptual issues relating the estimation of area-level effects can be found elsewhere (Diez-Roux 2004b; Oakes 2004; Subramanian 2004).

Life Course Socioeconomic Position

A life course approach to chronic diseases is particularly relevant in understanding how socioeconomic circumstances influence health. A life course approach in epidemiology investigates the long-term effects on health and chronic disease risk of physical and social hazards across generations and during gestation, childhood, adolescence, young adulthood, and later adult life. It explicitly incorporates time of exposure and can be conceptualized at the individual level, across generations, and through population disease trends (Lynch and Davey Smith 2005).

At the individual level, the indicators of SEP, measured at different stages of the life course, can be useful in examining how socioeconomic conditions operating at different stages of life influence disease risk to create the observed adult inequalities in health (Davey Smith 2003). Combinations of the indicators described in the first part of this chapter allow construction of a lifelong measure of one's SEP. Some indicators are only valid at specific ages; for example, education is mostly completed by young adulthood, whereas own occupation can only occur after the age of 16 in rich countries. The same indicator, for example an occupation-based indicator, can be measured at different times during the life course, however; for example, father's occupation characterizes childhood SEP, and first, longest, and last occupation characterize adult SEP. An indicator may be particularly appropriate for a given period of time, as is the case of wealth, which may better characterize SEP at old age. Figure 3.1 presents several indicators of SEP combined in a life course framework.

There are several theoretical models that help in conceptualizing how life course exposures influence disease risk (Kuh and Ben-Shlomo 2004). The critical period model argues that an exposure during a particular time window has lasting effects that result in higher disease risk. Barker's formulation of the fetal hypothesis is an example of this model, which has subsequently been modified to include later-life effect modifiers: low birth weight (reflecting poor intrauterine nutrition, which programs one's metabolism for a life of thrift) combined with later life obesity or accelerated growth (indicating the reality of a life of plenty—in terms of energy dense foods) seems to carry the highest adult coronary heart disease (CHD) risk (Eriksson et al. 1999; Frankel et al. 1996). In addition to critical periods, there may be "sensitive periods" when an exposure has a particularly marked but not unique effect. For example, infancy may be a particularly sensitive period for the effect of dietary salt intake on future intake of salty food and high blood pressure, but the liking for a high-salt diet may also develop at other times in the life course (Lawlor and Smith 2005). The other proposed life course models state that effects accumulate over the life course. In this scenario health

FIGURE 3.1. EXAMPLES OF INDICATORS MEASURING LIFE COURSE SOCIOECONOMIC POSITION.

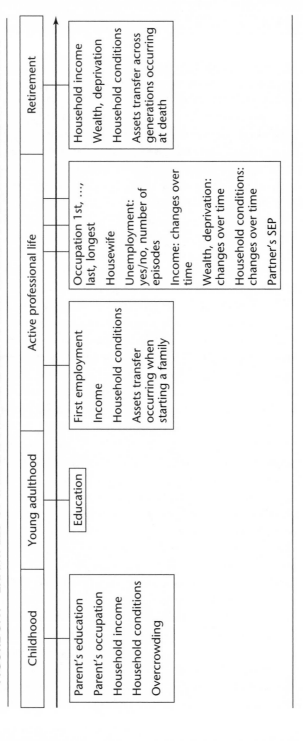

damage increases with the patterning, duration, or number of exposures (Ben-Shlomo and Kuh 2002). These exposures can occur independently due to uncorrelated insults, or they may be due to correlated insults, such as risk clustering or chains of risk (Kuh and Ben-Shlomo 2004). Understanding the specific life course model that affects a particular disease outcome is important, because this indicates the appropriate timing of any preventive intervention.

The contribution of childhood and adulthood SEP is specific to disease outcomes. In a systematic review, childhood SEP (often indexed by father's occupation) was particularly relevant in determining the risk of stomach cancer (Galobardes et al. 2004). This probably reflects the time in the life course during which the relevant etiological exposures causing these diseases take place, as is the case for Helicobacter pylori and stomach cancer. Childhood SEP contributed, together with socioeconomic conditions in adult life, to determining mortality from CHD, lung cancer, and respiratory-related deaths, although the relative contribution of child versus adult circumstances varied in different contexts. Worse childhood socioeconomic circumstances not only contribute to a higher risk of death due to CHD; they also determine a higher risk of developing CHD disease and, at least in women, seem to correlate with higher levels of atherosclerosis at pre-clinical phases of the disease (Galobardes et al., forthcoming). In the United States, a study of twins that had lived together until the age of 14 and thus matched on childhood socioeconomic circumstances found that levels of cardiovascular factors were more different among twins who had different as opposed to similar occupational levels in adulthood (Krieger et al. 2005). Among the pairs discordant for adult occupational class, risk factors were worse for twins classified as working-class in adulthood compared with those that belonged to the professional class. Other studies report additive effects between childhood and adulthood SEP in relation to CHD risk (Davey Smith et al. 1997; Lawlor et al. 2004), and longer or higher number of times experiencing poverty throughout one's life is associated with worse health (Lynch et al. 1997; McDonough et al. 2005), although the relationship might be complex and dependent on ethnicity or race, gender and age (McDonough et al. 2005). Thus, the role of life course socioeconomic circumstances in determining CHD risk is best explained under the accumulation of risks model (Davey Smith et al. 1997; Heslop et al. 2001). Accumulation of risks throughout life can also be due to clustering of exposures. For example, children from lower socioeconomic backgrounds are more likely to be of low birth weight, have poorer diets, be more exposed to passive smoking and some infectious agents, and have fewer educational opportunities (Ben-Shlomo and Kuh 2002). Finally, exposures may form chains of risk, where coming from a family background of low SEP leads to low educational attainment that in turn will increase the probability of working in an occupation with a high risk of toxic exposures and of having low income (Davey Smith 2003).

There is an intrinsic problem in differentiating life course processes, and it is most likely that different models will apply to different disease outcomes (Hallqvist et al. 2004). Whether critical period, social mobility, accumulation of risks, or combinations of these underlie the association between SEP and a health outcome requires prior knowledge of the specific causal mechanisms; however, comparing changes in the direction or magnitude of the association between a specific health outcome with different SEP indicators across the life course can point to specific exposures. As the role of SEP from across the life course in adult disease outcomes becomes more apparent, the need to adjust for these different life course SEP measures in observational studies of exposures and outcomes that are strongly socially patterned is increasingly acknowledged (Davey Smith et al. 2002; Lawlor et al. 2004).

Use of life course SEP indicators presents some methodological challenges. As mentioned before in regard to income, it would be desirable to have summary measures that indicated the entire income trajectory of an individual over time but, with few exceptions (McDonough et al. 2005), these data are both hard to obtain and only cover a certain portion of the life course. An extended array of life course indicators might include measures of parental SEP prior to birth and during childhood, own education, first job, and then subsequent occupational history, income over time, and asset accumulation and asset transfers from parents. Collecting such information then raises questions of how to create summary measures when each individual indicator is based on a different measurement scale as well as taken at different times and consequently different contexts. The use of latent variable and structural equation modeling may be helpful in capturing these complicated processes (Singh-Manoux et al. 2003).

The life course approach can also be applied to provide understanding of trends in population health. Studying long-term trends in socioeconomic circumstances as, for example, with income inequality and how these relate to long-term disease trends can test for plausible relationships between these trends. The income inequality hypothesis formulates that levels of income inequality is a better predictor of life expectancy in wealthy societies than absolute income (Wilkinson 1992). Problems with the original data used to formulate this hypothesis (Lynch et al. 2001) and a systematic review of the studies that have investigated the association between income inequality and health cast doubt on its relevance in explaining levels of population health (Lynch et al. 2004a). Lynch et al. (2004b), using a life course approach, assessed how time trends in income inequality correspond with trends in mortality in the United States. They showed that trends in income inequality to the end of World War II are coincidental with changes in poverty and initiation of welfare programs; thus disentangling the independent effects on mortality of income inequality from those of poverty is difficult. The continuous fall of infant mortality and stroke during the twentieth century is inconsistent with fluctuations in income inequality. Trends in CHD during the twentieth century are more compatible with what is known in trends of established risk factors than with income inequality trends. And trends in income inequality do not seem to correspond to trends of known CHD risk factors (for example, smoking rose at the same time income inequality decreased in the twentieth century) (Lynch et al. 2004b). Nevertheless, even if the life course perspective allows us to understand most of the trends in chronic diseases, such as CHD, with what is known from their established risk factors, we still lack understanding of the socio-environmental circumstances that determine changes in the distribution of these risk factors in different birth cohorts and social groups over time (Davey Smith 2003; Lynch and Davey Smith 2005).

Recommendations

The departure point for a more complete etiological understanding of socioeconomic health differentials should be based on mechanistic specificity of links between particular SEP indicators (as described in this chapter) and different health outcomes (Davey Smith 2003). Careful investigation of the associations of specific health outcomes with different indicators of SEP can provide insight into these mechanisms. The following are generic guidelines that summarize the main aspects to consider when deciding which measure of SEP to use and how to use it:

- Have a hypothesis of the mechanism relating SEP to the particular health outcome. For example, if the question is about socioeconomic differences in the prevalence of diabetes in men, it would be important to consider the socioeconomic influences on the main risk factors for the outcome—in this case, a range of socially determined behaviors involving diet, exercise, and medication as well as access to health services, together with indicators of early life (or parental SEP), given the considerable evidence regarding early life origins of diabetes risk.
- Tailor the SEP indicators more likely to capture or reflect etiological mechanisms. In the previous example, it might be important to measure early life SEP, individual adult SEP, and household income and education of both the man and his partner, given that it is reasonable to assume that education of the partner (if indeed he has one) may be important in understanding how well the man manages the array of self-care behaviors likely to influence progression of diabetes.

• Use several indicators of SEP; it is very unlikely that one single indicator from one period of the life course will characterize the whole spectrum of exposures experienced by different socioeconomic groups. In this regard, we should examine carefully how well lifetime SEP has been measured when controlling for its effects in studies of other exposures.

• When possible use theoretically grounded measures of SEP and interpret results according to this theoretical basis. In practice, the preferred indicators may not always be available, in which case the associations should be interpreted within the limitations of the available indicators.

• Always consider time by thinking about the social conditions experienced by the particular birth cohort being studied and how they played out across lifetime. For example, early-life social disadvantage for a cohort born in the 1920s may have implied very different exposures than for a cohort born in the 1950s and may, as a consequence, have very different associations with health outcomes. Considering time in this way will better contextualize the SEP indicators across the life course.

• Consider contextual (area-based) influences as well as individual socioeconomic characteristics. Think about the social processes that occur at different levels that influence the outcomes(s), and include indicators accordingly. For example, diabetes might be likely to progress more rapidly in men, independently of their individual SEPs, who live in poor neighborhoods where choice of food is less varied and health care facilities are poorer.

• If specific subgroups of the population are the focus of the research, modify the indicators and their interpretation to the particular subgroup of the population being studied.

• Where possible, interpret associations specifically between the particular indicator and the particular health outcome. In both multilevel and life course applications of SEP and health, greater specificity is more likely to produce meaningful explanations and mechanisms for understanding the genesis of socioeconomic inequalities in health.

• Think about measurement of the outcome, especially if this is likely to be differentially affected by SEP. The main focus of this chapter is on accurate measurement of indicators of SEP, but the association of SEP with outcomes can only be accurately interpreted with care in outcome assessment. In the previous example, it would be very important to use biological measures for this outcome (fasting blood glucose or glucose tolerance tests) rather than clinical diagnosis. This is because diabetes is largely asymptomatic, with estimates that up to 50 percent of cases are undiagnosed in industrialized populations and the likelihood of its diagnosis is greater in those from high socioeconomic groups (who are more likely to have routine health checks).

Thus, other things being equal, the use of clinical diagnoses as the outcome could result in a false positive association (greater risk in those from higher socioeconomic groups).

References

Abramson, J. H., Gofin, R., Habib, J., Pridan, H., Gofin, J. (1982). Indicators of social class. A comparative appraisal of measures for use in epidemiological studies. *Social Science & Medicine, 16,* 1739–1746.

Arber, S., Ginn, J. (1993). Gender and inequalities in health in later life. *Social Science & Medicine, 36,* 33–46.

Asthana, S., Halliday, J., Brigham, P., Gibson, A. (2002). *Rural deprivation and service need: A review of the literature and an assessment of indicators for rural service planning.* Bristol, UK: South West Public Health Observatory.

Avlund, K., Holstein, B. E., Osler, M., et al. (2003). Social position and health in old age: The relevance of different indicators of social position. *Scandinavian Journal of Public Health, 31,* 126–136.

Banguero, H. (1984). Socioeconomic factors associated with malaria in Colombia. *Social Science & Medicine, 19,* 1099–2104.

Bartley, M. (2004). *Health inequality: An introduction to theories, concepts and methods.* Cambridge, UK: Polity Press.

Beebe-Dimmer, J., Lynch, J. W., Turrell, G., et al. (2004). Childhood and adult socioeconomic conditions and 31-year mortality risk in women. *American Journal of Epidemiology, 159,* 481–490.

Ben-Shlomo, Y., Kuh, D. (2002). A life course approach to chronic disease epidemiology: Conceptual models, empirical challenges and interdisciplinary perspectives. *International Journal of Epidemiology, 31,* 285–293.

Benavides, F. G., Benach, J., Diez-Roux, A. V., Roman, C. (2000). How do types of employment relate to health indicators? Findings from the second European survey on working conditions. *Journal of Epidemiology and Community Health, 54,* 494–501.

Berkman, L. F., Macintyre, S. (1997). The measurement of social class in health studies: Old measures and new formulations. *IARC Scientific Publications,* 138, 51–64.

Blane, D. (2003). Commentary: Explanations of the difference in mortality risk between different educational groups. *International Journal of Epidemiology,32,* 355.

Blane D., Davey Smith G., Hart C. (1999). Some social and physical correlates of intergenerational social mobility: Evidence from the West of Scotland Collaborative Study. *Sociology, 33,* 169–183.

Breeze, E., Fletcher, A. E., Leon, D. A., et al. (2001). Do socioeconomic disadvantages persist into old age? Self-reported morbidity in a 29-year follow-up of the Whitehall Study. *American Journal of Public Health, 91,* 277–283.

Burstrom, B., Diderichsen, F., Smedman, L. (1999). Child mortality in Stockholm during 1885–1910: The impact of household size and number of children in the family on the risk of death from measles. *American Journal of Epidemiology, 149,* 1134–1141.

Carstairs, V., Morris, R. (1989). Deprivation and mortality: An alternative to social class? *Community Medicine, 11,* 210–219.

Chandola, T. (1998). Social inequality in coronary heart disease: A comparison of occupational classifications. *Social Science & Medicine, 47,* 525–533.

Chandola, T., Jenkinson, C. (1999). Social class differences in morbidity using the new UK National Statistics Socio-Economic Classification. Do class differences in employment relations explain class differences in health? *Annals of the New York Academy of Sciences, 896,* 313–315.

Chandola, T., Jenkinson, C. (2000). The new UK National Statistics Socio-Economic Classification (NS-SEC): Investigating social class differences in self-reported health status. *Journal of Public Health Medicine, 22,* 182–190.

Claussen, B., Davey Smith, G., Thelle, D. (2003). Impact of childhood and adulthood socioeconomic position on cause specific mortality: The Oslo Mortality Study. *Journal of Epidemiology and Community Health, 57,* 40–45.

Cohen, D., Spear, S., Scribner, R., et al. (2000). "Broken windows" and the risk of gonorrhea. *American Journal of Public Health, 90,* 230–236.

Cortinovis, I., Vella, V., Ndiku, J. (1993). Construction of a socio-economic index to facilitate analysis of health data in developing countries. *Social Science & Medicine, 36,* 1087–1097.

Currie, C. E., Elton, R. A., Todd, J., Platt, S. (1997). Indicators of socioeconomic status for adolescents: The WHO Health Behavior in School-Aged Children Survey. *Health Education Research, 12,* 385–397.

Davey Smith, G. (2000). Learning to live with complexity: Ethnicity, socioeconomic position, and health in Britain and the United States. *American Journal of Public Health, 90,* 1694–1698.

Davey Smith, G. (2003). *Health inequalities: Lifecourse approaches.* Bristol, UK: The Policy Press.

Davey Smith, G., Ben-Shlomo, Y., Hart, C. (1999). Re: "Use of census-based aggregate variables to proxy for socioeconomic group: Evidence from national samples." *American Journal of Epidemiology, 150,* 996–997.

Davey Smith, G., Ben-Shlomo, Y., Lynch, J. W. (2002). Life course approaches to inequalities in coronary heart disease risk. In S. A. Stansfeld and M. G. Marmot (Eds.), *Stress and the Heart.* London: BMJ Books.

Davey Smith, G., Blane, D., Bartley, M. (1994). Explanations for socio-economic differentials in mortality. Evidence from Britain and elsewhere. *European Journal of Public Health, 4,* 131–144.

Davey Smith, G., Harding, S. (1997). Is control at work the key to socioeconomic gradients in mortality? *Lancet, 350,* 1369–1370.

Davey Smith, G., Hart, C., Blane, D., Gillis, C., Hawthorne, V. (1997). Lifetime socioeconomic position and mortality: Prospective observational study. *British Medical Journal, 314,* 547–552.

Davey Smith, G., Hart, C., Hole, D., et al. (1998). Education and occupational social class: Which is the more important indicator of mortality risk? *Journal of Epidemiology and Community Health, 52,* 153–160.

Davey Smith, G., Hart, C. L., Watt, G., Hole, D. J., Hawthorne, V. M. (1998). Individual social class, area-based deprivation, cardiovascular disease risk factors, and mortality: The Renfrew and Paisley Study. *Journal of Epidemiology and Community Health, 52,* 399–405.

Davey Smith, G., Neaton, J. D., Wentworth, D., Stamler, R., Stamler, J. (1996a). Socioeconomic differentials in mortality risk among men screened for the multiple risk factor intervention trial: I. White men. *American Journal of Public Health, 86,* 486–496.

Davey Smith, G., Shipley, M. J., Rose, G. (1990). Magnitude and causes of socioeconomic differentials in mortality: Further evidence from the Whitehall Study. *Journal of Epidemiology and Community Health, 44,* 265–270.

Davey Smith, G., Wentworth, D., Neaton, J. D., Stamler, R., Stamler, J. (1996b). Socioeconomic differentials in mortality risk among men screened for the multiple risk factor intervention trial: II. Black men. *American Journal of Public Health, 86,* 497–504.

Dedman, D. J., Gunnell, D., Davey Smith, G., Frankel, S. (2001). Childhood housing conditions and later mortality in the Boyd Orr cohort. *Journal of Epidemiology and Community Health, 55,* 10–15.

Diez-Roux, A. V. (2002). A glossary for multilevel analysis. *Journal of Epidemiology and Community Health, 56,* 588–594.

Diez-Roux, A. V. (2004a). Estimating neighborhood health effects: The challenges of causal inference in a complex world. *Social Science & Medicine, 58,* 1953–1960.

Diez-Roux, A. V. (2004b). The study of group-level factors in epidemiology: Rethinking variables, study designs, and analytical approaches. *Epidemiologic Reviews, 26,* 104–111.

Diez-Roux, A. V., Nieto, F. J., Tyroler, H. A., Crum, L. D., Szklo, M. (1995). Social inequalities and atherosclerosis. The Atherosclerosis Risk in Communities Study. *American Journal of Epidemiology, 141,* 960–972.

Dohrenwend, B. P., Levav, I., Shrout, P. E., et al. (1992). Socioeconomic status and psychiatric disorders: The causation-selection issue. *Science, 255,* 946–952.

Dorling, D. (1999). Who's afraid of income inequality? *Environment and Planning A, 31,* 571–574.

Duncan, G. J., Daly, M. C., McDonough, P., Williams, D. R. (2002). Optimal indicators of socioeconomic status for health research. *American Journal of Public Health, 92,* 1151.

Ebrahim, S., Papacosta, O., Wannamethee, G., Adamson, J. (2004). Social inequalities and disability in older men: Prospective findings from the British regional heart study. *Social Science & Medicine, 59,* 2109–2120.

Ecob, R., Davey Smith, G. (1999). Income and health: What is the nature of the relationship? *Social Science & Medicine, 48,* 693–705.

Engels, F. (1958). *The condition of the working class in England.* (W. O. Henderson and W. H. Chaloner, Trans.). Stanford, CA: Stanford University Press. (Original work published 1845)

Eriksson, J. G., Forsen, T., Tuomilehto, J., et al. (1999). Catch-up growth in childhood and death from coronary heart disease: Longitudinal study. *British Medical Journal, 318,* 427–431.

Erikson, R., Goldthorpe, J. H. (1992). *The constant flux.* Oxford: Clarendon Press.

Filmer, D., Pritchett, L. H. (2001). Estimating wealth effects without expenditure data—or tears: An application to educational enrollments in states of India. *Demography, 38,* 115–132.

Forsdahl, A. (1977). Are poor living conditions in childhood and adolescence an important risk factor for arteriosclerotic heart disease? *British Journal of Preventive and Social Medicine, 31,* 91–95.

Frankel, S., Elwood, P., Sweetnam, P., Yarnell, J., Davey Smith, G. (1996). Birthweight, body-mass index in middle age, and incident coronary heart disease. *Lancet, 348,* 1478–1480.

Fuchs, V. R. (1979). Economics, health, and post-industrial society. *Milbank Memorial Fund Quarterly/Health and Society, 57,* 153–182.

Galobardes, B., Davey Smith, G., Lynch, J. W. (forthcoming). Systematic review of the influence of childhood socioeconomic circumstances on risk of cardiovascular disease in adulthood [Electronic version]. *Annals of Epidemiology.*

Galobardes, B., Demarest, S. (2003). Asking sensitive information: An example with income. *Sozial-und Präventivmedizin, 48,* 70–72.

Galobardes, B., Lynch, J. W., Davey Smith, G. (2004). Childhood socioeconomic circumstances and cause-specific mortality in adulthood: Systematic review and interpretation. *Epidemiologic Review, 26,* 7–21.

Galobardes, B., Morabia, A. (2003). Measuring the habitat as an indicator of socioeconomic position: Methodology and its association with hypertension. *Journal of Epidemiology and Community Health, 57,* 248–253.

Galobardes, B., Shaw, M., Lawlor, D. A., Lynch, J. W., Davey Smith, G. (2006a) Glossary: Indicators of socioeconomic position (Part 1). *Journal of Epidemiology and Community Health, 60,* 7–12.

Galobardes, B., Shaw, M., Lawlor, D. A., Lynch, J. W., Davey Smith, G. (2006b) Glossary: Indicators of socioeconomic position (Part 2). *Journal of Epidemiology and Community Health, 60,* 95–101.

Geronimus, A. T., Bound, J. (1998). Use of census-based aggregate variables to proxy for socioeconomic group: Evidence from national samples. *American Journal of Epidemiology, 148,* 475–486.

Goldthorpe, J. H. (1980). *Social mobility and class structure in modern Britain.* Oxford: Oxford University Press.

Gordon, D. (1995). Census based deprivation indices: their weighting and validation. *Journal of Epidemiology and Community Health, 49,* S39–S44.

Gordon, D., Pantazis, C. (1997). *Breadline Britain in the 1990s.* Aldershot, UK: Ashgate.

Grundy, E., Holt, G. (2001). The socioeconomic status of older adults: How should we measure it in studies of health inequalities? *Journal of Epidemiology and Community Health, 55,* 895–904.

Hadden, W. C. (1996). Annotation: The use of educational attainment as an indicator of socioeconomic position. *American Journal of Public Health, 86,* 1525–1526.

Hallqvist, J., Lynch, J., Bartley, M., Lang, T., Blane, D. (2004). Can we disentangle life course processes of accumulation, critical period and social mobility? An analysis of disadvantaged socio-economic positions and myocardial infarction in the Stockholm Heart Epidemiology Program. *Social Science & Medicine, 58,* 1555–1562.

Hart, C. L., Davey Smith, G. (2003). Relation between number of siblings and adult mortality and stroke risk: 25-year follow-up of men in the Collaborative Study. *Journal of Epidemiology and Community Health, 57,* 385–391.

Heslop, P., Davey Smith, G., Macleod, J., Hart, C. (2001). The socioeconomic position of employed women, risk factors and mortality. *Social Science & Medicine, 53,* 477–485.

Hollingshead, B. A., Redlick, F. C. (1958). *Social class and mental illness.* New York: John Wiley & Sons.

Horta, B. L., Victora, C. G., Menezes, A. M., Barros, F. C. (1997). Environmental tobacco smoke and breastfeeding duration. *American Journal of Epidemiology, 146,* 128–133.

Howden-Chapman, P. (2004). Housing standards: A glossary of housing and health. *Journal of Epidemiology and Community Health, 58,* 162–168.

Jarman, B. (1983). Identification of underprivileged areas. *BMJ, 286,* 1705–1709.

Kaufman, J. S. (2002). Whad'ya know? Another view on cultural literacy. *Epidemiology, 13,* 500–503.

Kaufman, J. S., Cooper, R. S. (2001). Considerations for Use of Racial/Ethnic Classification in Etiologic Research. *American Journal of Epidemiology, 154,* 291–298.

Kelleher, J. (2002). Cultural literacy and health. *Epidemiology, 13,* 497–500.

Krieger, N., Chen, J. T., Selby, J. V. (1999). Comparing individual-based and household-based measures of social class to assess class inequalities in women's health: A methodological study of 684 U.S. women. *Journal of Epidemiology and Community Health, 53*, 612–623.

Krieger, N., Chen, J. T., Coull, B. A., Selby, J. V. (2005). Lifetime socioeconomic position and twins' health: An analysis of 308 pairs of United States women twins. *Public Library of Science Medicine, 2*, 645–653.

Krieger, N., Chen, J. T., Waterman, P. D., et al. (2002). Geocoding and monitoring of U.S. socioeconomic inequalities in mortality and cancer incidence: Does the choice of area-based measure and geographic level matter?: The Public Health Disparities Geocoding Project. *American Journal of Epidemiology, 156*, 471–482.

Krieger, N., Waterman, P. D., Chen, J. T., Soobader, M. J., Subramanian, S. V. (2003). Monitoring socioeconomic inequalities in sexually transmitted infections, tuberculosis, and violence: Geocoding and choice of area-based socioeconomic measures—the public health disparities geocoding project (US). *Public Health Report, 118*, 240–260.

Krieger, N., Williams, D. R., Moss, N. E. (1997). Measuring social class in U.S. public health research: Concepts, methodologies, and guidelines. *Annual Review of Public Health, 18*, 341–378.

Kuate-Defo, B. (1994). Determinants of infant and early childhood mortality in Cameroon: The role of socioeconomic factors, housing characteristics, and immunization status. *Social biology, 41*, 181–211.

Kuh, D., Ben-Shlomo, Y. (2004). *A life course approach to chronic disease epidemiology* (2nd ed.) Oxford: Oxford University Press.

Kunst, A. E., Groenhof, F., Mackenbach, J. P., Health, E. W. (1998). Occupational class and cause specific mortality in middle aged men in 11 European countries: Comparison of population based studies. EU Working Group on Socioeconomic Inequalities in Health. *British Medical Journal, 316*, 1636–1642.

Lauderdale, D. S., Cagney, K. A. (1999). Limitations to the use of education as an SES indicator in studies of the elderly. Confounding by cognition. *Annals of the New York Academy of Sciences, 896*, 373–375.

Lawlor, D. A., Davey Smith, G., Patel, R., Ebrahim, S. (2005). Life-course socioeconomic position, area deprivation, and coronary heart disease: Findings from the British Women's Heart and Health Study. *American Journal of Public Health, 95, 91-97*.

Lawlor, D. A., Davey Smith, G., Ebrahim, S. (2004). Association between childhood socio-economic status and coronary heart disease risk among postmenopausal women: Findings from the British Women's Heart and Health Study. *American Journal of Public Health, 94*, 1386–1392.

Lawlor, D. A., Davey Smith, G., Kundu, D., Bruckdorfer, K. R., Ebrahim, S. (2004). Those confounded vitamins: What can we learn from the differences between observational versus randomised trial evidence? *Lancet, 363*, 1724–1727.

Lawlor, D. A., Ebrahim, S., Davey Smith, G. (2003). The association of socio-economic position across the life course and age at menopause: The British Women's Heart and Health Study. *British Journal of Obstetrics and Gynaecology, 110*, 1078–1087.

Lawlor, D. A., Emberson, J. R., Ebrahim, S., et al. (2003). Is the association between parity and coronary heart disease due to biological effects of pregnancy or adverse lifestyle risk factors associated with child-rearing? Findings from the British Women's Heart and Health Study and the British Regional Heart Study. *Circulation, 107*, 1260–1264.

Lawlor, D. A., Harro, M., Wedderkopp, N., et al. (2005). Association of socioeconomic position with insulin resistance among children from Denmark, Estonia, and Portugal: Cross sectional study. *British Medical Journal, 331,* 183.

Lawlor, D. A., Smith, G. D. (2005). Early life determinants of adult blood pressure. *Current Opinions in Nephrology and Hypertension, 14,* 259–264.

Lenz, R. (1988). Jakarta kampung morbidity variations: Some policy implications. *Social Science & Medicine, 26,* 641–649.

Liberatos, P., Link, B. G., Kelsey, J. L. (1988). The measurement of social class in epidemiology. *Epidemiologic Review, 10,* 87–121.

Lombardi, C., Bronfman, M., Facchini, L. A., et al. (1988). Operationalization of the concept of social class in epidemiologic studies [*Operacionalizacao do conceito de classe social em estudos epidemiologicos*]. *Revista de Saúde Pública, 22,* 253–265.

Lundberg, O. (1993). The impact of childhood living conditions on illness and mortality in adulthood. *Social Science & Medicine, 36,* 1047–1052.

Lynch, J. (2001). Social position and health. *Annals of Epidemiology, 6,* 21–23.

Lynch, J., Davey Smith, G., Harper, S., et al. (2004a). Is income inequality a determinant of population health? Part 1. A systematic review. *Milbank Memorial Quarterly, 82,* 5–99.

Lynch, J., Davey Smith, G., Harper, S., Hillemeier, M. (2004b). Is income inequality a determinant of population health? Part 2. U.S. National and regional trends in income inequality and age- and cause-specific mortality. *Milbank Memorial Quarterly, 82,* 355–400.

Lynch, J., Davey Smith, G., Hillemeier, M., et al. (2001). Income inequality, the psychosocial environment, and health: Comparisons of wealthy nations. *Lancet, 358,* 194–200.

Lynch, J., Kaplan, G. (2000). Socioeconomic position. In L. F. Berkman & I. Kawachi (Eds.), *Social epidemiology* (1st ed., pp. 13–35). Oxford: Oxford University Press.

Lynch, J. W., Kaplan, G. A., Shema, S. J. (1997). Cumulative impact of sustained economic hardship on physical, cognitive, psychological, and social functioning. *New England Journal of Medicine, 337,* 1889–1895.

Lynch, J., Davey Smith, G. (2005). A life course approach to chronic disease epidemiology. *Annual Review of Public Health, 26,* 1–35.

Macintyre, S., Ellaway, A., Cummins, S. (2002). Place effects on health: How can we conceptualise, operationalise and measure them? *Social Science & Medicine, 55,*125–139.

Macintyre, S., Ellaway, A., Der, G., Ford, G., Hunt, K. (1998). Do housing tenure and car access predict health because they are simply markers of income or self esteem? A Scottish study. *Journal of Epidemiology and Community Health, 52,* 657–664.

Mackenbach, J. P., Bos, V., Andersen, O., et al. (2003). Widening socioeconomic inequalities in mortality in six Western European countries. *International Journal of Epidemiology, 32,* 830–837.

Mackenbach, J. P., Kunst, A. E., Cavelaars, A. E., Groenhof, F., Geurts, J. J. (1997). Socioeconomic inequalities in morbidity and mortality in Western Europe. The EU Working Group on Socioeconomic Inequalities in Health. *Lancet, 349,* 1655–1659.

Macleod, J., Davey Smith, G., Metcalfe, C., Hart, C. (2005). Is subjective social status a more important determinant of health than material circumstances? Evidence from male workers occupying contradictory class locations in a prospective observational study of Scottish men. *Social Science & Medicine, 61,* 1916–1929.

Marsella, A. J., Escudero, M., Brennan, J. (1975). Goal-striving discrepancy stress in urban Filipino men: II. Housing. *International Journal of Social Psychiatry, 21,* 282–291.

Marshall, G., Rose, D., Newby, H., Vogler, C. M. (1989). *Social class in modern Britain.* Oxford: Routledge.

Martikainen, P., Valkonen, T. (1999). Bias related to the exclusion of the economically inactive in studies on social class differences in mortality. *International Journal of Epidemiology, 28,* 899–904.

McClements, L. D. (1977). Equivalence scales for children. *Journal of Public Economics, 8,* 191–210.

McDonough, P., Duncan, G. J., Williams, D., House, J. (1997). Income dynamics and adult mortality in the United States, 1972 through 1989. *American Journal of Public Health, 87,* 1476–1483.

McDonough, P., Sacker, A., Wiggins, R. D. (2005). Time on my side? Life course trajectories of poverty and health. *Social Science & Medicine, 61,* 1795–1808.

Modin, B. (2003). Born out of wedlock and never married—it breaks a man's heart. *Social Science & Medicine, 57,* 487–501.

Montgomery, M. R., Gragnolati, M., Burke, K. A., Paredes, E. (2000). Measuring living standards with proxy variables. *Demography, 37,* 155–174.

Morris, J. N., Blane, D. B., White, I. R. (1996). Levels of mortality, education, and social conditions in the 107 local education authority areas of England. *Journal of Epidemiology and Community Health, 50,* 15–17.

Muntaner, C., Borrell, C., Benach, J., Pasarin, M. I., Fernandez, E. (2003). The associations of social class and social stratification with patterns of general and mental health in a Spanish population. *International Journal of Epidemiology, 32,* 950–958.

Muntaner, C., Eaton, W. W., Diala, C., Kessler, R. C., Sorlie, P. D. (1998). Social class, assets, organizational control and the prevalence of common groups of psychiatric disorders. *Social Science & Medicine, 47,* 2043–2053.

Muntaner, C., Wolyniec, P., McGrath, J., Pulver, A. E. (1994). Psychotic inpatients' social class and their first admission to state or private psychiatric Baltimore hospitals. *American Journal of Public Health, 84,* 287–289.

Naess, O., Claussen, B., Thelle, D. S., Davey Smith, G. (2005). Four indicators of socioeconomic position: Relative ranking across causes of death. *Scandanavian Journal of Public Health, 33,* 215–221.

Naess, O., Leyland, A. H., Davey Smith, G., Claussen, B. (2005) Contextual effect on mortality of neighbourhood level education explained by earlier life deprivation. *Journal of Epidemiology and Community Health, 59,* 1058–1059.

Oakes, J. M. (2004). The (mis)estimation of neighborhood effects: Causal inference for a practicable social epidemiology. *Social Science & Medicine, 58,* 1929–1952.

Oakes, J. M., Rossi, P. H. (2003). The measurement of SES in health research: Current practice and steps toward a new approach. *Social Science & Medicine, 56,* 769–784.

O'Leary, S. R., Wingard, D. L., Edelstein, S. L., et al. (1996). Is birth order associated with adult mortality? *Annals of Epidemiology, 6,* 34–40.

Osler, M., Andersen, A-M. N., Due, P., et al. (2003). Socioeconomic position in early life, birth weight, childhood cognitive function, and adult mortality. A longitudinal study of Danish men born in 1953. *Journal of Epidemiology and Community Health, 57,* 681–686.

Pickett, K. E., Pearl, M. (2001). Multilevel analyses of neighborhood socioeconomic context and health outcomes: A critical review. *Journal of Epidemiology and Community Health, 55,* 111–122.

Pleck, J. H., Sonenstein, F. L. (1998). Adolescent sexual behavior, drug use, and violence: Increased reporting with computer survey technology. *Science, 280,* 867–873.

Prandy, K. (1999). Class, stratification and inequalities in health: A comparison of the Registrar-General's Social Classes and the Cambridge Scale. *Social Health & Illness, 21,* 466–484.

Reijneveld, S. A., Pearl, M., Pickett, K. E. (2001). Explanations for differences in health outcomes between neighborhoods of varying socioeconomic level. *Journal of Epidemiology and Community Health, 55,* 847.

Rose, D., O'Reilly, K. (1998). The ESRC Review of Government Social Classifications. London: Office for National Statistics.

Rose, M. (1995). Official Social Classifications in the UK. *Social Research Update, 9.*

Schwalbe, M. L., Staples, C. L. (1986). Class position, work experience, and health. *International Journal of Health Services, 16,* 583–602.

Schwartz, S. (1994). The fallacy of the ecological fallacy: The potential misuse of a concept and the consequences. *American Journal of Public Health, 84,* 819–824.

Shaun, M., Egger, M. (2002) Studies of the social causes of tuberculosis in Germany before the First World War: Extracts from Mosse and Tugendreich's landmark book. *International Journal of Epidemiology, 31,* 742–749.

Shaw, M. (2004). Housing and public health. *Annual Review of Public Health, 25,* 397–418.

Shaw, M., Dorling, D., Gordon, D., Davey Smith, G. (1999). *The widening gap: Health inequalities and policy in Britain.* Bristol, UK: The Policy Press.

Sihvonen, A. P., Kunst, A. E., Lahelma, E., Valkonen, T., Mackenbach, J. P. (1998). Socioeconomic inequalities in health expectancy in Finland and Norway in the late 1980s. *Social Science & Medicine, 47,* 303–315.

Singh-Manoux, A., Richards, M., Marmot, M. (2003). Leisure activities and cognitive function in middle age: Evidence from the Whitehall II Study. *Journal of Epidemiology and Community Health, 57,* 907–913.

Smith, J. P. (1995). Racial and ethnical differences in wealth in the Health and Retirement Study. *Journal of Human Resources, 30,* S158–S183.

Sorlie, P. D., Backlund, E., Keller, J. B. (1995). U.S. mortality by economic, demographic, and social characteristics: The National Longitudinal Mortality Study. *American Journal of Public Health, 85,* 949–956.

Subramanian, S. V. (2004). The relevance of multilevel statistical methods for identifying causal neighborhood effects. *Social Science & Medicine, 58,* 1961–1967.

Subramanian, S. V., Kawachi, I. (2004). Income Inequality and Health: What Have We Learned So Far? *Epidemiologic Reviews, 26,* 78–91.

Subramanian, S. V., Nandy, S., Kelly, M., Gordon, D., Davey Smith, G. (2004). Patterns and distribution of tobacco consumption in India: Cross-sectional multilevel evidence from the 1998–9 national family health survey. *British Medical Journal, 328,* 801–806.

Sydenstricker, E. (1933). *Health and environment.* New York: McGraw-Hill.

Townsend, P., Phillimore, P., Beattie, A. (1988). *Health and deprivation: Inequality in the North.* London: Croom Helm.

Tunstall, H.V. Z., Shaw, M., Dorling, D. (2004). Places and health. *Journal of Epidemiology and Community Health, 58,* 6–10.

Turrell, G. (2000). Income non-reporting: Implications for health inequalities research. *Journal of Epidemiology and Community Health, 54,* 207–214.

Vagero, D., Leinsalu, M. (2005). Health inequalities and social dynamics in Europe. *British Medical Journal, 331,* 186–187.

Villerme, L. R. (1830). *De la mortalite dans divers quarters de la ville de Paris.* Annales d'hygiene publique, *3*, 341.

Virchow R. (1848). Report on the typhus epidemic in Upper Silesia. In L. J. Rather (Ed.), *Rudolph Virchow: Collected essays on public health and epidemiology* (Vol. 1, 1988, pp. 205–220). Canton, MA: Science History Publications.

Wamala, S. P., Lynch, J., Kaplan, G. A. (2001). Women's exposure to early and later life socioeconomic disadvantage and coronary heart disease risk: The Stockholm Female Coronary Risk Study. *International Journal of Epidemiology, 30,* 275–284.

Wardle, J., Robb, K., Johnson, F. (2002). Assessing socioeconomic status in adolescents: The validity of a home affluence scale. *Journal of Epidemiology and Community Health, 56,* 595–599.

West, P., Sweeting, H., Speed, E. (2001). We really do know what you do: A comparison of reports from 11-year-olds and their parents in respect of parental economic activity and occupation. *Sociology, 35,* 539–559.

White, I. R., Blane, D., Morris, J. N., Mourouga, P. (1999). Educational attainment, deprivation-affluence and self reported health in Britain: A cross-sectional study. *Journal of Epidemiology and Community Health, 53,* 535–541.

Wilkinson, R. G. (1992). Income distribution and life expectancy. *British Medical Journal, 304,* 165–168.

Wohlfarth, T. (1997). Socioeconomic inequality and psychopathology: Are socioeconomic status and social class interchangeable? *Social Science & Medicine, 45,* 399–410.

Wohlfarth, T., van den Brink, W. (1998). Social class and substance use disorders: The value of social class as distinct from socioeconomic status. *Social Science & Medicine, 47,* 51–58.

Wright, E. O. (1997). *Class counts. Comparability studies in class analysis.* Cambridge: Cambridge University Press.

Wright, E. O. (1985). *Classes.* London: New Left Books.

Yen, I. H., Moss, N. (1999). Unbundling education: A critical discussion of what education confers and how it lowers risk for disease and death. *Annals of the New York Academy of Sciences, 896,* 350–351.

Acknowledgments

This chapter is based on previous work the authors have published in the *Journal of Epidemiology and Community Health* in the form of glossaries.

CHAPTER FOUR

MEASURING AND ANALYZING "RACE," RACISM, AND RACIAL DISCRIMINATION

Saffron Karlsen and James Yzet Nazroo

There are many potential problems associated with the measurement and analysis of "race," racism, and racial discrimination. This is at least partially a consequence of the variable conceptualization of "race" and "ethnicity" that may be seen in the differential treatment of racial and ethnic issues by researchers and in the way in which many commentators cannot bring themselves to use the term *race* without enclosing it in quotation marks. There are disagreements about what "ethnicity" and "race" are, how they relate to each other, and how they relate to wider social and economic circumstances and experiences. In particular, there are debates as to how far the characteristics ascribed to particular "ethnic"/"racial" groups signify group differences in innate, biological, or genetic ability, culture, social and economic power, or a combination of all three. For those who refuse to contemplate anything beyond "natural" (genetic or biological) or cultural differences between groups, there can be no role for racism in the social, economic, and health disadvantage experienced by members of ethnic minority groups. But racism may be the key to explaining the disadvantaged position in which many people from ethnic minority groups find themselves across the globe.

Genetic explanations for ethnic differentials in social position and health persist (Herrnstein and Murray 1994), despite a considerable lack of evidence and over one hundred years of contrary evidence exposing the limitations of such assumptions. On the whole, however, rather than being the focus of explicit investigation, genetic or cultural factors are alluded to—once other potential "confounders" have been statistically controlled for (Marmot, Adelstein, and Bulusu 1984; Harding and Maxwell 1997). Such explanations therefore assume that all other "confounders" have been both recognized and accurately accounted for, such that the remaining unexplained component of ethnic difference can only be attributable to unmeasured "innate" (that is, cultural or genetic) characteristics.

These interpretations fail to account for the complexity of the social and economic inequalities faced by people from ethnic minority groups, a complexity that cannot be fully captured by simple measures of socioeconomic position, such as class or education (Nazroo 1997, 1998). There is evidence that markers of social position are not sufficiently comparable across different ethnic groups to be used in this way (Kaufman et al. 1997, 1998, Nazroo 2001). The extent to which any residual effect in a statistical model can be assigned to (unmeasured) factors when social position is incompletely measured is therefore questionable.

There are also aspects of the relationship between ethnicity, social position, and health that have been generally ignored. In particular, measures of social position often fail to account for both the accumulation of disadvantage over the life course—measuring socioeconomic status only at one time point—and the role of ecological effects produced by the concentration of ethnic minority groups in deprived residential areas. A third aspect of this relationship ignored by many current approaches is the effect of being a victim of racism, in terms of its effect on group social identity, social status, and socioeconomic position (Bonilla-Silva and Baiocchi 2001). As a consequence, the investigation of the way in which social and economic disadvantage may structure the experiences of different ethnic groups has remained relatively superficial.

Discrimination has been shown to occur in almost every facet of public and private life—from the "daily hassles" experienced when going about one's normal life to major events, such as being the victim of a racist physical attack. For example, there is widespread evidence of intolerance toward immigrants and asylum seekers in the United Kingdom, and the United Nations Committee on Racial Discrimination has severely criticized race-relations in Britain (United Nations 2000). Responses to the British Social Attitudes surveys suggest that between one-quarter and two-fifths of people in the United Kingdom are racially prejudiced (Rothon and Heath 2003). But this is not a problem only apparent in the United Kingdom. Oakley (1992, p. 40) concludes that "there is prima facie (if often anecdotal) evidence that racial violence and harassment occur in all countries of Europe in which visible minorities of post-war immigrant origin are settled." This can be seen in the growth of far-right electoral parties across some countries of Europe during the 1990s, particularly France, Italy, Belgium, Germany, the Netherlands, and some parts of Eastern Europe (Bjorgo and Witte 1993; Oakley 1992). Similarly,

80 percent of black respondents to a U.S. study reported having experienced racial discrimination at some time in their lives (Krieger and Sidney 1996).

Racism can enter people's lives in a number of ways. It may be based on "race"/ethnicity, religion, or nationality and combine with other negatively stereotyped aspects of identity to produce experiences of multiple discrimination. It may be experienced directly though interpersonal discrimination or perpetuated via an institution's discriminatory policies. But whereas racism has repeatedly been shown to be associated with poor health outcomes (Brown et al. 2000; Karlsen and Nazroo 2002, 2004; Krieger 2000, 2003) and is considered to account for at least part of the socioeconomic disadvantage in which many people from ethnic minority groups are concentrated (Krieger 2000; Nazroo 1998, 2001), further exploration is required to fully understand how racism affects people's lives. Producing meaningful analyses requires a careful consideration of both measurement (discussed later in this chapter) and of conceptual issues.

Concepts

Research into "race"/ethnicity requires the investigation of a number of different concepts. This section contains a brief discussion of some of them.

"Ethnicity"

According to Weber (1922), the concept of **ethnicity,** and an **ethnic group,** implies: membership in a group, which in turn requires recognition of who is and is not a member of that group—a categorization that may be defined by personal choice by "members" of that group (internally) or by an external audience or both; the establishment of a common identity on the part of group members; and the development of perceived stereotypes related to that group that are imposed on them by other (external) social groups.

Bolaffi et al. (2003, p. 94) state that "it is preferable not to refer the concept of ethnicity to stable groups, but to groups which share certain economic, social, cultural and religious characteristics at a given moment in time." An ethnic group should not, then, be seen as something static or grounded in anything as inflexible as particular genes or historical or linguistic ancestry, although the common identity *may* be expressed as such. People *choose* what characteristics with which to define themselves that may or may not have recourse to ideas of color, language, history, or ancestry.

"The features that are taken into account are not the sum of 'objective' differences but only those that the actors themselves regard as significant . . . some cultural features are used by the actors as signals and emblems of differences; others are ignored, and in some relationships radical differences are played down and denied" (Barth 1969, p. 14).

But, as Weber (1922) argues, such choices are also influenced by the stereotypes that other social groups impose on them and by the (ethnic and other) group identities of those around them (Gilroy 1987; Smaje 1996). The experience of being a member of any particular ethnic group may also be affected by an individual's other social identities (relating to gender, age, social class, and so forth): being "African American" may mean different things to young African-American males than to older African-American females, for example. And these definitions will also change over time and circumstance.

Ethnic groups, then, rather than being definitive, timeless entities existing independent of the world around them, are entirely historically and spatially located. Considering and therefore exploring them as if they were otherwise is potentially meaningless. The process of ethnic identification is a means of defining yourself as part of an "us" in opposition to a "them" or an "other." "Ethnicity" provides a basis for the mobilization or exploitation of interests (Barth 1969). It can provide a means of social, political, or economic support. An ethnic "minority" obviously requires an ethnic "majority," even if that ethnic majority has sufficient power to ignore the ethnic dimension to its associations. Being "white" is as much a definition of ethnicity as being "non-white." "Ethnicity" is not then something only held by the "exotic." It is simply only mobilized under particular (usually threatening) circumstances, situations that are likely to occur more frequently among "minority" or less powerful groups. Differing circumstances may promote the mobilization of different forms of "ethnic" identification. "Blackness" (Miles 1994; Modood 1988), for example, was a term used in the United Kingdom in the 1970s and 1980s to describe the "expression of a common experience of exclusion and of a common political identity forged through resistance to that exclusion" (Miles 1994, p. 7), and in this way the term has been applied to the political struggles of people from all ethnic groups who experience racism. Certain individuals may therefore define themselves as "black" in some circumstances, (south) "Asian," "Bangladeshi," and "Sylheti" in others. This creates obvious problems for the collection of meaningful quantitative single-response data.

"Race" and the Evolution of Ideas of "Racial Difference"

In contrast to an understanding of **"ethnicity,"** the concept of **"race"** stems more from the apparent need of human beings to categorize, identify, and control others (Jenkins 1994). To an extent, the concepts of "ethnicity" and "race" are similar: both require the maintenance of both group boundaries and group identification based on perceived similarities between members of a group (Weber 1922); but "race" rather than ethnicity places emphasis on the external process of stereotyping and exclusion *at the expense of* internal processes of inclusion (Banton 1983). A further distinction is that "race" but not "ethnicity" inherently contains a judgment of value (Miles 1999): racial prejudice in the West generally conceiving non-white groups as inferior to "white" groups, which becomes justification for mistrust and the mistreatment of non-white groups.

In much the same way as members of an ethnic group are "free" to choose that with which they identify themselves, the characteristics emphasized in racial stereotyping are opportunistic; their wider significance, mythical. As discussed previously, Weber's (1922) definition of ethnic groups allows for the imposition of stereotyping by an external "other." Whereas a role for power is not necessary to a definition of ethnicity, the concept of "race" is, in some senses, dependent on the ability of certain social groups to exploit science, the media, and education to promote stereotypes relating to the "natural" inferiority of certain social groups compared with others, which become perceived as "common sense," "rational," and therefore unquestioned attitudes regarding differences between them—not only for those who may potentially gain from such negative stereotyping, but also among those whom they stereotype. Research suggests that the negative stereotyping of an ethnic/"racial" group has a significant effect on the self-perceptions of people considered (by themselves and others) part of that group. Furthermore, being a victim of racist stereotyping has been found to be one dimension in which (internal) "ethnic identity" may be defined (Karlsen 2004; Nazroo and Karlsen 2003). Discrimination on the grounds of "race" then provides us with a more convincing explanation for the persistence of inequalities between different ethnic/ "racial" groups than that based on "ethnicity" (Omi and Winant 1994). The continued assumption that "race" has a clear, unambiguous, neutral, and meaningful definition stems from this desire to categorize. The particular reasons for the pervasiveness of these ideas require an exploration of early interactions between "Europeans" and non-Europeans.

The idea of the existence of distinct biological "races" was used from the sixteenth and seventeenth centuries to explain the appearance and behavior of the (supposedly) "uncivilized" and "immoral" people "discovered" by early European explorers. Color symbolism—where white was seen to be associated with all things good and black with all things undesirable—had been evident at least since medieval times. This symbolism was exaggerated further, "blackness" coming to be associated with an inversion of everything European, Christian, and civilized (Jordan 1982).

"The Europeans who traveled in pursuit . . . of trade, military advantage, religious mission, and curiosity carried with them expectations about what and whom they might meet . . . a negative representation of the Other . . . [that] served to define and legitimate what was considered to be the positive qualities of the author and reader" (Miles 1999, pp. 20–21).

During the sixteenth century, "race" was perceived as a consequence of lineage or descent rather than biology, with differences a product of ignorance rather than inability—an idea that prompted the "civilizing mission" of Christianity from Europe around this time. From the end of the eighteenth century, however, ideas about the basis of perceived ethnic or racial differences became increasingly narrow and precise. Phrenology brought arguments that such differences were innate and that, in fact, certain "races" could not be "civilized" owing to their limited brain capacity. Certain groups were argued to be inherently more suited to carrying out certain tasks, such as heavy labor, and this argument was used to justify the systems of slavery that were being introduced to exploit the natural resources available in the newly "discovered" colonies.

Motivated by this idea of natural and unavoidable difference, western Europeans identified a "great chain of being" that organized the different groups that they recognized (including themselves) into a supposedly biological hierarchy. At the top were a group of what Miles (1999) describes as a "Nordic" people: white people from western Europe—with the exception of Irish (Curtis 1968, 1971) and Jewish (Mosse 1978) people, who were ranked further down. In the United States, Europeans—particularly migrants from Italy, Poland, or Russia and Jewish people—were also not included in this top stratum.

"Before the slave trade in Africa there was neither a Europe nor a European. Finally, with the European arose the myth of European superiority and separate existence as a special species or "race" . . . the particular myth that there was a creature called a European which implied, from the beginning, a "white" man" (Jaffe 1985, p. 46).

Groups exploited through slavery also had their post-emancipation treatment justified along this "great chain of being" (Eriksen 1993, 2002). Reducing the impact of the increased competition occurring with the movement of former slaves into the labor market involved the further implementation of the "great chain of being" to justify racial segregation in the paid labor market and ensuring that people from racialized minority groups were confined to the least advantaged positions. This also ensured that people from ethnic minority groups would be concentrated in those industries most affected by economic fluctuation, with its associated variation in demand for labor and consequent high levels of unemployment (Eriksen 1993).

So, the beginning of the nineteenth century saw a growing acceptance of science and its ability to explain the basis of nature and society. Ideas of biological determinism, which saw differences between human beings both as natural and unchangeable rather than environmental and therefore adaptable, became increasingly popular. Human beings were argued to be a species made up of number of races of different capacity and temperament, recognizable by group differences in appearance (phenotype). It followed that people could only be understood in light of their "racial" characteristics, in particular the supposed excessive sexuality of black people (Miles 1999), which "explained" why some groups were "naturally" inferior to others.

In essence though, as mentioned previously, rather than being based on any empirical research, these arguments were part of an ideological process to justify the exploitation of the less powerful by the powerful, by the colonial empires and in Nazi Germany, apartheid South Africa, post-emancipation southern United States, and elsewhere. And attempts to use scientific, particularly genetic, exploration to lend support to the existence of systematic relationships between phenotype and behavior have proved unproductive. As Krieger (2003, p. 195) puts it: "The fact that we know what 'race' we are says more about our society than it does our biology." But sadly this has not always meant an end to the prejudice that such arguments have justified.

Nation

Arguments about inherent "racial" differences also played a central role in the creation of myths of **national** origin during the twentieth century and still do today (Centre for Contemporary Cultural Studies 1982; Miles 1999). Labor shortages in Western Europe between the 1940s and 1970s saw the development of a contract migrant worker system that encouraged workers from Africa, the Caribbean, and Asia to move to the United Kingdom for employment. This migration was met with concern regarding a potential disruption of "national unity." Rather than returning to the biological superiority/inferiority arguments of previous centuries, however, the 1970s saw the development of ideas suggesting that it is "natural" for people to live amongst their "own kind" and that, as a response to the production of this unnatural situation, discrimination toward migrants—those not of this "common community"—was to be expected (Barker 1981). The British Conservative politician Enoch Powell's discourse, for example, was concerned with the destruction of cultural homogeneity caused by the influx of immigrants who would "swamp" the culture of England's "own people." So, although nations were not explicitly seen to be hierarchical, they were argued to be natural, and the promotion of ethnic boundaries was unavoidable (Miles 1999). It has been argued more recently that the supposed need for the "dispersal" of asylum-seekers arriving in the United Kingdom at the turn of the twenty-first century, as promoted by the Blair Labor government in Britain, is motivated by similar ideas relating to a "threshold of tolerance" of "outsiders" (Kundnani 2000).

In as far as **"nation"** indicates a geographically-based community, it may be seen simply as a particular form of ethnic group. It is described as having a collective name, a common myth of descent, a distinctive shared culture, and a sense of solidarity as well as an association with a specific territory (Smith 1986). Defining a nation is as problematic as defining an ethnic group, and the idea of the existence of a national character, or *folk,* is as potentially ethnocentric and racist as ideas of racial difference. In essence, the promotion of ideas of who is (and who is not) part of a nation could be seen as one of a number of examples of the "rebranding" of racist motivations into more socially acceptable forms. Lack of access to resources, mistrust, and mistreatment can now be justified along national as well as "biological" lines, and minority groups can continue to be associated and blamed for unwanted social change or for any lack of resources among those seen to be more "entitled" (Eriksen 1993; Miles 1999). People who wish to continue to hold a xenophobic standpoint can do so without feeling obliged to also label themselves **"racist."**

Race Relations and Racialization

This blaming of ethnic minority or migrant groups for unwanted social change, increased social tension (or reduced social stability), and economic shortage (housing or employment for example), where "racial" meanings are attached to non-racial social relations, is termed **"racialization."** It is used by authors wishing to discuss **race relations**—relations between different racialized groups—while emphasizing the socially constructed nature of "race." Racialization allows a refocus of social problems from those of inadequate supply to those of demand. The racialization of problems in the housing market, for example, occurs when certain ethnic groups are regarded as making inappropriate demands on the housing system—rather than there being recognition of a more *general* lack of suitable housing. The problems therefore become related to culturally-based housing preferences rather than housing supply. Overdemand is the principle justification for racist discourse by individuals, social organizations, political parties, and governments today. A further example is the supposed need to control immigration, mentioned previously, which has tended to employ an ethnically-/ "race"-specific focus to related policies and panic.

Racism, Racial Discrimination, and Racial Harassment

The unequal treatment or exploitation of social groups stemming from the racialization of a social relationship, with its associated assumptions of the inherent superiority or inferiority of different social groups is described as **racial discrimination** or **racism.** As Krieger (2003, p. 195) states: *"[R]acism refers to institutions and individual practices that create and reinforce oppressive systems of race relations whereby people and institutions engaging in discrimination adversely restrict, by judgment and action, the lives of those against whom they discriminate."

Racism is often, particularly in the United Kingdom, assumed to refer solely to the exclusion of non-white groups by white groups, largely in response to the negative treatment of black and Asian groups migrating to the United Kingdom during the second half of the twentieth century. In reality, though, white migrants have also been (and still are [Fekete 2001]) victims of racism, and so a broader focus is often taken when using this term.

Racial discrimination is sometimes divided into intentional (or direct) and unintentional (or indirect) discrimination (Krieger 2000). Direct discrimination occurs when one is treated unequally as a consequence of one's "racial group." Indirect discrimination occurs when a person is either unable to comply with a requirement that cannot be justified on other than racial grounds or is less likely to be able to do so compared with people from other "racial groups." In this way, it is possible for someone who is non-prejudiced to be discriminatory, often as a consequence of **institutional racism.** Institutional racism refers to the continued (conscious or unconscious) adherence of large-scale enterprises to racially discriminatory policies, assumptions, or procedures.

"Racial harassment" is often used to denote demeaning, derogatory, threatening, violent, or other forms of offensive, racially motivated behavior by individuals from one ethnic group toward those of another. Research suggests that simply the awareness of such behavior may affect ethnic minority communities, regardless of the actual experience (Chahal and Julienne 1999; Karlsen and Nazroo 2004; Virdee 1995, 1997), partly as a consequence of a failure to condemn such behavior by the wider community (including institutions with a responsibility to deal with complaints of victimization) (Sibbitt 1997; Virdee 1995). Racial harassment (or **interpersonal discrimination**) and institutional discrimination are not, as this would suggest, unrelated experiences.

"The individual acts of bias and interpersonal discrimination that grow out of racism represent its latter-day, or surface (Williams 1997, p. 328), manifestations. They are salt in wounds previously inflicted by a host of negative life events whose relationship to racism is often cloaked. Indeed, it is likely that, at the point at which people encounter these individual forms of racism, other racist forces already have encroached on their lives." (Harrell et al. 2003, p. 243)

Measurement

In addition to recognizing the conceptual issues influencing analyses of "race," racism, and racial discrimination, investigators must also be mindful of the various measurement issues they face.

Interpersonal (Individual) Racism

Perhaps the major problem associated with measuring incidents of racism and racial discrimination concerns recognition, both for those exploring issues of racism and for its victims. Defining exactly what does and does not constitute racism is complex, and this often leads to inconsistencies in data collection. Studies exploring self-reports of actual experiences of interpersonal racism, for example, may collect information on criminal incidents (such as the British Crime Survey) or those reported to and recorded by the police or "low-level" experiences, such as racial abuse or insulting behavior (like the Fourth National Survey of Ethnic Minorities [FNS] in the United Kingdom) (Modood et al. 1997). Or the time frame may vary—exploring, for example, experiences over the past year or a lifetime or the frequency with which someone is generally exposed to racism.

The FNS (Virdee 1997) asked respondents whether they had, in the year prior to interview, been verbally abused or experienced a physical attack to either their person or their property for reasons that they perceived related to their race or color. The Coronary Artery Risk Development in Young Adults (CARDIA) and other studies asked respondents about experiences "at some time" in their lives (Krieger 1990; Krieger and Sidney 1996). "The National Survey of American Life" (NSAL) (Jackson et al. 2004), in contrast, asked "how often" respondents experienced a variety of forms of disrespect, from "almost everyday" to "less than once a year" or "never," similar to the "Daily Life Experiences" and "Racism and Life Experiences" scales used elsewhere (Harrell 1997; Scott 2003). The forms of disrespect explored in the NSAL include: being treated with less courtesy or respect than other people; receiving poorer service compared with other people; people acting as if they think you are not smart; people acting as if they are afraid of you; people acting as if they think you are dishonest; people acting as if they think they are better than you are; being called names or insulted; being threatened or harassed; and being followed while shopping.

During a study conducted by Noh and Kaspar (2003) with Korean immigrants residing in Toronto, Canada, respondents were told: "when people insult other people, make fun of them or treat them unfairly because they belong to a certain racial/ethnic group, this is called discrimination. This may happen to people who are not born in Canada, or who speak another language, or look different. The next few questions are about this type of discrimination." They were then asked how often they had been discriminated against in terms of having been: hit or handled roughly; insulted or called names; treated rudely; treated unfairly; threatened; refused services in a store or restaurant or subjected to delays in services; and excluded or ignored.

As these questions show, studies may supplement more "general" questions about experiences of verbal or physical harassment by asking about experiences in relation to specific circumstances. So, the FNS, for example, asks respondents if they have ever experienced discrimination in regard to accessing paid employment or promotion (Modood 1997). The NSAL (Jackson et al. 2004) asks a series of questions exploring:

- ever having been unfairly fired, not hired, or denied promotion;
- ever having been unfairly stopped, searched, questioned, physically threatened, or abused by the police;
- ever having been unfairly discouraged by a teacher or advisor from continuing education;
- ever having been unfairly prevented from moving into a neighborhood because the landlord or a realtor refused to sell or rent you a house or apartment;
- ever having moved into a neighborhood where neighbors made life difficult for you or your family;
- ever having been denied a bank loan; and
- ever having received poorer service, compared with others, from a plumber or car mechanic.

A particular issue related to the definition of racism in research is the distinction between what have been called "major" or "life" events, "chronic stressors," and "daily hassles" (Williams et al. 2003). Life events are described as discrete, observable stressors: actual experiences that can (it is assumed) be directly perceived and reported, such as those described in the preceding bulleted list. Chronic stressors (such as persistent noise, air pollution, and overcrowding) are ongoing problems, exposure to which is often related to people's roles—their occupation, for example. Daily hassles, also called "everyday discrimination" (Essed 1992), are chronic or episodic events considered part of everyday life, the impact of which is perceived to be minor and relatively short-term: negative treatment or hostility that is not seen as serious enough to constitute "racial harassment."

Unlike more "major" experiences, information regarding daily hassles is often not collected in surveys. There is evidence, however, that racially motivated daily hassles may have a greater impact (on mental health, for example) than other forms of daily hassles, as they can evoke painful memories relating to past racist experiences and communal histories of prejudice in a way that other daily hassles may not (West 1993; Williams et al. 1999). Racially motivated daily hassles may have more of a cumulative effect or combine with other racist experiences to produce more severe consequences. Ignoring these aspects of experience may, then, seriously underestimate the impact of racism on people's lives. Williams et al. (2003) also describe three additional distinctive types of stressors (traumas, "macrostressors," and non-events) that may be promising areas to investigate. Traumas are described as "acute or chronic stressors, such as sexual assault or natural disasters"; macrostressors refer to "large-scale systems related stressors such as economic recessions"; and "non-events are desired and expected experiences that fail to occur" (Williams et al. 2003, p. 203), discussed later in the chapter.

It is argued that when collecting data, questions should be direct and address the multiple facets of discrimination, ask about distinct types of unfair treatment in particular situations and locations, and avoid global questions about experiences or awareness (Krieger 2000). Also important are assessments of the domain in which the racism occurs, the magnitude and temporal characteristics of the event, the associated threat, and the impact of other individual characteristics and stressors (Williams et al. 2003). At the same time, it has been argued that "approaches to the assessment of discrimination that involve long lists of questions in which a respondent is repeatedly asked whether a particular event occurred 'because of your race' can produce demand characteristics that lead to either overreports or underreports of exposure" (Williams et al. 2003, p. 204).

Studies have also suggested that, unlike other criminal acts, racism need not have been experienced personally for it to produce a sense of threat, interpersonal incidents being viewed as "an attack on the community as a whole" (Virdee 1995, p. 284). As Oakley (1992, p. 11) points out: the distinguishing feature of *racial* violence and harassment is not simply that it involves members of different racial groups or ethnic groups; it is that the action is racially *motivated*. . . . Racially motivated behavior, therefore, is not an attack aimed at a person purely as an individual, but an attack on a member of a category or group.

This may be seen in findings that suggest that those living with the threat or fear of racism are more numerous than those reporting actual personal experience of racism (Virdee 1995, 1997). To explore this, some studies also ask about respondent knowledge of other people's (in this case, family members') experiences of racism (Noh and Kaspar 2003). Other studies have asked more directly about people's concerns about being the victim of racism (Virdee 1997). Measuring only an individual's actual experience may fail to explore the effects of the threat produced by knowledge of racism in a community if this is not reflected in the actual experience of study respondents.

Responses, Reactions, and Coping

Each of these measures assumes experiences of interpersonal racism to be real and observable phenomena, recognition of which is unrelated to the appraisal processes applied by an individual as a consequence of the relationship between them and their environment. Unfortunately, from a measurement perspective at least, many individual psychological and demographic consequences may affect the perception and reporting of prejudice, which may confound the analyses.

Therefore, one problem with measuring racial discrimination is related to difficulties associated with people's ability to recognize and report their experiences of racism. Further problems may be related to disclosure: one British-based study found that people who initially denied any experience of racial discrimination later shared such experiences (Chahal and Julienne 1999). There is also evidence that people may be motivated to ignore evidence of discrimination by a wish to avoid unnecessarily disrupting social relations and undermining life satisfaction (Contrada et al. 2000). Alternatively, people may simply not remember individual incidents of harassment or negative treatment.

People's interpretations of an experience will vary: whether an experience is seen to be a function of an individual's social category or something else will be a consequence of their own history of intergroup interactions as well as a response to the "objective" experience. Research suggests, for example, that the perception or reporting of discrimination may be associated with gender (with women reportedly more likely to underreport experiences of racism compared with men [Armstead et al. 1989]), social class (with more underreporting occurring among those with fewer socioeconomic resources [Krieger 2000; Ruggiero and Taylor 1995]), or particular historical cohorts (with those coming of age during or after the civil rights and women's movements of the 1960s more likely to identify discrimination than older cohorts [Davis and Robinson 1991; Essed 1992]).

There is also evidence that there may have been a change in the nature of racial prejudice over time, such that experiences of racism may be more difficult to recognize today. Dovidio and Gaertner (2000, p. 315) describe the rise of "aversive racism," characterized by people who "endorse egalitarian values, who regard themselves as non-prejudiced, but who discriminate in subtle rationalizable ways." As Cooper (1993, p. 137) puts it: "The lynch mob was an effective instrument of social policy in its day, but too clumsy for a time when appearances count for more than reality." So, in addition to more overt, traditional forms, discrimination may also be expressed in indirect and rationalizable ways, which will be more difficult to recognize and report. The rise of aversive racism, Dovidio and Gaertner (2000) argue, has led to a decline in self-reported experiences of discrimination.

Research has also repeatedly shown that people report perceiving greater discrimination directed toward their group as a whole than toward themselves, personally, as members of that group—what has been called the "personal/group discrimination discrepancy" (Taylor et al. 1990). That an individual may consciously not wish to discuss or simply not recognize the discrimination they experience is one possible explanation for this. Alternatively, this phenomenon may result from unconscious reactions to personal experiences of discrimination.

Some people have been shown to *internalize* their experiences of discrimination, perceiving themselves to be in some way deserving of their negative treatment (Essed 1992; Krieger 1990; Krieger and Sidney 1996). It has also been suggested that individuals may exaggerate experiences of discrimination to avoid blaming themselves for failure (Neighbors et al. 1996).

Ruggiero and Taylor (1995) describe several theories that suggest that effective coping is achieved through an internal sense of control over one's experiences, maintenance of which requires minimizing the role of external forces, which may limit their negative impact but also lead to the denial of influences such as discrimination. But, other studies have suggested that the health effects of such internalization may vary, that although it may have self-protective qualities under some circumstances, it has also been shown to be related to hypertension (James et al. 1987; Krieger 1990; Krieger and Sidney 1996). Part of this contradiction may stem from variations related to coping style. Problem-focused coping styles (sometimes called "confrontation"), for example, have been found to be more effective in reducing the mental and physical health impact of perceived discrimination and other forms of social stress, compared with emotion-focused coping (passive acceptance or emotional distraction), which has serious consequences for mental health (Krieger 1990; Noh and Kaspar 2003). There is also evidence that people who actively cope with prejudice are more likely to notice, recall, and report experiences of prejudice (Contrada et al. 2000). The coping response options available are highly structured by social context, however (Noh and Kaspar 2003).

One possibility for overcoming the problem of potential underreporting involves including more abstract questions alongside the more direct ones described previously—relating more explicitly to people's perceptions of racism rather than their experiences. The FNS (Modood et al. 1997), for example, asked what proportion of British employers the respondent felt would discriminate against someone on the grounds of race, religion, color, or cultural background when recruiting (Virdee 1997). Perceptions of British employers as racist were more widely reported than actual experiences of interpersonal discrimination. This discrepancy may have occurred because only interpersonal experiences within the previous year were explored, whereas a sense of institutional or societal racism is likely to be developed over a longer period, in response to repeated institutional and interpersonal experiences of racism. Alternatively, responses relating to societal racism may explore a "sense" of being a victim of discrimination, which might not develop from direct, reportable experiences. Other studies have asked similar questions exploring perceived discrimination in terms of access to housing or equal wages (Sigelman and Welch 1991). It is important to recognize that these problems may be related to an overreporting as well as an underreporting of experiences.

Rather than simply an artifactual problem, though, people's responses to racism may allow important insight into the severity and intensity of their experiences of racism. A number of studies, for example, have explored the way in which victims of racism may adapt their lives in an attempt to avoid further harassment (Chahal and Julienne 1999; Virdee 1997). The NSAL (Jackson et al. 2004) asked respondents reporting themselves to be victims of racism how they responded to their experiences. In particular, they were asked whether they had: tried to do something about it; accepted it as a fact of life; worked harder to prove them (the perpetrators) wrong; realized that they had brought it on themselves; talked to someone about how they were feeling; expressed anger or got mad; or prayed about the situation.

The FNS found that people that worried about being the victim of racism had constrained their lives in a number of ways, including avoiding going out at night and to certain places, improving home security, stopping their children playing outside, and changing travel routines (Virdee 1997). The researchers also found that around one-half of respondents felt that "black and Asian people should organize self-defense groups to protect themselves from racial attacks" (Virdee 1997). Noh and Kaspar (2003) asked respondents who reported themselves to be victims of racism whether they: did not react, took it as a fact of life, ignored it, or pretended not to be offended (indication of a *passive acceptance* form of emotion-focused coping response); screamed, cried, took it to someone else, watched television, or played games to forget (indication of an *emotional distraction* form of emotion-focused coping response); protested verbally or talked or reasoned with the offender (indication of a *personal confrontation* form of problem-focused coping response); reported the incident to the authorities or went to the media (indication of a *taking formal action* form of problem-focused coping response); or talked to family or friends (indication of a *social support seeking* form of problem-focused coping response). They were also asked how often their experiences made them feel angry, scared, sad, unwanted, revengeful, rejected, frustrated, intimidated or frightened, humiliated, puzzled, discouraged, helpless, weak, stupid, foolish, or ashamed.

There are also more general avenues for the exploration of the impact of racial discrimination. Some of these will be explored in the following sections.

Institutional (Organizational) Racism

Individual-level measures of exposure and responses to direct interpersonal discrimination can, at best, only describe one aspect of the way in which discrimination may affect people's lives. Other forms of discrimination relate to more institutional and structural processes. Institutional racism typically refers to the discriminatory policies or practices of institutions, although both institutional and interpersonal discrimination will be legitimized by the ingrained discriminatory attitudes persistent in the wider social structure (Krieger 2000). Institutional racism has been described as thwarting prosperity, self-esteem, honor, power, and influence (Adams 1990). As a process of structural limitation, then, institutional discrimination is almost impossible to perceive at an individual level. An individual is likely to be unable to detect whether they have been a victim of discrimination in gaining access to employment or housing, for example, largely because the perpetrator is likely to have made efforts (either as an individual or as part of organizational policy) to disguise the discriminatory nature of the decision or policy. Exploring these aspects of discrimination, then, require population-level analyses and "indirect" methods (Krieger 2003), through ethnic differences in distributions of deleterious exposures or socioeconomic or health disadvantage, which, it can be inferred, are a consequence of racism. What must be emphasized, though, is that indirect measures can provide nothing more than indirect evidence.

There is considerable evidence demonstrating the concentration of people from ethnic minority groups in socioeconomic, residential, and occupational disadvantage in the United States, United Kingdom, and elsewhere (Lillie-Blanton and Laveist 1996; Massey and Denton 1989; Modood et al. 1997; Navarro 1990; Nazroo 2001; Williams and Collins 2001). Evidence linking this socioeconomic disadvantage with racism has been less forthcoming, however. There is evidence that experiences of discrimination have a negative impact on income (Herring et al. 1998) and that not only are there pay disparities between black-dominated and white-dominated occupations but that black workers are paid less than white workers—in both black-dominated and higher-paid occupations (Huffman 2004). There is also evidence that racism in housing and mortgage markets produces the concentration of ethnic minority groups in disadvantaged residential areas (Logan and Alba 1995; Yinger 1995).

Despite this, the impact of social position on the relationship between, for example, racism and health was until fairly recently, in the United Kingdom at least, largely ignored in favor of more biological approaches (Nazroo 2003). Research often involved statistically adjusting models exploring the relationship between ethnicity and health for the effects of socioeconomic status. As Kaufman et al. (1997, 1998) point out, the process of standardization is, in essence, an attempt to deal with the non-random nature of samples used in cross-sectional population studies. But whereas controlling for all relevant "extraneous" explanatory factors introduces the *appearance* of randomization, attempting to introduce randomization into cross-sectional studies by adding "controls" has a number of problems: "When considering socioeconomic exposures and making comparisons between racial/ethnic groups . . . the material, behavioral, and psychological circumstances of diverse socioeconomic and racial/ethnic groups are distinct on so many dimensions that no realistic adjustment can plausibly simulate randomization" (Kaufman et al. 1998, p. 147).

Traditionally, the social class measure most frequently used in the United Kingdom is the Registrar General's (RG) measure of occupational class, which classifies occupations into six groups: professional, intermediate, skilled non-manual, skilled manual, partly skilled, and unskilled (Office of Population Censuses and Surveys 1991). Close inspection has suggested serious problems associated with its suitability for use in adjusting for socioeconomic inequality when comparing across ethnic groups. In particular, research by Nazroo (1997, 2001) has suggested that the internal heterogeneity of the RG class groupings masks the concentration of people from ethnic minority groups in lower-income occupations compared with white people in the same class. Data from the FNS shows, for example, that Pakistani and Bangladeshi people in the RG professional and intermediate (most affluent) classes in the United Kingdom have average weekly incomes similar to that of white people in partly skilled and unskilled (least affluent) occupations (Nazroo 2001). Relying on such measures to deny the impact of socioeconomic disadvantage on the experiences and circumstances of people from ethnic minority groups would therefore seem mistaken. Perhaps not surprisingly, more appropriate measures of social position have been shown to have significant effects on the relationship between ethnicity and health (Krieger 2000; Nazroo 1997, 2001).

This lack of measurement comparability may also occur when discriminatory practices prevent similar levels of resources from commanding access to similar levels of socioeconomic return. Exploring evidence of unequal rewards, then, may be both a further means of improving the cross-ethnic appropriateness of our measures and a means of exploring the existence and impact of racism in itself. Kaufman et al. (1997) describe the relationship between income values and average living costs. People from ethnic minority groups have been shown to be more likely to live in areas where basic food, housing, and other living expenses are higher, suggesting that comparable control over resources requires more than simply comparable incomes. Analyses exploring the effects of income across different ethnic groups may therefore fail to explore key aspects of the disadvantage occurring as a result of the residential and occupational segregation of ethnic minority groups.

Studies exploring the relationship between ethnicity, education, and health suggest that, as education increases, black adults do not have the same improvement in health as white adults. This may provide support for the "diminishing returns" hypothesis, where experiences of racial discrimination prevent black people, or people from non-white ethnic minority groups more generally, from fully benefiting from the capital accumulating as a consequence of their educational achievement (Bowles and Gintis 1976; Farmer and Ferraro 2005) or from other socioeconomic gains (Farley 1984). It has also been suggested that increased education, income, and occupational prestige may bring higher expectations in terms of standards of living, which, if not realized, would increase levels of distress and potentially enhance the opportunity to recognize the discrimination faced by members of ethnic minority groups. As well as exploring the impact of socioeconomic status on the relationship between racism and other indicators, residential and occupational segregation and the existence of diminishing returns in income and education are in themselves important indicators of the existence and experience of institutional racism (for more discussion of the measurement of residential segregation, see Massey and Denton 1988, 1989, and Massey et al. 1996).

Further exploration of socioeconomic status as a proxy for the impact of institutional racism may be achieved through the investigation of ethnic differences in: power over economic resources, particularly in the share of earned income measured as the proportion of people from ethnic minority groups who are economically active and their average wage, compared with society in general; exposure to toxic substances and hazardous conditions as a consequence of occupational and residential segregation (Lanphear et al. 1996; Moore et al. 1996; Northridge and Shepard 1997); political empowerment (LaVeist 1993), expressed as the number of people from ethnic minority groups in political office—either as an absolute number (Bevins 1999) or as a proportion of people from ethnic minority groups of voting age (Bobo and Gilliam 1990)—voter registration, voting patterns, and the existence, membership, and strength of political, civic, and other social organizations that focus particularly on issues pertaining to people from ethnic minority groups; and perceptions of life constraints and restricted opportunities among members of ethnic minority groups, similar to the ideas around unequal rewards or "diminishing returns" described earlier.

Perpetrators

Studies have also asked self-reported victims of racism about the characteristics of the perpetrators of racist incidents. The FNS, for example, asked whether the most serious incident of racial harassment experienced by the respondent had been perpetrated by neighbors, acquaintances, people at work, in a store or place of entertainment, by police officers or other officials, or by complete strangers. Respondents were also asked about the ethnicity, age, gender, and the number of perpetrators (Virdee 1997).

Although the majority of investigations exploring the existence and effects of racism look to the experience of the victim, there are also ways to explore the existence of racially discriminatory attitudes. Investigating experiences of racially motivated crime or discrimination is, obviously, one way of doing this. Studies have also asked people directly about their attitudes toward other ethnic groups. The British Social Attitudes (BSA) survey asked whether respondents were "very," "a little," or "not prejudiced at all against people of other races" (Rothon and Heath 2003). One-quarter of white people to the FNS (Modood et al. 1997) reported that they were racially prejudiced against (South) Asian and Muslim people, and one-fifth reported themselves to be racially prejudiced against Caribbean people (Virdee 1997). Such figures should be interpreted with caution, however, as there is evidence that people underreport negative social attitudes and deny the existence of discrimination, particularly when it is no longer legal (Essed 1996). One way of avoiding such potential bias may be through more indirect questioning, related to specific practices or policies. The BSA also asked respondents, ". . . there is a law in Britain against racial discrimination, that is against giving unfair preference to a particular race in housing, jobs and so on. Do you generally support or oppose the idea for this purpose?" (Rothon and Heath 2003). The 2002 European Social Survey asked British respondents, "To what extent do you think Britain should allow people of the same race or ethnic group as most British people to come and live here? . . . And how about people of a different race or ethnic group from most British people?" (Rothon and Heath 2003).

Area-level indicators of racial disrespect have also been used to explore the relationship between racism and ethnic differences in mortality. Kennedy et al. (1997) explored the relationship between attitudes toward collective disrespect (using data from thirty-nine U.S. states) and black and white mortality across the United States. Collective disrespect was measured using responses to the question: "On average blacks have worse jobs, income, and housing than white people. Do you think the differences are: mainly due to discrimination? (yes/no); because most blacks have less in-born ability to learn? (yes/no); because most blacks don't have the chance for education that it takes to rise out of poverty? (yes/no); because most blacks just don't have the motivation or will power to pull themselves out of poverty? (yes/no)" A 1 percent increase in the prevalence of those believing that black people lacked innate ability was found to be associated with an increase in the age-adjusted black mortality rate of 359.8 per 100,000 (Kennedy et al. 1997). It could be argued, however, that rather than the fact of living in an environment where these attitudes are present *in itself* causing increased ethnic disparity in mortality, they are more a means for people to explain (away) the ethnic disparities in employment, income, and housing that they see, which are produced by institutional racism and will directly affect mortality. Exploring the impact of racism, then, requires a consideration of complex potential causal pathways as well as appropriate measures.

There may also be opportunities to explore institutional racism from the perspective of the perpetrator, particularly the actions of an institution's representatives. For example, evidence of ethnic bias in the behavior of the British police force has been reported, particularly in relation to and motivated by the governmental inquiry into the racist murder of Stephen Lawrence, lead by Sir William Macpherson (Macpherson 1999). Fewer than two-thirds of respondents from ethnic minority groups to the FNS felt that "black and Asian people can rely on the police to protect them from racial harassment" (Virdee 1997). And over one-third of white FNS respondents felt that "[British] police harass young black people more than young white people." Similar reports have also been forthcoming from the United States. There may be opportunities to conduct similar analyses in the education and justice systems, mental and physical health services, and other public and private organizations.

There is evidence, for example, that people may experience discrimination in their interactions with health services (Einbinder and Schulman 2000; Etchason et al. 2001; Fiscella et al. 2002; Oddone et al. 2002; Smedley et al. 2002). Van Ryn and Fu (2003; see also Van Ryn 2002) provide a summary of the current evidence supporting the hypotheses that the behaviors of health and human service providers contribute to ethnic differences in health and therefore to institutional racism. This includes:

- the way in which providers may influence help-seekers' views of themselves and the world around them, including reinforcing societal messages regarding their value, self-reliance, competence, and deservingness;
- the communication of providers' lower expectations of people in disadvantaged social positions affecting help-seekers' expectations regarding chances of a positive outcome;
- the way in which providers' attitudes may affect help-seekers' health-related cognition and behavior, and;
- incomprehensive provider–seeker communication affecting both the uptake of health promotion and disease-prevention behavior as well as ability to access treatments and services.

The attitudes of politicians and the media may also be indicative of the racist climate of a society. Bashi (2004), for example, describes political attitudes toward non-white immigration to Canada, Britain, and the United States, whereas Bourne (2001) describes the rebranding of "racist" British government policies, particularly those relating to immigration in recent years. Coverage or lack of coverage by the media of topics relating to ethnicity or immigration-related issues (as numbers of stories or column-space allocated, for example) may also give us a picture of attitudes toward different ethnic groups within a society.

Conclusions

Discrimination is multidimensional, so its assessment should provide comprehensive coverage of all of its relevant domains. In terms of interpersonal experiences, we require direct and indirect investigation that can explore its multiple facets—from low-level harassment, daily hassles, or "everyday" discrimination, through chronic stressors and traumas, to major life events and macro stressors—and its cumulative effects. We need to develop ways to investigate how people's reactions to the racism they experience affect both the impact of racism on their lives and their reports of their experiences. The exploration of institutional racism requires further assessment, including the way in which racism may produce ethnic differences in returns on educational, social, economic, and other forms of capital. This may offer the most promising means by which to enlighten others as to the limited opportunities afforded people from ethnic minority groups and the limitations of the measures traditionally used. Perhaps this, in particular, provides the best opportunity for the negative role of racism on the lives of people from ethnic minority groups to be finally given the voice it requires. Another avenue may be through the continued recognition of the racist attitudes of the powerful. Without thorough investigation, we cannot hope but to underestimate racism's widespread nature and impact. We also cannot begin to understand its consequences.

References

Adams, P. L. (1990). Prejudice and exclusion and social traumata. In J. D. Noshpitz & R. D. Coddington (Eds.), *Stressors and the adjustment disorders* (pp. 362–391). New York: John Wiley and Sons.

Armstead, C., Lawler, K., Gordon, G., Cross, J., & Gibbons, J. (1989). Relationship of racial stressors to blood pressure responses and anger expression in black college students. *Health Psychology, 8,* 541–556.

Banton, M. (1983). *Racial and ethnic competition.* Cambridge: Cambridge University Press.

Banton, M., & Harwood, J. (1975). *The race concept.* Newton Abbot, U.K. David and Charles.

Barker, M. (1981). *The new racism.* London: Junction Books.

Barth, F. (1969). *Ethnic groups and boundaries: The social organsation of culture difference.* Oslo: Universitetsforlaget.

Bashi, V. (2004). Globalised anti-blackness: Transnationalizing Western immigration law, policy, and practice. *Ethnic and Racial Studies 27*(4), 584–606.

Bevins, A. (1999). No blacks, please, we're MPs. (1999, August 2). *New Statesman.* 15–16

Bjorgo, T., & Witte, R. (1993). *Racist violence in Europe.* London: Macmillan Press.

Bobo, L., & Gilliam, F. D. (1990). Race, sociopolitical participation and black empowerment. *American Political Science Review, 84,* 377–393.

Bolaffi, G., Bracalenti, R., Braham, P., & Gindro, S. (2003). *Dictionary of race, ethnicity and culture*. London: Sage.

Bonilla-Silva, E., & Baiocchi, G. (2001). Anything but racism: How sociologists limit the significance of racism. *Race and Society, 4*, 117–131.

Bourne, J. (2001). The life and times of institutional racism. *Race and Class, 43*(2), 7–22.

Bowles, S., & Gintis, H. (1976). *Schooling in capitalist America: Educational reform and the contradictions of economic life*. New York: Basic Books.

Brown, T. N., Williams, D. R., Jackson, J. S., Neighbors, H. W., Torres, M., Sellers S. L., et al. (2000). Being black and feeling blue: The mental health consequence of racial discrimination. *Race and Society 2*, 117–131.

Centre for Contemporary Cultural Studies (CCCS) (1982). *The empire strikes back: Race and racism in 70s Britain*. London: Hutchinson.

Chahal, K., & Julienne, L. (1999). *"We can't all be white!": Racist victimisation in the UK*. London: YPS.

Contrada, R. J., Ashmore, R. D., Gary, M. L., Coups, E., Egeth, J. D., Sewell, A., et al. (2000). Ethnicity-related sources of stress and their effects on well-being. *Current Directions in Psychological Science, 9*, 137–139.

Cooper, R. S. (1993). Health and the social status of blacks in the United States. *Annals of Epidemiology, 3*(2), 137–144.

Curtis, L. P. (1968). *Anglo-Saxons and Celts*. Bridgeport, CT: University of Bridgeport Press.

Curtis, L. P. (1971). *Apes and angels: The Irishman in Victorian caricature*. Washington, DC: Smithsonian Institution Press.

Davis, N. J., & Robinson, R. V. (1991). Men's and women's consciousness of gender inequality: Austria, West Germany, Great Britain and the United States. *American Sociological Review, 56*, 72–84.

Dovidio, J. F., & Gaertner, S. L. (2000). Aversive racism and selection decisions: 1989 and 1999. *Psychological Science, 11*(4), 315–319.

Einbinder, L. C., & Schulman, K. A. (2000). The effect of race on the referral process for invasive cardiac procedures. *Medical Care Research Review, 57*(Suppl. 1), 162–180.

Eriksen, T. H. (1993). *Ethnicity and nationalism: Anthropological perspectives*. London: Pluto Press.

Eriksen, T. H. (2002). *Ethnicity and nationalism: Anthropological perspectives* (expanded version). London: Pluto Press.

Essed, P. (1992). *Understanding everyday racism: An interdisciplinary theory*. London: Sage.

Essed, P. (1996). *Diversity: Gender, colour and culture*. Amherst: University of Massachusets Press.

Etchason, J., Armour, B., Ofili, E., Rust, G., Mayberry, R., Sanders, L., et al. (2001). Racial and ethnic disparities in health care. *JAMA, 285*, 883.

Farley, R. (1984). *Black and white: Narrowing the gap?* Cambridge, MA: Harvard University Press.

Farmer, M. M., & Ferraro, K. F. (2005). Are racial disparities in health conditional on socioeconomic status? *Social Science & Medicine, 60*, 191–204.

Fekete, L. (2001). The emergence of xeno-racism. *Race and Class, 43*(2), 23–40.

Fiscella, K., Franks, P., Doescher, M. P., & Saver, B. G. (2002). Disparities in health care by race, ethnicity, and language among the insured: Findings from a national sample. *Medical Care, 40*, 52–59.

Gilroy, P. (1987). *There ain't no black in the Union Jack: The cultural politics of race and nation*. London: Routledge.

Harding, S., & Maxwell, R. (1997). Differences in the mortality of migrants. In F. Drever, & M. Whitehead (Eds.), *Health inequalities: Decennial supplement* (Series DS No. 15). London: The Stationery Office.

Harrell, S. P. (1997). *The racism and life experiences scales (RaLES)* (Self-administration version). Unpublished manuscript.

Harrell, J. P., Hall, S., & Taliaferro, J. (2003). Physiological responses to racism and discrimination: An assessment of the evidence. *American Journal of Public Health, 93*(2), 243–428.

Herring, C., Thomas, M. E., Durr, M., & Horton, H. D. (1998). Does race matter? The determinants and consequences of self-reports of discrimination and victimization. *Race and Society, 1*(2), 109–123.

Herrnstein. R. J., & Murray, C. (1994). *The bell curve: Intelligence and class structure in American life.* New York: The Free Press.

Huffman, M. L. (2004). More pay, more inequality? The influence of average wage levels and the racial composition of jobs on the Black-White wage gap. *Social Science Research, 33,* 498–520.

Jackson, J. J., Torres, M., Caldwell, C. H., Neighbors, H. W., Ness, R. M., Taylor, R. J., et al. (2004). The National Survey of American Life: A study of racial, ethnic and cultural influences on mental disorders and mental health. *International Journal of Methods in Psychiatric Research, 13*(4), 196–207.

Jaffe, H. A. (1985). *History of Africa.* London: Zed Books.

James, S. A., Strogatz, D. S., Wing, S. B., & Ramsey, D. L. (1987). Socioeconomic status, John Henryism and hypertension in blacks and whites. *American Journal of Epidemiology, 126*(4), 664–673.

Jenkins, R. (1994). Rethinking ethnicity: Identity, categorization and power. *Ethnic and Racial Studies, 17*(2), 197–223.

Jordan, W. D. (1982). First impressions: Initial English confrontations with Africans. In C. Husband (Ed.), *'Race' in Britain.* London: Hutchinson.

Karlsen, S. (2004). Black like Beckham? Moving beyond definitions of ethnicity based on skin colour and ancestry. *Ethnicity and Health, 9*(2), 107–137.

Karlsen, S., & Nazroo, J. Y. (2002). Agency and structure: The impact of ethnic identity and racism in the health of ethnic minority people. *Sociology of Health and Illness, 24*(1), 1–20.

Karlsen, S., & Nazroo, J. Y. (2004). Fear of racism and health. *Journal of Epidemiology and Community Health, 58*(12), 1017–1018.

Kaufman, J. S., Cooper, R. S., & McGee, D. L. (1997). Socioeconomic status and health in Blacks and White: The problem of residual confounding and the resiliency of race. *Epidemiology, 8,* 621–628.

Kaufman, J. S., Long, A. E., Liao, Y., Cooper, R. S., & McGee, D. L. (1998). The relation between income and mortality in U.S. blacks and whites. *Epidemiology, 9*(2), 147–155.

Kennedy, B., Kawachi, I., Lochner, K., Jones, C., & Prothrow-Stith, D. (1997). (Dis)respect and black mortality. *Ethnicity and Disease, 7,* 207–214.

Krieger, N. (1990). Racial and gender discrimination: Risk factors for high blood pressure? *Social Science & Medicine, 30*(12), 1273–1281.

Krieger, N. (2000). Discrimination and health. In L. Berkman & I. Kawachi (Eds.), *Social epidemiology* (pp. 36–75). Oxford: Oxford University Press.

Krieger, N. (2003). Does racism harm health? Did child abuse exist before 1962? On explicit questions, critical science and current controversies: An ecosocial perspective. *American Journal of Public Health, 93*(2), 194–199.

Krieger, N., & Sidney, S. (1996). Racial discrimination and blood pressure: The CARDIA study of young black and white adults. *American Journal of Public Health, 86*(10), 1370–1378.

Kundnani, A. (2000). 'Stumbling on': Race, class and England. *Race and Class, 41*(4), 1–18.

Lanphear, B. P., Weitzman, M., & Eberly, S. (1996). Racial differences in urban children's environmental exposures to lead. *American Journal of Public Health, 86,* 1460–1463.

LaVeist, T. A. (1993). Segregation, poverty, and empowerment: health consequences for African Americans. *Milbank Quarterly, 71*(1), 41–64.

Lillie-Blanton, M., & Laveist, T. (1996). Race/ethnicity, the social environment, and health. *Social Science & Medicine, 43*(1), 83–91.

Logan, J. R., & Alba, R. D. (1995). Who lives in affluent suburbs? Racial differences in eleven metropolitan regions. *Sociological Focus, 28,* 353–364.

Macpherson, W. (1999). *The Stephen Lawrence inquiry: Report of an inquiry by Sir William Macpherson of Cluny Cmnd 4262-I.* London: The Stationery Office.

Marmot, M. G., Adelstein, A. M., & Bulusu, L. (1984). *Immigrant mortality in England and Wales 1970–78: Causes of death by country of birth* (Office of Population Censuses and Surveys). London: The Stationery Office.

Massey, D. S., & Denton, N. A. (1988). The dimensions of residential segregation. *Social Forces, 67,* 281–315.

Massey, D. S., & Denton, N. A. (1989). Hypersegregation in U.S. metropolitan areas: Black and Hispanic segregation along five dimensions. *Demography, 26,* 373–391.

Massey, D., White, M., & Phua, V. (1996). The dimensions of segregation revisited. *Sociological Methods Research, 25,* 172–206.

Miles, R. (1994). Explaining racism in contemporary Europe. In A. Rattansi & S. Westwood (Eds.), *Racism, modernity and identity: On the Western Front* (pp. 189–221). Oxford: Polity Press.

Miles, R. (1999). *Racism.* London: Routledge.

Modood, T. (1988). "Black," racial equality and Asian identity. *New Communit, 14*(3), 397–404.

Modood, T. (1997). Employment. In T. Modood, R. Berthoud, J. Lakey, J. Nazroo, P. Smith, S. Virdee, et al. (Eds.), *Ethnic minorities in Britain: Diversity and disadvantage.* London: Policy Studies Institute.

Modood, T., Berthoud, R., Lakey, J., Nazroo, J., Smith, P., Virdee, S., et al. (1997). *Ethnic minorities in Britain: Diversity and disadvantage.* London: Policy Studies Institute.

Moore, D. J., Williams, J. D., & Qualls, W. J. (1996). Target marketing of tobacco and alcohol-related productes to ethnic minority groups in the United States. *Ethnicity and Disease, 6,* 83–98.

Mosse, G. L. (1978). *Toward the final solution: A history of European racism.* London: Dent and Sons.

Nazroo, J. Y. (1997). *The health of Britain's ethnic minorities.* London: Policy Studies Institute.

Nazroo, J. Y. (1998). Genetic, cultural or socio-economic vulnerability? Explaining ethnic inequalities in health. *Sociology of Health and Illness, 20(5),* 710–730.

Nazroo, J. Y. (2001). *Ethnicity, class and health.* London: Policy Studies Institute.

Nazroo, J. Y. (2003). The structuring of ethnic inequalities in health: Economic position, racial discrimination and racism. *American Journal of Public Health, 93*(2), 277–284.

Nazroo, J. Y., & Karlsen, S. (2003). Patterns of identity among ethnic minority people: Diversity and commonality. *Ethnic and Racial Studies, 26*(5), 902–930.

Navarro, V. (1990). Race or class versus race and class: Mortality differentials in the United States. *The Lancet, 336,* 1238–1240.

Neighbors, H. W., Jackson, J. S., Broman, C., & Thompson, E. (1996). Racism and the mental health of African Americans: The role of self and system blame. *Ethnicity and Disease, 6,* 167–175.

Noh, S., Kaspar, V. (2003). Perceived discrimination and depression: Moderating effects of coping, acculturation and ethnic support. *American Journal of Public Health, 93*(2), 232–238.

Northridge, M. E., & Shepard, P. M. (1997). Environmental racism and public health. *American Journal of Public Health, 87*, 730–732.

Oakley, R. (1992). *Racial violence and harassment in Europe.* Strasbourg, FR: Council of Europe.

Oddone, E.Z., Petersen, L. A., Weinberger, M., Freedman, J., & Kressin, N. R. (2002). Contribution of the Veterans Health Administration in understanding racial disparities in access and utilization of health care: A spirit of inquiry. *Medical Care, 40*(Suppl. 1), I3–I13.

Office of Population Censuses and Surveys. (1991). *Explanation of the Occupational Classification Scheme.* London: The Stationery Office.

Omi, W., & Winant, H. (1994). *Racial formation in the United States: From the 1960s to the 1990s.* New York: Routledge.

Parker, H., Botha, J. L., & Haslam, C. (1995). "Racism" as a variable in health research—can it be measured? (abstract). *Journal of Epidemiology and Community Health, 48*, 522.

Rothon, C., & Heath, A. (2003). Trends in racial prejudice. In A. Park, J. Curtice, K. Thomson, L. Jarvis, & C. Bromley (Eds.), *British social attitudes: The 20th Report—continuity and change over two decades.* London: Sage.

Ruggiero, K. M., & Taylor, D. M. (1995). Coping with discrimination: How disadvantaged group members perceive the discrimination that confronts them. *Journal of Personality and Social Psychology, 68*(5), 826–838.

Scott, L. D., Jr., (2003). The relation of racial identity and racial socialization to coping with discrimination among African American adolescents. *Journal of Black Studies, 33*(4), 520–538.

Smaje, C. (1996). The ethnic patterning of health: New directions for theory and research. *Sociology of Health and Illness, 18*(2), 139–171.

Sibbitt, R. (1997). *The perpetrators of racial harassment and racial violence.* (Home Office Research Study 176) London: Home Office and Statistics Directorate.

Sigelman, L., & Welch, S. (1991). *Black Americans' views of racial inequality: The dream deferred.* New York: Cambridge University Press.

Smedley, B. D., Stith, A. Y., & Nelson, A. R. (2002). *Unequal treatment confronting racial and ethnic disparities in health care.* Washington, DC: National Academy Press.

Smith, A. D. (1986). *The ethnic origins of nations.* Oxford: Blackwell.

Taylor, D. M., Wright, S. C., Maghaddam, F. M., & Lalonde, R. N. (1990). The personal/group discrimination discrepancy: Perceiving my group, but not myself, to be a target of discrimination. *Personality and Social Psychology Bulletin, 16*, 254–262.

Tuckson, R. (1989). Race, sex, economics and tobacco advertising. *Journal of the National Medical Association, 47*, 1363–1375.

United Nations (2000). *Report of the Committee on the Elimination of Racial Discrimination.* New York: United Nations.

Van Ryn, M. (2002). Research of the provider contribution to race/ethnicity disparities in medical care. *Medical Care, 40*(Suppl. 1), I140–I151.

Van Ryn, M., & Fu, S. S. (2003). Paved with good intentions: Do public health and human service providers contribute to racial and ethnic disparities in health? *American Journal of Public Health, 93*(2), 248–255.

Virdee, S. (1995). *Racial violence and harassment.* London: Policy Studies Institute.

Virdee, S. (1997). Racial harassment. In T. Modood, R. Berthoud, J. Lakey, J. Nazroo, P. Smith, S. Virdee, et al., (Eds.), *Ethnic minorities in Britain: Diversity and disadvantage.* London: Policy Studies Institute.

Weber, M. (1922). *Wirtschaft und Gesellschaft.* Mohr, GR: Tubingen.

West, C. (1993). *Race Matters.* Boston: Beacon Press.

Williams, D. R. (1997). Race and health: Basic questions, emerging directions. *Annals of Epidemiology, 7,* 322–333.

Williams, D. R., & Collins, C. (2001). Racial residential segregation: A fundamental cause of racial disparities in health. *Public Health Reports, 116,* 404–416.

Williams, D. R., Neighbors, H. W., & Jackson, J. S. (2003). Racial/ethnic discrimination and health: findings from community studies. *American Journal of Public Health, 93*(2), 200–208.

Williams, D. R., Spencer, M. S., & Jackson, J. (1999). Race, stress and physical health: The role of group identity. In R. J. Contrada & R. D. Ashmore (Eds.), *Self, social identity and physical health: Interdisciplinary explorations* (pp. 71–100). New York: Oxford University Press.

Yinger, J. (1995). *Closed doors, opportunities lost: The continuing costs of housing discrimination.* New York: Russell Sage Foundation.

CHAPTER FIVE

MEASURING POVERTY

David M. Betson and Jennifer L. Warlick

"A nation one-third ill-housed, ill-clad, ill-nourished"

FRANKLIN D. ROOSEVELT (1937)

Every fall, the Census Bureau releases their statistical report describing the size and composition of the poverty population and those individuals without health care insurance. Both of these closely watched statistics are anticipated by the research community, policymakers, and the press, because they reflect how society's most vulnerable members fared during the previous year. The purpose of this chapter is to provide the reader with a summary of the measurement issues underlying this important statistic.

We begin with a discussion of the concept of interest—poverty—and the efforts in the United States to measure the extent and nature of poverty. We then will turn to the work of the National Research Council (NRC) Panel on Poverty Measurement and Family Assistance.[1] The Panel's report provides a blueprint for improving the official poverty measure that has been in use since 1969. The final sections of the chapter document how the Panel's recommendations would affect our statistical picture of poverty in the United States, especially the relative success and failure of addressing elderly and child poverty.

---

[1]Dr. Betson was a member of the NRC Panel on Poverty Measurement and Family Assistance. The report (Citro and Michael 1995) still provides the most comprehensive description of the statistical issues surrounding the measurement of poverty.

What Does It Mean to Be Poor?

The adjective *poor* is used to describe any individual characteristic or condition that is below average or could be viewed as socially unacceptable. It signifies a deficiency or deficit. For example, we could say that she was in poor health or he was in poor spirits or the student received poor grades. We can use the adjective to describe a group of individuals—they live in a poor neighborhood. Yet note how easy it is to substitute the adjective bad for poor in each of these phrases. She was in bad health. He earned a bad grade in the class. They live in a bad community.

The adjectives are interchangeable when used to describe the condition in which an individual can find himself or herself, but when the adjectives are used to refer to the individual they are no longer interchangeable. When referring to the individual, *poor* and *bad* stir quite different emotions in society. A poor individual is to be viewed as deserving of pity or compassion, whereas a bad person is one to be scorned because they are viewed as the source of their own condition. It is quite possible to think of "good" poverty and "bad" poverty. American social policy has avoided the use of "good" and "bad" poor but has adopted the terms "deserving" and "undeserving" poor to arrive at the same distinction between individuals who find themselves in the same condition. The remainder of the chapter is concerned with identifying a condition that individuals may find themselves in and not delineating who is and is not deserving of compassion and assistance.

We will define the poor as those individuals who live in conditions that are both below the conditions of the average citizen and deemed as socially unacceptable. Social deprivation and alienation can manifest themselves in many forms. One can be deprived of one's psychological or social well being by suffering from heightened anxiety and stress or feelings of social isolation. A chronic illness or threat to one's physical security may reflect a deprivation of physical well-being. An inability to acquire goods and services that are viewed as necessities to participate in society reflects economic deprivation. Poverty or being poor encompasses all of these dimensions, yet it will be forms of economic deprivation that command center stage in the discussions of poverty measurement.

Economic deprivation is when an individual does not have access to the necessities of life. Whereas in most cases, poverty measurement relies on the concept of income to measure an individual's ability to access consumption, what is meant by the much harder-to-define "necessities of life"? Adam Smith (1776, Book V, Chapter II, Point II, Article 4) stated that the necessities of life included "not only the commodities which are indispensably necessary for the support of life, but whatever the custom of the country renders it indecent for creditable people, even of the lowest order, to be without." Two centuries later, Townsend (1979, p. 31) built upon the Smithian view that the necessities of life were more than the minimum amount of goods needed to sustain life by concluding that the necessities of life are those goods that allow individuals to "play the roles, participate in the relationships, and follow the customary behavior which is expected of them by virtue of their membership in society."

Smith's and Townsend's views of the necessities of life or poverty budget suggest that what is considered economic deprivation or poverty in one society may not be considered so in another society or in the same society but at another point in time. To be poor in the United States does not take on the same meaning as it does in China or India. Being poor in the United States in 1900 as opposed to being poor in 2000 is more than reflected in the differences in consumer prices over the century. As societies become wealthier, the cost of fully participating in that society rises.

Unfortunately the implementation of the concept of relative poverty appears to be quite arbitrary. A common threshold for economic deprivation is set at one-half of the median income in the population. One can always question and quibble why we should focus our definition of poverty at 50 percent of the median income and not at either one- or two-thirds of the median. Given its construction, the median household can never be poor and hence the maximum poverty rate would be 50 percent. Why constrain the poverty rate in this fashion? The British "solved" this problem by adopting a poverty threshold that reflects one-half of the average income of the population.

A relative view of poverty is not universally accepted. For some, poverty is an absolute concept where necessities should be framed by a "scientific" determination or expert judgment of individual needs that are invariant to changes in social wealth if not also social context. Examples of absolute definitions of poverty abound. The World Bank's and United Nations' poverty definition of $1 per day varies across developing countries accounting for only differences in the domestic prices needed to "buy" one dollar's worth of goods. Similarly, the real purchasing power of the official U.S. poverty thresholds has not changed since their inception in 1969.

The use of an absolute measure of economic deprivation may reflect the practical problems of agreeing on what constitutes poverty conditions across different societies. The choice of an absolute standard for economic deprivation in a developed country might be driven by the political needs of policy makers who wish to succeed at reduction of poverty. Relative poverty thresholds become a moving policy goal and consequently reduce the chances of successes in poverty alleviation programs.

Early Attempts at Constructing Poverty Budgets (Thresholds)

Fisher (2000) notes that the first statistical attempt to define a poverty population in a government report was the Manly Report of 1916 as part of the work of the Commission on Industrial Relations. Basil Manly wrote that based on available budget studies "that the very least that a family of five persons can live upon in anything approaching decency is \$700" (annual income, \$12,131 in 2004 dollars). Manly concluded that an annual income of \$500 relegated the family to "abject poverty." He estimated that at least one-third and perhaps up to one-half of those individuals employed by manufacturing failed to achieve a "decent" level of income. The report was mute on exactly how Manly arrived at his levels of income, defining neither economic deprivation nor whether or how these thresholds varied by family size.

It is not until the 1930s and the Depression that the question of income adequacy and economic deprivation reemerges in federal government documents. For the Works Progress Administration, Margaret Stecker produced a set of income levels denoted as "maintenance" and "emergency" budgets that varied by family size. The White House Conference on Children and the National Resources Planning Board used these thresholds in their reports (Fisher 2000).

After the end of World War II and the creation of the Congressional Joint Committee on the Economic Report (later renamed the Joint Economic Committee [JEC]), a congressional subcommittee was formed to examine the plight of low-income families who were unable to afford rental properties and a nutritious diet. Without any explanation, the subcommittee designated urban families as low-income if their incomes were less than \$2,000 (\$15,676 in 2004 dollars). Farm families and individuals were deemed low-income if their incomes were less than \$1,000 (\$7,838 in 2004 dollars). The subcommittee continued to issue reports until it was disbanded in 1956.

Interest in the poor again awoke in the early 1960s leading up to Lyndon Johnson's proclaiming the War on Poverty (Fisher 2000). In 1962, Michael Harrington published his acclaimed book, *The Other America,* which sought to show the reader that, despite the growth in the U.S. economy, poverty persisted throughout America. Harrington set a poverty threshold at somewhere between \$3,000 and \$3,500 for an urban family of four (\$19,145 to \$22,336 in 2004 dollars). Also outside of government, the Conference on Economic Progress set a poverty line of \$4,000 (\$25,527 in 2004 dollars) for families of all sizes and \$2,000 for individuals (\$12,763 in 2004 dollars).

Within government, Robert Lampman of the Council of Economic Advisors (CEA) documented the relationship between growth in the economy and the poor, who he defined as anyone making less than \$3,000 per year (\$19,145 in 2004 dollars). Lampman's analysis showed that the reduction in poverty between 1957 and 1961 had slowed. Walter Heller, then-Chair of the CEA, used Lampman's analysis to demonstrate to President Kennedy the cost of economic slack and why a tax cut was needed to stimulate the economy (Fisher 2000).

Lampman's poverty thresholds did not vary with the size of the household—a single individual's poverty threshold was identical to that for a family of four or eight. Mollie Orshansky, a research analyst at the Social Security Administration, was worried about the impact the Lampman analysis would have on the public's perception of who was poor (Fisher 2000). She reasoned that by adopting a threshold that did not vary with the size and composition of the family, the incidence of poverty among children relative to the elderly and individuals would be understated. Orshansky developed a series of poverty thresholds that varied by family size, the number of children, the age of the head of the family, and whether the family lived in a rural or an urban setting. She then compared the composition of the poverty populations based on her thresholds and those based on the thresholds of the CEA. The analysis presented in Orshansky's 1965 paper, "Counting the Poor: Another Look at the Poverty Profile," was in direct contradiction to the CEA's report that expressed the belief that the characteristics of the poverty population would not be affected by the choice of the poverty threshold.

When the War on Poverty was announced, the Office of Economic Opportunity was established to coordinate the government's efforts. As noted in a memorandum, the government needed a poverty index in order to measure its successes and its failures. The poverty measure that the Office of Economic Opportunity chose to adopt was the Orshansky poverty measure—the measure that in large part is the official poverty measure of the federal government.

Current Methods of Poverty Measurement

On August 29, 1969, the U.S. government adopted an official poverty measure when the Bureau of the Budget (now the Office of Management and Budget) issued an executive order requiring all government agencies to use the poverty measure developed by Mollie Orshansky of the Social Security Administration. In December of the same year, the Census issued their first statistical report devoted to poverty in the United States. This publication series known as the P60 series continues to be published annually by the Bureau.

Identifying individuals and families that live in economic poverty requires that the analyst determine whether the family exceeds their poverty threshold or, in other words, has insufficient resources to meet their needs. Prior to the work of Orshansky, poverty thresholds did not recognize differences in family size or, if they did, they reflected only the difference between the needs of single individuals and all families (families with two or more individuals). The setting of the thresholds appears to reflect more personal judgment than methodology. Orshansky's methodology for setting the poverty threshold lent a semblance of credibility to her work that could not be summoned by previous researchers. Drawing on the work of other agencies, Orshansky developed thresholds that were based on reason and empirical assumptions.

The foundation for the Orshansky poverty thresholds is food requirements. She used census data to estimate the age and gender composition of all family sizes with a given number of children. For example, for a family of four composed of two adults and two children, Orshansky would produce a two-way table of the gender and ages of the family members. Using the food budgets developed for the U.S. Department of Agriculture's Economy food plans that varied by the gender and age of the family member, she computed the expected food requirements by family sizes, the number of children and the sex and age of the head of the family. To estimate the total needs of the family, Orshansky adopted a proportional multiplier approach. Her analysis of the 1955 Consumer Expenditure Survey led her to conclude that the average family spent one-third of their budget on food. Consequently, she reasoned that total consumption needs of the family would be three times her estimates of food requirements. For individuals living alone, she reasoned that their needs would be 80 percent of those of a childless couple. Farm families could be expected to meet a certain proportion of their needs from their farm production, and she applied a constant proportional reduction for farm families. In later revisions to the poverty thresholds, the gender-specific thresholds and the distinction based on farm and non-farm residence were eliminated; so today the only differences in thresholds are based on family size, the number of children, and the age of the head in single individuals and childless couples.

To measure the family's resources, the Census Bureau collects annual data on various sources of income from the March Supplement to the Current Population Survey (CPS). The income concept, known as "Census Money Income," reflects the wage, salaries, self-employment income, farm and business income, rental income, dividends, royalties, and interest income. In addition, Census Money Income includes transfers from other households in the form of alimony and child support, social insurance payments from Social Security, workers' compensation, and unemployment insurance. Finally, Census Money Income includes all cash payments from means-tested welfare programs, including Supplemental Security Income, General Assistance, and Temporary Assistance to Needy Families (formally Aid to Families with Dependent Children). These forms of income reflect the primary sources of cash or money income to families at the time of the development of poverty thresholds.

With the annual economic and demographic data from the March CPS, the Census Bureau determines whether the family's Census Money Income meets their needs. If there is a shortfall, then the family is denoted as poor. On the basis of this determination, the Census Bureau constructs annual profiles of the poverty population, the incidence of poverty among various subgroups of the population, and the extent of poverty in terms of the poverty gap—the amount of shortfall of the family's income relative to their needs.

FIGURE 5.1. CENSUS POVERTY RATE BY AGE: 1966 TO 2003.

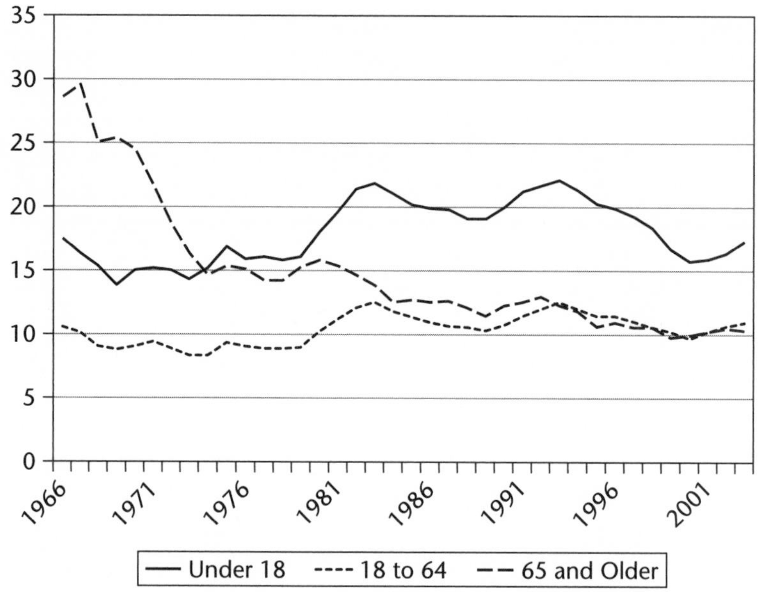

Source: Census Bureau (2004).

Although the Census Bureau's report documents many interesting facets of poverty over the past three-plus decades, we chose to highlight the same comparison that caught Orshansky's attention—the incidence of poverty among children relative to that among the elderly. Figure 5.1 documents the success that society has had in reducing poverty among the elderly while, at the same time, seeing rising child poverty rates. One might question, just as Orshansky did in the mid-1960s, how much of this picture is being determined by how we measured poverty?

NRC Panel Recommendations

The official poverty measure has remained virtually unchanged since its inception in the late 1960s. The only changes that have been implemented by the Census Bureau have been the elimination of the thresholds differences based on gender of the head of the family and the lower thresholds for farm households. The durability of the original Orshansky poverty measure does not reflect the extent of criticism the measure has received over the decades. During the 1970s as the number of poverty programs that directly delivered their services instead of providing cash grants increased, analysts began questioning the adequacy of Census Money Income as a measure of the family's resources. The work of Timothy Smeeding (1982) is one of the first that addressed this issue in a rather complete and rigorous manner. Later the Census Bureau began publishing a series of experimental poverty measures that reflected Smeeding's research (United States Bureau of the Census, 1993).

In her book *Drawing the Line: Alternative Poverty Measures and Their Implications for Public Policy,* (1990) Ruggles provides a comprehensive critique of the Census Bureau's poverty measure. All of this work culminates in the 1995 report of the NRC Panel on Poverty Measurement and Family Assistance (Citro and Michael 1995). The Panel concluded that the current measure of poverty has failed to reflect important economic trends as well as policies aimed to alleviate the condition it attempts to measure—economic poverty.

The NRC Panel identified four problems with the current specification of the poverty thresholds. First, the current thresholds display an erratic pattern of implicit equivalence scales. For example, in two-parent families the economic cost of the second child exceeds the cost of the first, third, fourth, or fifth child. The Panel recommended that the poverty thresholds be adjusted with an explicit set of equivalence scales that would capture the relative needs of families.[2] Second, the thresholds for families headed by someone sixty-five years or older are lower than for families headed by younger individuals. This difference reflects the relatively smaller food requirements of the elderly, and the Panel did not find sufficient rationale that this difference should be retained. Third, the current thresholds ignore geographic differences in the cost of living; for example, the cost of housing in New York City is 162 percent higher than in rural Mississippi. The Panel proposed that thresholds should be adjusted for the differences in the geographic cost of living.

Finally, since 1969 there has been no adjustment in the real value of the threshold, despite a nearly 30-percent increase in median after-tax incomes of

---

[2]The specific scales proposed by the Panel were defined by the following

$$S(A, C) = (A + cC)^e$$

where A and C are the number of adults and children in the family and c and e are constants. The proposed values of c and e were .70 and .75, respectively. Since the Panel's report has been released, further research has led the Census Bureau to adopt a three-parameter set of scales (Iceland 2005).

four-person families. Since 1947, the Gallop organization has been asking Americans, "What is the smallest amount of money a family of four would need to get along in your community?" During the 1960s, the official poverty threshold for a family of four, one-half of median after-tax income, and the average response from the Gallop "get along" question were equal. In years prior to the setting of the threshold, both the relative threshold based on median after-tax income and the Gallop question were less than the value of the official poverty threshold for a family of four, whereas in the years after, they both exceeded the official poverty threshold. The Panel concluded that although in the 1960s the official poverty threshold may have been "right" in mirroring what Americans believed poverty was, today the thresholds are too low and that some upward adjustment in the poverty thresholds is warranted. To set the thresholds today, they should reflect current social reality and not what a nutritionist believes is needed. To accomplish this goal, the Panel proposed that the threshold for a family of four should reflect what Americans spend on food, clothing, and shelter and that changes over time in the thresholds should reflect changes in American spending patterns on these necessities.

Families are officially classified as being in poverty if their available resources (annual Census money income before taxes and other deductions) fall below official poverty thresholds. The Panel examined the adequacy of Census Money Income as a measure of the family's ability to meet their needs and found it deficient in four specific areas. Whereas, in principle, many if not all of these proposals could have been made as changes to the official thresholds, the Panel explicitly proposed to make changes to the Bureau's resource measure.

Census money income does not include the value of services from numerous government transfer programs to low-income families, such as food stamps, school breakfast and lunch programs, Women Infants and Children (WIC), Energy Assistance, and public housing. Their omission from the Bureau's resource measure could be explained either by the technical difficulty of valuing in-kind as opposed to cash transfers or the fact that these programs didn't constitute a major source of assistance for low-income families. The Panel proposed that the market value of any in-kind program that assisted families in meeting their food, clothing, and shelter needs should be included in the measure of the family's available resources.

In the 1960s, the poor were practically exempted from federal income taxation and very few states taxed low-income families. The only tax they paid on their income was the Social Security Payroll tax at three percent of earnings. In the 1960s, there was very little error introduced into poverty measurement by not subtracting the family's tax liability even though a poverty level before tax income would not be enough to purchase the family's income. Today the poor are subject to considerably higher taxes at both the federal and state levels. At the same time, today's IRS is also one of the largest providers of cash assistance to the low-income population. Through the refundable Earned Income Tax Credit, over 30 billion dollars of cash assistance is provided annually. The NRC Panel recommended that these higher taxes should be taken into account in measuring poverty by subtracting the family's net tax liability from available resources.

The growth in multiple earner households, reflecting the rise in women's labor force participation, has been dramatic; however, only the earnings minus the cost of employment are available to meet the family's consumption needs. The Panel recommended that a limited amount of child care as well as other work-related expenses should be deducted from the family's available resources.

Of all the Panel's recommendations, its proposed treatment of medical needs and expenditures in the poverty measure has received the most attention and criticism. Although medical needs may seem to be comparable to other nonmedical needs, such as food and housing, the Panel rejected their inclusion in the poverty thresholds. The Panel reasoned that the nonmedical needs of any family of a given size and composition could be assumed to be roughly equal across families. The same could not be said of their medical needs. The large variation in medical spending, after holding family size and income constant, was believed to reflect differences in the needs of families rather than personal choices. To designate the medical needs of a family of a given size as the average or median level of spending would misrepresent the true needs of the family. For some families, the figure used to represent medical needs would overstate their needs, whereas for others it would understate their true needs. Given the highly skewed distribution of medical spending amounts, it was not evident that these errors would balance out.

The use of health care insurance shields the family against the risk of variations in medical needs, and the past four decades have seen dramatic changes in both private and public insurance policy. Faced with rising health care costs, employers have been shifting larger shares of premium cost to their employees as well as adopting larger deductibles and co-payments requirements. In the mid- 1960s, governments created the Medicare and Medicaid programs that provided protection for the elderly and poor from the risk of the cost of their medical needs. But the public sector has not been immune from the pressure of rising medical costs, and so they too have been retrenching the coverage of their programs while asking recipients to pay a portion of their use of health care services. The consequence has been that the rapid rise in health care expenditures directly financed by family has affected the family's ability to meet their nonmedical needs (Acs and Sablehaus 1995). This line of reasoning led the NRC Panel to recommend that the definition of family resources be altered to reflect the burden imposed by medical expenses by subtracting the amount of medical out-of-pocket spending from the family's available resources. It was the Panel's intention that the poverty measure would reflect the ability of families to meet their nonmedical needs and that a separate measure would be constructed to reflect the family's risk of not meeting their medical needs.

After the release of the Panel's report in 1995, the Census Bureau undertook an internal examination of the recommendations. Beginning in June 1999, the Bureau began publishing a series of experimental poverty measures reflecting the NRC Panel's recommendations as well as some other alternatives (Short et al 1999). The most significant alternatives to the NRC Panel recommendations address the question of the treatment of medical needs. The leading alternative proposes the addition of an expected amount of medical out-of-pocket spending to the poverty thresholds and subtracting the actual amount of spending from the family's resources.

During the summer of 2004, with Census Bureau funding, the NRC held a workshop to discuss the future of the current poverty measure as well as the experimental poverty measures (see Iceland 2005 for a summary of the workshop). The hope of the workshop was to examine the areas where broad agreement existed and discuss what research could be undertaken to narrow the areas where disagreement still existed after almost ten years since the report's release. In many respects, the workshop was successful by highlighting the broad consensus that exists on the vast majority of the Panel's proposals. But the treatment of health care still represents a major stumbling block to adoption of a new poverty measure. The difficulty in achieving a consensus is that there does not appear to be a clear best solution but a variety of second-best ones, where no single option can muster a significant majority of supporters. The deadlock on this issue stands in contrast to another recommendation—the adjustment of the poverty thresholds to reflect geographic differences in the cost of living. Although there is almost unanimous agreement that these cost-of-living differences should be reflected in the thresholds, there is concern over the potential deficiencies of any cost-of-living index. These concerns are magnified by the impact this change would have on distribution of intergovernmental grants based on the number of poor, such as the Title One educational grants to local school districts. In many respects, the political misgivings about this recommendation seem to trump any technical concerns.

Impact on Elderly and Child Poverty

The NRC Panel's contention was that the official poverty measure was flawed not merely because of technical concerns but because it had failed to capture important economic trends and the impact of government programs targeted on the population it was intended to determine. The NRC report and subsequent research has attempted to document this point of contention. The official poverty measure has been used to document two important poverty trends, the decline of poverty among the elderly and the rise in the relative importance of child poverty. It is estimated that in 1950 one of every two elderly individuals were poor but as the real value of Social Security benefits rose and with the adoption of a minimum income program for the elderly (Supplement Security Income [SSI]), elderly poverty rates declined to the point that today the incidence of poverty among the elderly is 10 percent and is lower than the rate for all individuals. Although the war on elderly poverty may not be completely won, the major battle appears to be over. Since the mid- 1980s, the poverty rate of the elderly has roughly equaled the poverty rate among other adults.

In 1966, the poverty rate for children was 17.6 percent, whereas the poverty rate for the elderly was 28.5 percent. In the next eight years, both children and the elderly saw their risk of poverty reduced. But given the significant gains of the elderly, by 1974 the two groups faced roughly the same risk of poverty—15.1 percent for children and 14.6 percent for the elderly. Since 1974, the experiences of the two groups began to diverge. Whereas the elderly have seen their incidence of poverty continue to decline, child poverty has risen. In 1993, the poverty rate of children reached 22 percent, a level that had not been experienced since the beginning of the War on Poverty. Although children shared in economic gains of the 1990s, their poverty rate as measured by the Census Bureau continues to be significantly higher than any other age group.

Forty years ago, Mollie Orshansky was concerned that child poverty would be understated relative to other groups, especially the elderly, because of the choice of an identical threshold for all family sizes. Today, the opposite concern may be raised. Is our progress in addressing child poverty being understated because of how we measure the family's available resources to meet their needs? The current poverty measure considers, as an available resource, the family's before-tax market income plus their receipt of means-tested transfers given in cash and payments from social insurance programs. Abstracting from the effect of taxes, the cost of working, and out-of-pocket medical spending, this definition of available resources captures the majority of resources available to the elderly population but not for children. Families with children have, over time, received a growing proportion of their governmental assistance not in the form of cash but through programs that directly provide specific goods and services. Food Stamps, public housing, housing and energy assistance, school breakfast and lunch, and subsidized child care are just some examples of programs that are counted as available resources for the families that receive these forms of assistance. Because the IRS and not a welfare agency administers the Earned Income Tax Credit, it is not counted even though it is received in the form of cash.

Although the neglect of in-kind benefits will overstate the poverty rate of all groups that receive assistance in this form, the growing reliance of children on these sources of resources could seriously affect their poverty relative to the elderly. Inclusion of the value of in-kind subsidies was not the only proposed change to the measure of available resources made by the NRC Panel. The subtraction of work-related expenses and the net tax liability of the family would increase children poverty rates both in absolute level and relative to the elderly. The subtraction of medical out-of-pocket spending from the measure of the family's available resources could be expected to have a larger effect on the poverty rates of the elderly than on the poverty rate of children. To examine the impact of alternative resource measures, we have analyzed their impact on four years of data (1979, 1983, 1989, and 1994[3]). We have chosen to examine two alternatives to the official resource measure, Census Money Income. The "Expanded Census Money Income" adds to the current resource measure the value of nonmedical in-kind assistance and the value of the Earned Income Tax Credit. The "NRC Panel's Resource" subtracts from the previous measure the amount of tax paid, work-related expenses incurred, and the amount of medical out-of-pocket spending. We have maintained the level of Census Bureau's thresholds for each of the respective years, and consequently the Panel's recommendations for changes in the thresholds are not reflected in the following estimates.

Table 5.1 presents the impact on the poverty rate of children, persons 18 to 64 years old, and the elderly when implementing two alternative measures of a family's available resources. Based on the Census Money Income measure of resources, being a child meant that you faced a heightened relative risk of being poor, especially when compared to the elderly. In 1979, children were 8 percent more likely to be poor than an elderly individual. By 1994, children were 86 percent more likely to be poor. Over time, the risk of poverty for elderly adults declined. In 1979, the elderly faced a significantly higher risk of being poor than a younger adult; by 1994 both age groups faced roughly equal poverty risks.

Including the value of nonmedical in-kind benefits and the family's Earned Income Tax Credit reduces the poverty rates for all age groups. Including the value of these transfers had the largest effect on children. In 1979, the number of poor children is reduced by 23 percent, and the elderly poor fell by 11 percent. The net effect of adding these sources of income is to reverse the relative poverty risks of these two groups of vulnerable citizens. In 1983 and later years, the relative poverty risks of

---

[3]The years 1979 and 1989 reflect the troughs in the overall poverty rates, whereas the other two years represent peaks.

TABLE 5.1. IMPACT OF ALTERNATIVE RESOURCE MEASURES ON POVERTY RATES.

	1979	1983	1989	1994
Children Poverty Rates:				
Census Money Income	16.4%	22.3%	19.6%	21.8%
Expanded Census Money Income	12.6%	19.7%	16.0%	16.6%
NRC Panel's Resources	18.2%	27.4%	23.7%	25.3%
Poverty Rates of Persons 18 to 64:				
Census Money Income	8.9%	12.4%	10.2%	12.0%
Expanded Census Money Income	7.3%	11.2%	8.7%	9.8%
NRC Panel's Resources	11.0%	16.1%	14.4%	15.6%
Elderly Poverty Rates:				
Census Money Income	15.2%	13.8%	11.4%	11.7%
Expanded Census Money Income	13.5%	12.0%	9.6%	9.7%
NRC Panel's Resources	22.4%	20.4%	19.4%	20.9%

Source: Betson and Warlick, 1998.

children and the elderly remain similar to what was documented in the official poverty statistics. The addition of the in-kind and tax credits does not alter the relative poverty comparisons between the elderly and younger adults.

The NRC Panel recommended not only the addition of these government transfers but the subtraction from available family resources the amount of taxes paid by the family, the amount of work-related expenses including child care, and the amount of the family's medical out-of-pocket spending. The difference between the NRC Panel and the previous resource measure can be expected to raise the poverty rates of all groups. The marginal effect of these changes is the greatest on the poverty rates of the elderly. In 1979, these net subtractions from available family resources resulted in 66 percent more elderly poor. By 1994, they resulted in 115 percent more poor among the elderly. For children and younger adults, the marginal impact was smaller but still significant.

Compared with the official poverty measure, the use of the NRC Panel's resource definition does affect how one views child poverty relative to the elderly. In 1983 and later years, children would still be seen to face a higher risk of poverty than the elderly, but the gap between the two groups is not only smaller but is becoming smaller over time. Compared with younger adults, the elderly face elevated risks of poverty. In summary, the picture of the poverty risk of the elderly is not as rosy as the one created by the official statistics.

Although the major focus of poverty analysis is on the head count of those in poverty (expressed as the poverty rate), researchers have long recognized that the distribution of the poor's unmet needs (needs minus available resources) should be reflected in our view of the extent of poverty in the population. Many poverty researchers have developed poverty indexes that attempt to capture both the risk of being poor as well as the depth of poverty (see Foster 1984, Sen 1988). The Census Bureau reports the average and aggregate poverty gap (unmet needs of the poverty population) as well as the distribution of poor individuals by the percentage of their unmet need. Although lacking the sophistication of the poverty indexes, this latter statistic provides additional information not contained in the simple head count of the poor.

Table 5.2 presents, the distribution of poor children, young adults, and the elderly in 1994 by two different resource definitions, Census Money Income and the NRC Panel's resource measure.

Extreme poverty has been defined as having less than 50 percent of your needs met. When using Census Money Income as the resource measure, the serious plight of children is reflected in the 45 percent of poor children that face extreme poverty. A much smaller proportion of the elderly poor (21.8 percent) find themselves in extreme poverty, whereas 52 percent of the elderly poor have more than 75 percent of their needs met by this resource measure. But this picture changes dramatically if we adopt the NRC Panel's resource measure; 27.5 percent of poor children and 41.7 percent of elderly poor find themselves in extreme poverty. Betson (2001) found that when the Sen poverty measure (a poverty index

TABLE 5.2. DISTRIBUTION OF THE POOR BY THE AMOUNT OF THEIR UNMET NEEDS (1994).

	Percentage of Unmet Needs			
	76–100%	51–75%	26–50%	0–25%
Children:				
Census Money Income (21.8%)	16.7%	28.3%	39.1%	25.8%
NRC Panel's Resources (25.3%)	12.3%	15.2%	32.8%	39.7%
Age 18 to 64 Years Old:				
Census Money Income (11.9%)	20.4%	20.0%	28.9%	30.7%
NRC Panel's Resources (15.6%)	20.1%	15.3%	27.7%	37.0%
Elderly:				
Census Money Income (12.1%)	12.1%	9.7%	26.0%	52.0%
NRC Panel's Resources (20.9%)	27.7%	14.0%	23.2%	35.1%

Source: Betson, 2001.

Note: The percentage in parentheses represents the poverty rate for that group when using a specific resource measure.

that combines the group's overall risk of being poor with a measure of the depth of poverty of the group) is employed, the poverty of children relative to the elderly was dependent on which resource measure was employed. Census Money Income resource definition provided a picture of rising child poverty over time and relative to poverty of the elderly population. The use of the NRC Panel's resource measure produced a picture of rising child poverty that was now equal to a consistently high extent of poverty among the elderly.

The NRC Panel also was of the belief that the composition of the poverty population would be affected by the implementation of their proposed poverty measure. Betson, Citro, and Michael (2000) produced estimates that showed the adoption of the NRC Panel's recommendation would produce a different picture of who is poor. Poor children would be more likely to be found in two-parent families where the parents worked. The poor would be less likely to receive assistance from the government. They would be more likely to be white and Hispanic. The poor would be more likely to live in the Northeast and the Western regions of the country.

Progress Toward Adoption of a New Poverty Measure

Since the 1995 release of the NRC Panel report, poverty analysts both inside and outside of government have been examining the Panel's recommendations. Beginning in 1999, the Census Bureau has issued annual reports implementing versions of the Panel's recommendations denoted as "Experimental Poverty Measures." The variants explored by the Census Bureau could be divided into two sets of alternatives. In the category that could be called technical alternatives, the Bureau examined alternative methods of setting the thresholds and adjustment over time, alternative equivalence scales, and imputation of work-related expenses, including childcare. The more substantive alternatives considered by the Census Bureau included not adjusting for geographic differences in the cost of living and alternative treatments of medical needs, specifically including an amount in the poverty thresholds for expected out-of-pocket medical spending.

Both of the substantive variations examined by the Census Bureau provide interesting insights on the political dimensions of statistical measurement of poverty. The adjustment of the poverty thresholds to reflect geographic differences in the cost-of-living would alter the geographic distribution of the poor—higher proportions of the poor in the Western and Northeastern regions and significantly smaller proportions of the poor living in the South. Even though the NRC Panel's recommendation would only affect how the Census Bureau determines who is poor for "statistical" purposes, it would be difficult to maintain one set of poverty thresholds for counting the poor for statistical and evaluations purposes that recognized geographic difference in the cost of living and another set of thresholds used to count the poor for the determination of amount provided for income transfer programs and intergovernmental grants. Eventually there would be pressure to change the grant formula to reflect the geographic differences in cost of living and consequently the federal flow of funds. To avoid this potential political problem, some analysts have argued that because of difficulties of constructing a geographic cost of living, no adjustment should be made.

The treatment of medical care in the measurement of poverty has been the most controversial recommendation. Many analysts argue that not including an amount for the medical needs of the family in the poverty threshold is plainly a mistake. Every family can be expected to require health care during the year, and it should be reflected in the thresholds. A secondary concern is that some of the medical care used by the family reflects their discretion of how to spend their money. To subtract the family's out-of-pocket spending on medical care is permitting families to spend themselves into poverty. We don't allow this for other family needs, such as shelter; why should we allow this for its medical needs?

Although this argument may be convincing, it ignores what the Panel felt was an important distinction between the need for medical care and the need for other necessities. What families need is an ability to pay for the access to medical care when they are ill. But all families need food, clothing, and shelter, whether they are ill or not. Consequently, the healthy family is more likely to be able to afford their nonmedical needs than a family whose members require medical attention. Placing an expected amount of medical out-of-pocket spending in the threshold could produce types of errors in the determination of families unable to financially meet their needs. Healthy families who do not have spend the average or expected amount on medical care could be falsely labeled as poor, even though they had enough resources to meet both their medical and nonmedical needs during the year. Conversely, the extremely ill whose health care coverage is inadequate could face higher-than-average out-of-pocket medical spending and not have enough resources to meet their nonmedical needs. Many of these types of families would not be classified as poor. The combined effect of the two classification errors would lead to a poverty population that is significantly healthier than the poverty population determined by the NRC Panel's recommendations.

The failure to arrive at a consensus on the appropriate treatment of medical care is most likely the single reason that the Census Bureau has not formally adopted a new poverty measure. Given how the current poverty thresholds were constructed, it is not clear whether any amount for medical care is reflected in the thresholds. To understand why this proposal, above all others, has been so controversial, it is instructive to examine the consequences of the Panel's recommendation. As noted previously, the Panel's recommendation to subtract medical out-of-pocket from the family's resources is the primary factor altering our perception of the level and trend in elderly poverty from the one presented in the current poverty reports. To disturb the idea that the elderly do not face an elevated risk of poverty is to question the need for addressing programs aimed at the elderly population.

Conclusions

Statistical measures are reflections of the underlying currents and trends in our society. Early attempts to identify those individuals with resources insufficient to meet their needs were undertaken to document a social ill that was not expected to exist in a nation with such wealth. Poverty measurement provides a statistical face to the portion of the population in need. That portrait provides the impetus for the nation to address poverty, but at the same time it provides a standard by which progress is measured. As society and poverty programs changed, our poverty measure remained fixed in time. The result was that it failed to reflect changes in what poverty means in society and chronicle the success of our programs to alleviate poverty.

A decade after the NRC Panel released its report, the Census Bureau has published numerous variations of poverty measures based on the Panel's recommendations. Yet no official decision has been made to elevate these experimental poverty measures to a more official status. As time progresses, concerns arise among the policy community that these experimental poverty measures will soon disappear from the Bureau's reports in a manner similar to the experimental poverty series developed in the 1970s that modified the definition of Census Money Income to include the value of all in-kind benefits and subtract taxes.

The 2004 NRC workshop, mentioned previously in this chapter, was convened to examine the progress toward adoption of a new poverty measure and determine what could be done to bring the research to fruition. The published summary of the workshop (Iceland 2005) suggests that many of the initial concerns about the Panel's recommendations have been mitigated by the research done in the intervening years; however, concerns still remain with the treatment of medical needs and the role that assets (home ownership in particular) should play in poverty measurement. Both of these issues have a significant impact on the extent of poverty in the population, but especially on elderly poverty.

Whether these issues can be resolved in the near future is purely a matter of speculation. It is clear that changes to official statistics are difficult to obtain even when there are obvious shortcomings of the current measure. The difficulty of rectifying the problems seen in our official poverty measure is only heightened by the close relationship between what is being measured and the demands on government action that will be created. All of the current research suggests that the adoption of the NRC Panel recommendations would increase the number of poor. Politicians would not welcome this message as they seek to rein in government spending. Ultimately, and unfortunately, the political considerations will dictate whether sensible changes will be made to what should be a politically neutral picture of our society.

References

Acs, G., & Sablehaus, J. (1995, December). Trends in out-of-pocket spending on health care, 1980–92. *Monthly Labor Review, 35–45.*

Betson, D. M., & Warlick, J. L. (1998, May). Alternative historical trends in poverty. *American Economic Review,* 348–351.

Betson, D. M., Citro, C., & Michael, R. T. (2000). Recent developments for poverty measurement in U.S. official statistics. *Journal of Official Statistics, 16*(2), 87–112.

Betson, D. M. (2001). Estimating the relative poverty status of children and the elderly using a comprehensive measure of poverty. In A. K. Dutt & K. P. Jameson (Eds.), *Crossing the mainstream: Ethical and methodological issues in economics.* Notre Dame, IN: University of Notre Dame Press.

Citro, C., & Michael, R. T. (1995). *Measuring poverty: A new approach.* Washington, DC: National Academy Press.

Fisher, G. M. (2000). *Reasons for measuring poverty in the United States in the context of public policy— A historical review, 1916–1995.* (Department of Health and Human Services). Online paper available at http://aspe.hhs.gov/poverty/papers/reasmeaspov.htm

Foster, J. (1984). On economic poverty: A survey of aggregate measures. *Advances in Econometrics, 3,* 215–251.

Iceland, J. (2005). Experimental poverty measures: Summary of workshop. Washington, DC: National Academy Press.

Ruggles, P. (1990). *Drawing the line: Alternative poverty measures and their implications for public policy.* Washington, DC: The Urban Institute Press.

Sen, A. (1988). *Poverty and famines: An essay on entitlement and deprivation.* Oxford: Oxford University Press.

Short, K., Garner, T., Johnson, D., & Doyle P. (1999). *Experimental poverty measures: 1990 to 1997.* (US Census Bureau, Current Population Report, Consumer Income, P60–205). Washington, DC: US Government Printing Office.

Short, K., & Garner, T. (2002). *A decade of experimental poverty thresholds 1990 to 2000.* Retrieved Demember 28, 2006, from http://www.census.gov/hhes/poverty/povmeas/topicpg3.html.

Smeeding, T. (1982). *Alternative methods for valuing selected in-kind transfer benefits and measuring their effect on poverty.* (Technical Report No. 50). Washington, DC: Bureau of the Census, Department of Commerce.

Smith, A. ([1776]1993). *Wealth of nations* (Modern Library ed). New York: Random House. (Original work published 1776)

Townsend, P. (1979). *Poverty in the United Kingdom: A survey of household resources and standard of living.* Harmondsworth, United Kingdom: Penguin Books.

United States Bureau of the Census (1993). *Measuring the effect of benefits and taxes on income and poverty, 1992.* (Current Population Report, P60–186RD). Washington, DC: Government Printing Office.

APPENDIX: Some Practical Advice on Implementing a Poverty Measure

Identifying families who are poor by comparing their needs to their income appears to be quite simple; however, the information required to perform this comparison as recommended by the NRC panel is extensive. It is anticipated that not all data sets will contain sufficient information to implement the panel's poverty measure and some compromises will have to be made.

The unit or group of individuals, for the purpose of determining the poverty status of any individuals, comprises those individuals who can be assumed to be sharing resources for the purpose of consumption. The NRC Panel recommended that a "broadened" definition of family—all persons living together who are related by blood or marriage with the inclusion of cohabiting couple—be the primary unit of analysis; that is, the determination of whether an individual is poor is based on whether the resources available to the individual's family exceed its needs. If an individual is either living alone or living with other unrelated adults (with the exception of cohabiting couples) then the poverty determination is based solely on the individual's needs and resources.

The NRC panel recommended that a poverty threshold be first developed for the reference family of four (two adults and two children) and then adjusted for differences in family composition from the reference family and geographic differences in the cost of living. The NRC panel examined data from the Consumer Expenditure Survey to determine the distribution of annual spending on food at home, shelter, and clothing in families of four. The poverty threshold would be determined by selecting the level of spending at a given percentile of this distribution of spending. The panel suggested a range between the 30th and 35th percentiles. To account for other nonmedical related needs, the panel recommended using a small (15 to 25 percent) multiple of the amount determined for the basic food, shelter, and clothing needs. Over time, the poverty threshold for the reference family would be adjusted based on changes in the median spending of families of four on food, shelter, and clothing estimated using the Consumer Expenditure Survey. Table 5.A.1 contains the official poverty threshold and the panel's threshold as computed by Short and Garner (2002) for the reference family from 1989 to 2003.

To adjust for differences in family size and composition, the panel recommended a two-parameter set of equivalence scales based on the number of adults (A) and the number of children (C) in the family. Since the publishing of the panel's report, additional research (see Short et al 1999) has been undertaken, and the Census Bureau now favors a three-parameter set of equivalence scales. We would

TABLE 5.A.1.   OFFICIAL AND RECOMMENDED
POVERTY THRESHOLD FOR THE REFERENCE FAMILY
OF FOUR (TWO ADULTS AND TWO CHILDREN).

Year	Official	Recommended
1989	$12,575	$12,734
1990	13,254	13,398
1991	13,812	13,917
1992	14,228	14,284
1993	14,654	14,806
1994	15,029	15,169
1995	15,455	15,514
1996	15,911	15,710
1997	16,276	15,985
1998	16,530	16,517
1999	16,895	17,036
2000	17,463	17,884
2001	17,960	18,709
2002	18,244	19,329
2003	18,660	19,778

Source: Short and Garner, 2002, updated by Short.

recommend the use of this set of scales. The recommended adjustment factors that would be applied to the threshold for a family of four are:

$$(1.80 + .5[C - 1])^{.70}/2.1577 \quad \text{if } A = 1 \text{ and } C > 0$$
$$.6554 \quad \text{if } A = 2 \text{ and } C = 0$$
$$(A + .5C)^{.70}/2.1577 \quad \text{if } A > 1 \text{ and } C > 0 \text{ or } A > 2 \text{ and } C = 0.$$

To adjust the thresholds for the geographic differences in the cost of living, the panel recommended the development of a geographic price index. In its report (see Citro and Michael 1995), the NRC panel did construct an index that varied by Census division and metropolitan size. The panel's index has drawn some criticism, and because it is now almost fifteen years out of date, we would recommend not making an adjustment for differences in the cost of living, with knowledge that poverty in metro areas will be understated while poverty in the southern region will likely be overstated.

The panel's recommended measure of available resources requires considerably more information on the family than was used in the determination of their needs. Most researchers will identify the family's available resources with its income. While some may wish to consider also the asset holdings of the family as available for spending, the NRC panel chose to recommend the family's income with some modifications aimed to make it compatible with the panel's definition of the family's needs. Currently the Census uses a measure of income that reflects the *cash* receipt of income from employment, assets, pensions, and public transfers. The panel recommended the following modifications be made to this basic definition of income (Census Money Income):

- Add the value of nonmedical in-kind benefits received from either private or public sources that could be used to acquire food, clothing, or shelter (includes utilities) for the family;
- Deduct federal, state, and local income taxes and Social Security payroll taxes;
- For families with two working parents, deduct actual child care expenses per week worked, not to exceed the earnings of the parent with lower amount of earnings;
- For each working parent, deduct a flat amount per week worked (but not to exceed the amount of earnings of the working parent) to reflect transportation and other costs of working;
- Deduct child support payments from the income of the payer; and
- Deduct out-of-pocket medical care expenditures including health insurance paid by the family.

The likelihood that the researcher will have sufficient data to make many (if any) of these modifications is low. The most likely scenario will be that the researcher will have only limited information on the family's cash income. Although one could attempt to impute the needed information to make all of the above modifications, we do not recommend this approach. We would, however, strongly recommend deducting from the family's income an expected (average) amount of out-of-pocket medical expenditures. Average amounts of out-of-pocket medical expenditures can be found in the annual reports on consumer expenditures from the Bureau of Labor Statistics Consumer Expenditure Survey.

The poverty status of the individual or family can be represented either as a dichotomous variable (poor versus non-poor) or as a continuous variable of the form of the income-to-needs ratio.

CHAPTER SIX

MEASURING HEALTH INEQUALITIES

Sam Harper and John Lynch

There is widespread research and policy interest in understanding and reducing health inequalities across social groups characterized by their socioeconomic position, race or ethnicity, gender, sexual orientation, disability status, and geographic location. Many countries now have explicit public health goals related to reducing or even eliminating social inequalities in health. Reliable measurement of progress toward such goals, if it is to be of value in policymaking, requires a framework for conceptualizing and measuring inequalities in health. As Amartya Sen (Sen 2002, p. 60) has argued, "The central step, then, is the specification of the space in which equality is to be sought, and the equitable accounting rules that may be followed in arriving at aggregative concerns as well as distributive ones."

Despite an emerging consensus on the moral and public health importance of addressing health inequalities, there appears to be a lack of consensus about how health inequalities should be defined and how they should be measured (Carter-Pokras and Baquet 2002; Oliver et al. 2002). Others have written about the importance of distinguishing between health inequality and health inequity (Braveman and Gruskin 2003; Murray et al. 1999; Whitehead 1992), and such discussion is crucial for clarifying the purpose of health inequality initiatives. In this chapter we focus on reviewing ways of measuring health inequalities—that is, observable differences in health among individuals of different social groups. We also show, however, that measures of inequality may inherently reflect, to a greater or lesser extent, different ethical and value judgments about what aspects of health inequality are important to capture, such as how much value to give to health improvements among the poor compared with rich or whether inequalities should be measured on an absolute or relative scale. So at the outset, it is worthwhile to note that any choice of health inequality statistic implicitly or explicitly reflects a choice over what is important to measure. There is a range of inequality statistics that have more or less desirable properties (depending on the value position held), and so different measures can give qualitatively and quantitatively different assessments of the direction, size, and trend in health inequality. There is thus no "correct" way to measure health inequality.

There have been some notable past (Mackenbach and Kunst 1997; Wagstaff et al. 1991) and contemporary efforts (Kakwani et al. 1997; Regidor 2004a, 2004b; Wagstaff and Van Doorslaer 2004) to review methods for measuring health inequalities, but despite the clarity and utility of these presentations, many of the recommended methods have yet to find widespread application in social inequalities research. In addition, most of the methods laid out in the cited reviews deal with summary measurement of socioeconomic inequalities in health. There has been less attention to issues involving summary measurement of health inequalities across social groups that have no inherent ordering, such as race or ethnicity or geographic areas. It is also interesting to note in this regard that, although the majority of the empirical work in the health inequalities field is done by epidemiologists, we could not find a description of methods for measuring health inequality in any general texts on epidemiology (Rothman and Greenland 1998; Szklo and Nieto 2000), social epidemiology (Berkman and Kawachi 2000), or in a recent volume on methods for monitoring population health (Brookmeyer and Stroup 2004). A book on epidemiologic methods for health policy, however, devotes a number of pages to the issue of health inequality measurement (Spasoff 1999, pp. 95–103).

The basic premise of this chapter is that the measurement strategies applied to health inequalities have implications for setting policy goals and understanding the extent of progress toward the reduction of health inequalities. It is therefore important to understand the advantages and disadvantages of different methods for measuring health inequalities and how the measures chosen reflect ethical conceptualizations and concerns about what constitutes health inequality and which aspects of inequality we are trying to capture. This chapter does not address the important and fundamental question of how we should measure the social position of individuals, a question dealt with in detail elsewhere in this volume. The methods described here presume a theoretically and scientifically defensible choice of social group indicators to characterize individuals, which is no easy task. The purpose of this chapter is to give an overview of the various metrics for expressing health differences between individuals and social groups—their strengths and weaknesses, assumptions, and utility for the purpose of measuring health inequalities and monitoring health inequality trends.

Issues

Choosing a measure (or measures) of health inequality necessarily involves the consideration of a number of important conceptual, pragmatic, and technical issues. Various measures of inequality differ in how they incorporate the issues outlined in this section.

Total Inequality versus Social Group Inequality

What is the quantity we want to measure when we measure health inequalities? The fundamental distinction here is between measuring total inequality, or total variation in health, and measuring inequality between social groups. The former involves measuring the univariate distribution of health across all individuals in a population without regard to their group membership, whereas the latter involves measuring health differences between individuals from certain *a priori* chosen social groups. The World Health Organization (WHO) initiative to measure health inequality has advocated for an approach to the measurement of health inequality as total health inequality among individuals that is blind to social groups, at least as an initial measure (Gakidou et al. 2000; Murray et al. 1999). This may seem at odds with our notion of why we are measuring health inequality in the first place (Braveman et al. 2000). It was the persistent presence of social group differences in health that led to the current initiatives to reduce or eliminate health inequalities, not a concern for a widening overall distribution of health among individuals. But a deeper understanding of the overall task of measuring variation in population health requires an appreciation of the concept of total health inequality. It is likely that the amount of health inequality between social groups that we often seek to measure is relatively small compared with the total inequality that exists between individuals in a population.

Figure 6.1 shows the average body mass index (BMI) for five education groups in the 1997 U.S. National Health Interview Survey (NHIS). It is clear that there is a gradient of decreasing BMI with increasing education when we compare average BMI across education groups; however, the plots of the 10th through the 90th percentiles of BMI in each education group show that there is far greater variation in BMI *within* education groups than *between* them. Thus, basing our measure of health inequality on between-group average differences will not capture very much of the total health inequality among individuals. This is not in itself problematic, but it

FIGURE 6.1.   MEAN AND 10TH–90TH PERCENTILES OF BODY MASS INDEX BY EDUCATION, 1997 U.S. NATIONAL HEALTH INTERVIEW SURVEY.

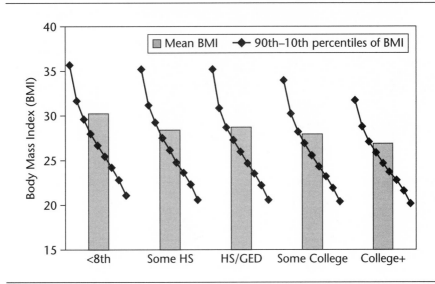

should be understood, and it the reason indicators of total health inequality can be informative. Thus, based on the group averages and a desire to reduce obesity in the population, focusing a health intervention on the "high risk" social group (those with less than an eighth-grade education) will, in practice, only target a very small proportion of those at high risk, because high-risk individuals exist in every educational group. Nevertheless, measures of total health inequality may mask substantial social group inequalities (Asada and Hedemann 2002), and there is no necessary relationship between the extent of total inequality and the extent of between-social-group inequality. Thus far, the evidence seems to indicate that total inequality and social-group inequality measure different aspects of population health. Two cross-national studies found little correspondence between measures of total inequality and measures of socioeconomic inequality for either child (Braveman et al. 2001) or adult (Houweling et al. 2001) mortality.

Absolute Inequalities

The most frequent method of communicating information about social inequalities in public health and epidemiology today is in relative terms—through measures

FIGURE 6.2.   ABSOLUTE AND RELATIVE RACIAL INEQUALITY IN INFANT MORTALITY (THREE-YEAR MOVING AVERAGES), U.S. 1900–2000.

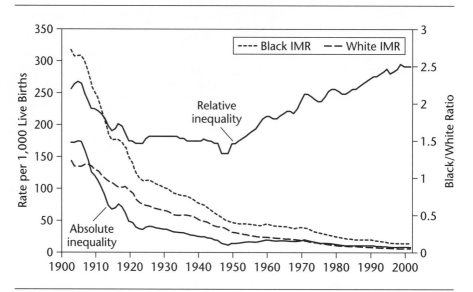

of association such as the relative risk. In epidemiology, relative risks are the most common measures of "effect size" partly because they have some advantageous properties not shared by absolute risk differences (Rothman and Greenland 1998; Walter 2000). Relative and absolute health differences between social groups are the primary language of health inequalities, but they often give different information, especially when monitoring changes over time. Figure 6.2 shows trends in absolute and relative inequality between U.S. blacks and whites in infant mortality over the past hundred years. Clearly there has been enormous progress in reducing infant mortality rates among both groups. But as the rates for both groups declined, absolute inequality between blacks and whites declined steadily while the ratio of black-to-white mortality (that is, the relative inequality) steadily increased. This chart illustrates the possibility that one might arrive at different conclusions about trends in this health inequality depending on which measure—the absolute or relative inequality—or time period is selected. Both absolute and relative inequality declined in the early part of the century; absolute inequality declined, and relative inequality remained about the same from around 1920 to 1950, and they have moved in opposite directions since mid-century.

Reference Groups

The language of inequality—defined literally as "difference"—implies a comparison group (that is, different from what?). Thus, a major question in choosing inequality measures is the choice of comparison group. Different definitions of inequality often imply different comparison groups, and thus the answer one would get about the extent and patterning of inequality may differ depending on the groups compared. Figure 6.3 shows the simplest situation for U.S. cervical cancer incidence rates among several race and ethnic groups. Hispanic women clearly have the highest incidence of cervical cancer, but how large is the inequality in cervical cancer incidence? The answer depends on the choice of the reference group. If Hispanic inequality is measured relative to the general population (that is, the total population rate) then the relative inequality is 1.75. If we focus on inequality in regard to the majority population—non-Hispanic whites—the relative inequality is 2.21. Or, if we choose the rate in the best-off group (American Indian and Alaska Natives) as the reference group, we obtain a relative inequality of 2.43.

FIGURE 6.3.   RELATIVE RISK (RR) OF INCIDENT CERVICAL CANCER (1996–2000) AMONG HISPANICS ACCORDING TO VARYING REFERENCE GROUPS.

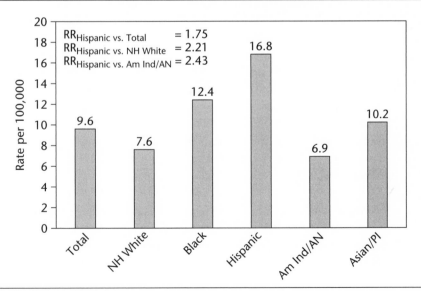

$RR_{Hispanic\ vs.\ Total} = 1.75$
$RR_{Hispanic\ vs.\ NH\ White} = 2.21$
$RR_{Hispanic\ vs.\ Am\ Ind/AN} = 2.43$

Source: Ries et al. 2003.

There is no "correct" reference group, but several choices are possible, and it is perhaps most important to make the rationale for the choice of referent clear.

Average Population Member. One logical reference group might be the population average, where the inequality measure reflects the gap between the health of different social groups and the population average. Although one potential disadvantage of using the population average is the fact that it changes over time, it is an intuitive and often explicit norm used when discussing health inequalities.

Best-Off Group or Rate. One might also measure inequality as a difference between each social group compared with the healthiest group. This is similar to Amartya Sen's concept of shortfalls (Sen 1992), where it is implicitly assumed that every social group in the society has the potential to achieve the health of the best-off group. One potential problem with this approach is when the "best-off" group is a small proportion of the population rates in that group can be unstable, so that wide swings in inequality could be recorded that are simply due to the instability of the rate in the comparison group (Keppel 2004).

All Those Better Off. It is also possible to measure inequalities by comparison with all those individuals or groups better off than a particular group or person. This may seem similar to the "best-off group" reference point, but it differs in a subtle way that may best be illustrated with an example. Figure 6.4 shows cancer incidence from 1996 to 2000 by race and ethnicity for two different cancers, kidney (renal pelvis) and myeloma. In both cases there is a substantial difference between the group with the highest incidence rate, blacks, and the group with the lowest or "best" rate, Asian and Pacific Islanders; however, when we look at the incidence rates of other groups, we see two different situations. In the case of kidney cancer, Hispanics and whites have rates more similar to blacks, whereas in the case of myeloma, they have rates more similar to Asian and Pacific Islanders. Relative to all of those better off than blacks, most people might judge the inequality to be greater in the case of myeloma compared with kidney cancer; yet, if measured relative to the "best-off" group, we would not be able to capture this nuance.

Fixed (Target) Rate. The prior three reference groups are inherently relative as they change over time, which may make assessments of trends in inequalities inconclusive if using pairwise comparisons. One advantage of a fixed or target rate is that the reference level does not change over time unless a new target is adopted.

FIGURE 6.4.   AGE-ADJUSTED INCIDENCE OF KIDNEY/RENAL PELVIS CANCER AND MYELOMA BY RACE AND ETHNICITY, 1996–2000.

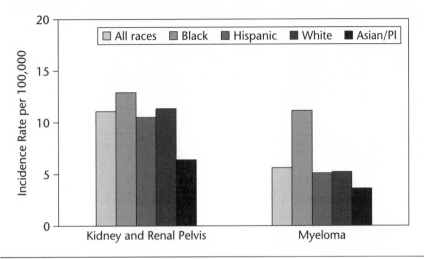

Source: SEER Cancer Statistics Review, 1975–2000.

Social Groups and "Natural" Ordering

We are often concerned with health inequalities across different normative social groups. For example, the U.S. *Healthy People 2010* initiative mandates eliminating health inequalities within categories of a number of different types of social groupings: gender, income and education, disability, geographic location, sexual orientation, and race and ethnicity. Such groups capture important normative dimensions of U.S. society but also differ in ways that may have implications for monitoring health inequalities. The social groups that measure dimensions of socioeconomic position (for example, education and income) have an inherent ordering *regardless of the health status of their members.* Individuals with less than a high school education unambiguously have less formal education than do individuals with a college degree. The same cannot be said for the other social groups targeted by the *Healthy People 2010* initiative. There is simply no inherent way to rank individuals by their race, ethnicity, geographic area, disability status, or sexual orientation. This has implications for measuring health inequality, because some inequality measures cannot be used to measure health inequality among unordered social groups.

Number of Social Groups

Many empirical studies measure health inequality by comparing the extreme groups (for example, the lowest income group compared with the highest), despite the fact that this ignores the health status of other groups. But it is worth asking whether the measure of inequality should include information from all social groups (that is, the entire population), especially when the two groups at the extreme ends of the social distribution may only reflect the health of a small fraction of the total population. For example, in 2000, there was a four-fold relative difference in deaths rates from ischemic heart disease across the U.S.; however, the states with the lowest (Alaska, 65 per 100,000) and the highest (Rhode Island, 255 per 100,000) rates collectively accounted for only 0.6 percent of the U.S. population in that year. Eliminating this inequality would have little impact on reducing the population burden of heart disease mortality, because only a fraction of deaths occurred in these two states. Additionally, although there are good reasons for focusing attention on specific comparisons, such as the inequality between blacks and whites in the receipt of treatment for cancers of similar stage (Bach et al. 1999), such pairwise comparisons do not quantify the inequality across *all* race or ethnic groups, which is precisely the goal of initiatives to reduce or eliminate health inequalities. For example, the gap between white and black men in the recent use of fecal occult blood test (FOBT) screening for colorectal cancer narrowed between 1987 and 1998 (Breen et al. 2001); however, this pairwise comparison conceals the fact that the gap between Hispanics and whites and between Hispanics and blacks increased (see Figure 6.5). Despite the utility of measuring inequalities between two groups, pairwise comparisons may conceal important heterogeneity and thus provide a limited view in monitoring progress toward eliminating health inequalities across the entire range of social group category.

Population Size

Should the inequality measure incorporate the size of the groups being compared? If we use a pairwise comparison of extreme groups, should it matter that one or both of those groups comprise a very small proportion of the population? Although this may seem relatively non-controversial, it has important implications for monitoring inequalities and is another case where a statistical choice reflects an ethical choice. That is, the decision of whether to account for the population size of social groups is implicitly a decision of how much weight to give individuals within each social group (Firebaugh 2003). For example, if we measure the inequality in mortality among American states in 2000 without weighting states by their population size, California and Wyoming receive equal weight despite the

FIGURE 6.5.   PROPORTION OF MEN REPORTING RECENT USE OF SCREENING FECAL OCCULT BLOOD TESTS (FOBT), BY RACE AND ETHNICITY, 1987–98.

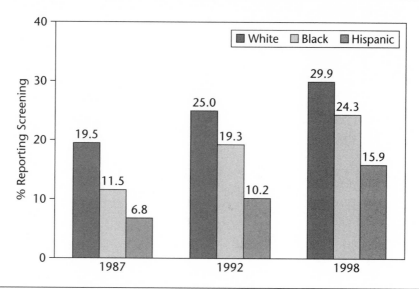

Source: Breen et al., *J Natl Cancer Inst* 2001; 93:1704–1713.

fact that California has nearly 70 times as many people as Wyoming. Thus in an unweighted analysis of the states, *individuals* in California receive approximately one-seventieth the weight of individuals in Wyoming. It is important to ask whether we want this unequal weighting of individuals reflected in our inequality measure.

Another difficulty in using unweighted measures of health inequality is their inability to incorporate the demographic changes that inevitably occur over time. For example, Figure 6.6 shows the percentage increase in population sub-groups between the 1980 and 2000 Census (Hobbs and Stoops 2002). These demographic shifts potentially have enormous impact on the population's health and should be factored into our assessment of health inequality. For a measure of health inequality to allow for an unambiguous comparison across time, it should be sensitive to changes in the distribution of social groups over time.

This sensitivity to changes in the proportion of people exposed to disadvantageous social positions is especially important when one thinks about the so-called "upstream" determinants of health inequalities. It is commonplace in health inequality research to discuss how distal social policy affects health and health

**FIGURE 6.6.   PERCENT CHANGE IN POPULATION SIZE BY RACE
AND HISPANIC ORIGIN: 1980–2000.**

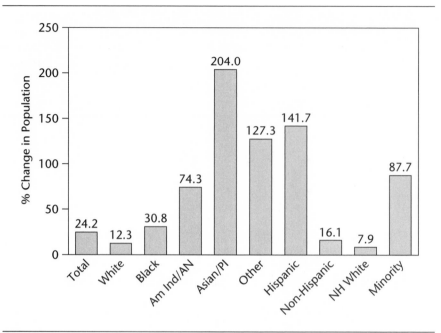

Source: Hobbs, F., Stoops, N., *Demographic Trends of the Twentieth Century,* 2002.

inequality. The policies and programs that define the nature of stratification in a society create educational opportunity, allocate income, and affect the types of jobs that are available. When these "upstream" social policy factors affect the nature of social stratification, for instance, by reducing the number of minimally educated individuals and thus reducing the number of individuals exposed to that form of social disadvantage, then measures of health inequality should account for that change. The same situation exists when the proportion of a particular population sub-group changes over time, as in the case of migration of Hispanics and Asians or Pacific Islanders shown in Figure 6.6.

Socioeconomic Dimension

Another potential criterion for a measure of health inequality, first articulated by Adam Wagstaff et al. (1991), is whether the measure is able to capture the direction of health gradients associated with ordered social group categories such as socioeconomic position. By health gradients, we mean a situation where a measure of health status either increases or decreases with increasing socioeconomic position. For instance, if at one time (or for one health outcome) health status increases across a particular social group ordering and at another time (or for another health outcome) health decreases with the same social group ordering, it would be advantageous if the inequality measure reflected this difference. Of necessity, this criterion is only applicable for measuring inequality between social groups that have an inherent ranking. The lack of an inherent ordering among race or ethnic groups, for example, means that the "socioeconomic dimension" criterion cannot be applied to inequality measures used to monitor race or ethnic or geographic health inequalities.

Distributional Sensitivity

One of the major reasons for the increasing focus on health inequalities is not simply that some individuals are healthy whereas others are sick. It is that some *kinds* of individuals or the members of some social groups are healthy whereas other kinds are sick. It is the normative distinction between the kinds of healthy or unhealthy individuals that drives our concern. For instance, we may be particularly concerned about ill-health in some socially disadvantaged groups (for example, the homeless or the unemployed) more than in others (Sen 2002; Wagstaff 2002). Not all inequality measures are able to reflect this ethical position. Similarly, all else being equal, if we would prefer a 10-percent improvement among those with the worst health rather than the same improvement among those with average health, then it would be advantageous if our measure of inequality could reflect this.

Measures

This section reviews many of the statistics that are available to measure health inequalities. Our goal is to provide the method of calculation and a brief statistical interpretation. It is important to note that there are methods to calculate indicators of precision (for example, 95 percent confidence interval) for all the measures reviewed here. These can be found in the source publications detailed in the references. Although issues of variability and precision are important, they are not germane to the choice of inequality measure, because they ultimately derive from the precision of the underlying rates and proportions that are used to generate a particular inequality measure.

Measures of Total Inequality

A measure of "total inequality" in health is a summary index of health differences across a population of individuals. Generally, measures of total inequality do not account for social grouping and have been chiefly used by health economists (for example, Gakidou et al. 2000; Illsley and Le Grand 1986). They are an important first step in understanding the scope of health variation in a population and have some advantageous properties for monitoring trends, particularly for cross-country comparisons where social groups may not be comparable. They do not, however, inform us about systematic variation in health among population sub-groups, which is inherent in many health inequality initiatives (Braveman et al. 2000, 2001; Houweling et al. 2001; Navarro 2001). Additionally, empirical investigations using measures of total inequality thus far appear difficult to interpret (Houweling et al. 2001; Wagstaff and Van Doorslaer 2004; Wolfson and Rowe 2001). Those endorsing this measure often cite as their primary justification the normative choices that must be made to measure health differences between social groups and note that the absence of such *a priori* choices makes inequality between individuals a more "objective" measure of health inequality (Murray et al. 1999). Whereas most health inequality initiatives specifically call for monitoring inequality among social groups, we explicate measures of total group inequality because they are prominent in the overall framework of efforts to monitor global health inequality and because they provide an essential context for understanding the "decomposition" of health inequality measures described later.

Individual-Mean Differences. Individual-mean difference (IMD) measures of health inequality sum-up the difference between the health of every individual in the population and the population average. The general formula for the class of individual-mean difference measures is given by Gakidou et al. (2000) as:

$$IMD(\alpha, \beta) = \frac{\sum_{i=1}^{n}|y_i - \mu|^{\alpha}}{n\mu^{\beta}} \tag{1}$$

where an individual i's health is y_i, μ is the mean health of the population, and n is the number of individuals in the population. The parameters α and β specify, respectively, the significance attached to health differences at the ends of the distribution relative to the mean and whether the individual-mean difference is absolute or relative to the mean health of the population. Larger values of α emphasize greater deviations from the mean, and larger values of β emphasize relative inequality because of heavier weighting of the mean. Those familiar with basic statistics will note that when $\alpha = 2$ and $\beta = 0$, the IMD is the variance and when $\alpha = 2$ and $\beta = 1$, the IMD is the coefficient of variation (Gakidou et al. 2000).

Inter-Individual Differences. The inter-individual differences (IID) measures health differences between all individuals in the population and is consistent with the Gini coefficient (defined later in this chapter) but may be weighted in accordance with differential aversion to inequality. These measures are different from the IMD class because they compare every individual in the population with every other individual in the population, whereas the IMD measures inequality relative to the population average. The class of inter-individual difference measures is (Gakidou et al. 2000):

$$IID(\alpha, \beta) = \frac{\sum_{i=1}^{n}\sum_{j=1}^{n}|y_i - y_j|^{\alpha}}{2n^2\mu^{\beta}} \qquad (2)$$

where y_i is individual i's health, y_j is individual j's health, μ is the mean health of the population, and n is the number of individuals in the population. The parameters α and β are defined as for the IMD above, and it is worth noting that when $\alpha = 2$ and $\beta = 1$, the IID is equal to the more well-known Gini coefficient. Gakidou and King (2002) have used this inequality measure (with $\alpha = 3$ and $\beta = 1$) in a comparative study of total inequality in child survival among fifty countries. Weighting $\alpha = 3$ implies that the measure should be more sensitive to larger rather than smaller pairwise deviations between individuals and thus reflects additional concern about larger health differences between individuals.

Measures of Social Group Inequality

The measures of total variation described in the preceding section have a number of merits, including their ability to make unambiguous health inequality comparisons between populations at a single time point and longitudinally. The ethical goals of many health inequality initiatives, however, are explicitly goals related to social group differences in health. It is an open question as to whether measures of total inequality and social group inequality are "better" or "worse" inequality measures, but the concern among many health policymakers is specifically expressed in terms of social group differences in health.

Pairwise Comparisons. Simple comparisons of some health indicator between two groups in a population (so-called pairwise comparisons) are one of the most straightforward ways to measure progress toward eliminating inequalities between them. For example, age-adjusted incidence rates of lung cancer for U.S. black and white females in 1973 were, respectively, 23.6 and 20.4 per 100,000. By 1999 rates for both groups had increased, to 57 for blacks and 52.3 for whites (Ries et al. 2002). It would seem easy enough to answer the question: did black-white inequality grow from 1973 to 1999? The answer, however, depends on the measure of inequality. If the inequality measure is the absolute difference between the black and white rates, then we would conclude that the black-white inequality increased from 3.2 to 4.7; however, if our inequality measure is the relative difference between the black and white rates (that is, black rate ÷ white rate), we would conclude the opposite, because the relative inequality decreased from 1.16 to 1.09. Both answers are correct. This has been a source of continuing confusion and sometimes unresolved debate in the health inequalities literature (Ebrahim 2002; Mackenbach et al. 1997; Oliver et al. 2002; Vågerö and Erikson 1997) and, whereas most of the empirical work in health inequalities has been in terms of "relative inequality," it should always be kept in mind that large relative differences can mask small differences in absolute terms.

Regression-Based Measures. One drawback of the pairwise comparison measures of inequality is that when a social group has more than two subgroups (as most do), information on the other groups is ignored. Normally it is desirable to use as much of the information present in the data as possible. One possible solution would be to calculate a series of $(j - 1)$ pairwise comparisons for j groups with one group as the reference point or j pairwise comparisons with an external reference point. The major difficulty with this strategy is that as the number of groups or time periods increases, attempting to evaluate the inequality trend may become complicated in terms of summarizing many pairwise comparisons. To overcome this limitation and to make use of the information for all groups, one might consider calculating a summary measure of inequality; however, this choice undoubtedly involves additional complexity and assumptions that must be traded off against the insights about inequality gleaned from the use of a summary measure (Mackenbach and Kunst 1997).

Slope Index of Inequality. If one is willing to assume that the relationship between social group and health status is linear (that is, that each step up an inherently ordered social group scale results in an equivalent health gain or loss), then one potential way to include information on all of the groups is to calculate a summary measure of inequality using regression. Although regression-based methods work well for calculating a summary measure of health inequality at a single point in time, it is likely that over time the distribution of the population in various social groups change, and it would be advantageous for a measure of health inequality to be sensitive to such changes. One measure that does so is the Slope Index of Inequality (SII). To calculate the SII, the social groups are first ordered from lowest (rank) to highest. The population of each social group category covers a range in the cumulative distribution of the population and is given a score based on the midpoint of its range in the cumulative distribution in the population. For example, in the 2001 U.S. NHIS, those with an income-to-poverty ratio of less than 0.5 (approximately $<$ \$9,000 for a family of four) were 3.45 percent of the population and those in the next highest income group—with an income-to-poverty ratio of 0.5 to 0.74—comprised 3.02 percent, in which case the lowest group is assigned a score of $(0 + [.0345 - 0]/2) = .0173$, whereas the next lowest group is assigned a score of $(.0345 + [.0647 - .0345]/2) = .0496$.

Health status is then plotted against this midpoint socioeconomic category variable, and a regression line is fit to the data. The SII thus uses the midpoint of the cumulative social group distribution and, because it is based on grouped data and is a *weighted* index, the weights are the share of the population in each social group. By weighting social groups by their population share, the SII thus is able to incorporate changes in the distribution of social groups over time that affect the population health burden of health inequalities. Figure 6.7 shows the observed data and predicted slope for the income-related inequality (based on income-to-poverty ratio) in current smoking for the United States in 2001. Note that the location of the data points on the *x*-axis is based on the group's share of the cumulative population, whereas the size of each point reflects each group's population share. Formally the

**FIGURE 6.7.   INCOME-BASED SLOPE INDEX OF INEQUALITY
IN CURRENT SMOKING, NHIS 2002.**

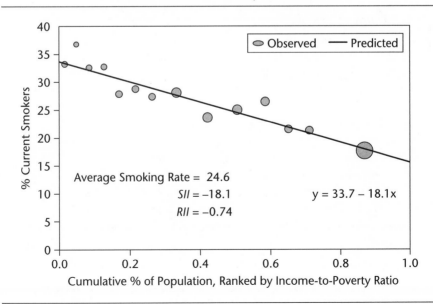

SII, which was introduced by Preston et al. (1981), may be obtained via regression of the mean health variable on the mean relative rank variable:

$$\bar{y}_j = \beta_0 + \beta_1 \bar{R}_j \qquad (3)$$

where j indexes social group, $\bar{y}_j$ is the average health status and $\bar{R}_j$ the average relative ranking of social group j, β_0 is the estimated health status of a hypothetical person at the bottom of the social group hierarchy (that is, a person whose relative rank R_j in the social group distribution is zero), and β_1 is the difference in average health status between the hypothetical person at the bottom of the social group distribution and the hypothetical person at the top (that is, $R_j = 0$ versus $R_j = 1$). Because the relative rank variable is based on the cumulative proportions of the population (from 0 to 1), a "one-unit" change in relative rank is equivalent to moving from the bottom to the top of the social group distribution. Because this regression is run on grouped data, it is estimated via *weighted* least squares, with the weights equal to the population size n_j of group j. The coefficient β_1 in equation 3 is the SII, which is interpreted as the absolute difference in health status between the bottom and top of the social group distribution. Thus, the regression equation in Figure 6.7 shows that the absolute difference in the prevalence of smoking across the entire distribution of income is -18.1 percentage points. The same regression may also be run on individual data, where R_i would be an individual's relative rank in the social group distribution. In this case the data would be self-weighting and could be estimated by ordinary least squares.

Relative Index of Inequality. The SII discussed in the previous section is a measure of absolute inequality; however, dividing this estimated slope by the mean population health gives a relative inequality measure, the Relative Index of Inequality (Pamuk 1988) or RII:

$$RII = SII/\mu = \beta_1/\mu \qquad (4)$$

where μ is mean population health and the SII is the estimate of β_1 from equation 3. Its interpretation is similar to the SII, but it now measures the proportionate (in regard to the average population level) rather than absolute increase or decrease in health between the highest and lowest socioeconomic group. In the income and smoking example seen in Figure 6.7, the RII is thus calculated as $-18.1/24.6 = -0.74$, indicating that a move from the bottom to the top of the income distribution is associated with a 74-percent decline in the prevalence of smoking. Kunst and Mackenbach (1995) modified this definition of the RII slightly by dividing the estimated health of the hypothetical person at the bottom of the social group distribution by the estimated health of the hypothetical person at the top of the social group distribution (that is, $\beta_0 \div [\beta_0 + \beta_1]$). Thus, the Kunst-Mackenbach

RII is more like a traditional relative risk in that it compares the health of the extremes of the social distribution, but it is estimated using the data on all social groups and is weighted by group size.

As we noted previously, the use of the SII and RII indices (as well as the Concentration Index discussed later in this chapter) depends on having a social group classification scheme that is hierarchical. This seems uncontroversial with respect to education and income, but social group classifications based on occupation may be somewhat more challenging because there is inherently more ambiguity in the ranking of occupations (Liberatos et al. 1988). In their international study of occupational mortality differences Kunst and Mackenbach (1994) note this difficulty as a possible explanation for the lack of consistency of their results with those of Wagstaff et al. (1991) for the size of inequality in Finland versus England and Wales.

Population Impact Measures

The Population Attributable Risk (PAR) and its relative analogue, the *PAR percent*, are epidemiologic measures of the population burden associated with differential health between groups. Although typically applied to groups defined by their exposure status (for example, comparing smokers with non-smokers), it may also be applied in the context of health differences between social groups. It is a summary of differences between each social group's health and the health of the best group. For example, it indicates the absolute (or relative) population health improvement that would be obtained if all educational groups had the health of the healthiest education group. The basic formulas for PAR and PAR percent as health inequality indicators (Kunst and Mackenbach 1995) are:

$$PAR = r_{pop} - r_{ref} \tag{5}$$

$$PAR\% = (r_{pop} - r_{ref})/r_{pop} \tag{6}$$

where r_{pop} is the rate in the total population and r_{ref} is the rate of health or disease in the reference group, typically the best-off social group. Although not immediately clear from the above formula, the PAR percent is in fact a population-weighted (by social group size) sum of the relative risks (RRs) for each group (Szklo and Nieto 2000) and may also be written as:

$$PAR\% = \frac{\sum p_j (RR_j - 1)}{\sum p_j (RR_j - 1) + 1} \tag{7}$$

where p_i is the group's population share and RR_i is the relative rate of group j compared with the reference group (to see this, note that we could substitute r_j/r_{ref} for RR_j and r_{ref}/r_{ref} for 1 in equation [7]). The PAR percent varies from 0 to 1 and is interpreted as the percent improvement in the health of the total population that would be achieved if all social groups had the rates of health in the best-off social group, an empirical expression of a common argument for reducing health inequalities. For example, Vicente Navarro argues that "the intervention that would add the most years to life to the populations of Spain or the USA . . . would be one that would lead to all social classes having the same mortality rates as those at the top." (Navarro 2001, p. 1701)

Index of Disparity

The Index of Disparity (ID_{isp}) summarizes the difference between several group rates and a reference rate and expresses the summed differences as a proportion of the reference rate. This measure was formally introduced by Pearcy and Keppel (2002) and is calculated as:

$$\left(\sum |r_j - r_{ref}|/\mathcal{J} \right) \Big/ r_{ref} \times 100, \tag{8}$$

where r_j indicates the measure of health status in the jth group, r_{ref} is the health status indicator in the reference population, and $\mathcal{J}$ is the number of groups compared. In principle any reference group may be chosen, but the authors recommend the best group rate as the comparison, because that represents the rate desirable for all groups to achieve.

Between-Group Variance

The variance is a commonly used statistic that summarizes all squared deviations from a population average. In the case of grouped data this is the Between-Group Variance (BGV), and it is calculated according to the following formula that squares the differences in group rates from the population average and weights by their population sizes:

$$BGV = \sum_{j=1}^{\mathcal{J}} p_j(y_j - \mu)^2, \tag{9}$$

where p_j is group j's population size, y_j is group j's average health status, and μ is the average health status of the population. The BGV may be a useful indicator of absolute inequality for unordered group data because it weights by population group size and is sensitive to the magnitude of larger deviations from the population average. As an example, Figure 6.8 shows trends in age-adjusted lung cancer mortality among U.S. Census divisions.

The between-region variance in lung cancer mortality in 1968 was 7.1 deaths per 100,000, but in 1998 the BGV was 22.8 deaths per 100,000. This larger

FIGURE 6.8. AGE-ADJUSTED LUNG CANCER MORTALITY BY U.S. DIVISION, 1968–1998.

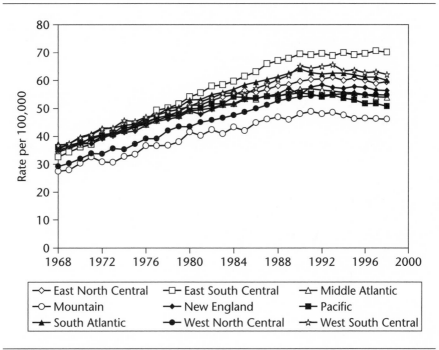

Source: NCHS. Compressed Mortality Files, 1968–1998. Data available from www.cdc.gov/nchs/products/elec_prods/subject/mcompres

absolute inequality in regional mortality indicates divergent regional trends in lung cancer over time (see Figure 6.8). The use of the variance as a measure of inequality in economics is sometimes discouraged because it is not "scale invariant" (Sen and Foster 1997). In other words, it is sensitive to absolute changes, as in the case where everyone's income doubles over time. In this case some economists feel that it is undesirable for the inequality measure to also double, because relative inequality is maintained. Although this may be an undesirable property when dealing with income inequality, we believe this is not necessarily a limitation for discussing health inequality where we may be interested in absolute inequality burdens. In addition, squaring the deviations from the mean gives additional weight to differences further from the mean (that is, changes in health among the groups furthest from the mean increase inequality to a greater extent than similar changes among those closer to the mean). So in this case, using the variance (where it squares the absolute deviations from the population average) is consistent with a particular value perspective (though it could reasonably be argued that squaring the deviations is arbitrary). In the previous example of changes in regional lung cancer inequality, the overall rates increase by 70 percent, the coefficient of variation (the variance divided by the mean) increases by 89 percent (indicating that relative inequality increases as well), but the BGV increases by 320 percent. Thus, choosing this as the measure of inequality reflects our concerns with widening absolute differences among the regions.

Measures of Average Disproportionality

When describing health inequalities, public health researchers and policy-makers often use what might be called the "language of disproportionality." For example, in the context of arguing for the importance of measuring health inequalities between socially meaningful population groups, Braveman et al. stated that "a disproportionate share of ill-health and premature mortality is borne by the socially disadvantaged" (p. 233). Terms such as "disproportionate share" and "unequal burden" are important qualifiers because they communicate the ethical notions inherent in collective concerns over health inequalities. That is, they capture the notion that it is unfair that some groups experience more ill-health than others; a just distribution of health implies that ill-health should be experienced proportionately by different social groups. A more explicit example can be found in the *Guidance for the U.S. National Health-care Inequalities Report* where, in discussing the inequality in cardiac catheterization rates between blacks and whites, LaVeist states that the "degree to which the predicted percentage of catheterization deviates from the observed percentage indicates the degree of inequality," and concludes that "African Americans received 67 percent of the catheterizations that they should have received, and whites received 14 percent more than their share" (LaVeist 2002, p. 90).

The preceding quote makes clear that health inequality is often equated with the concept of disproportionality. What is perhaps less clear is that in the context of the commonly used "language of disproportionality" there is usually an implied reference group, which is the general population (that is, the population average). In fact, in the catheterization example, LaVeist was explicitly arguing against measuring health inequality with a risk ratio or odds ratio, because doing so means using a particular social group (in this case, whites) as the reference group, which necessarily assumes that the rate in the reference group is most desirable. Thus, he argued that inequality measures that use whites as the reference group would not be able to identify their "over-utilization" of cardiac catheterization.

The intuitive ethical notion expressed in the preceding quotations is that the amount of ill-health in a disadvantaged social group is far greater than would be expected if ill-health were evenly distributed with respect to all social groups. An even distribution of ill-health across all social groups implies that the number of individuals of each social group with condition y is proportionate to that group's share of the total population. If this were the case, then the rate of ill-health in each group would be exactly the same and would necessarily equal the rate in the total population. Thus, the proportional distribution of condition y among J groups implies that $Y_j = \overline{Y}$ (the mean of y) for all groups.

This is an important point because many commonly used measures of income inequality and residential segregation, some of which are currently employed to measure health inequalities, may be conveniently expressed as measures of average disproportionality (Firebaugh 1999, 2003; Reardon and Firebaugh 2002). For each social group j, we can define a health (or ill-health) ratio as the ratio of measure y in the jth group to that of the mean of y for the whole population, so that $r_j = Y_j/\overline{Y}$ for each group. Note that this makes such measures relative rather than absolute inequality indicators. In this framework, measures of inequality take the general form

$$I = \sum_j p_j f(r_j), \tag{10}$$

where p_j is group j's proportion of the total population and $f(r_j)$ is some disproportionality function of the ratio $r_j = Y_j|\overline{Y}$. It should be clear that equation (10) is a population-weighted inequality measure, because each group's disproportionality function $f(r_j)$ is multiplied by its population share p_j. Thus, measures of this type of inequality indicator only differ because they implement different disproportionality functions. Perhaps one of the appealing features of such measures is that they provide a rather direct correspondence between the commonly-used language of health inequality in terms of "disproportionality" and the operationalization of the measurement.

Figure 6.9 shows a graphical depiction of the concept of "disproportionality" with data on all deaths in the United States, by gender and education, for the year 2000. Among males, those with less than twelve years of education bear a disproportionate burden of all deaths, as they account for 24 percent of all male deaths but only account for 12 percent of the male population. Conversely, males with greater than twelve years of education account for 55 percent of the total population, but only 32 percent of all deaths. The level of disproportionality for females with less than twelve years of education is slightly smaller.

Table 6.1 shows some commonly used statistical measures and their disproportionality functions. The table makes clear that the measures differ only in how they express the difference between shares of health and shares of population.

FIGURE 6.9.   GRAPHICAL EXAMPLE OF THE "DISPROPORTIONALITY" OF DEATHS AND POPULATION, BY GENDER AND EDUCATION, 2000.

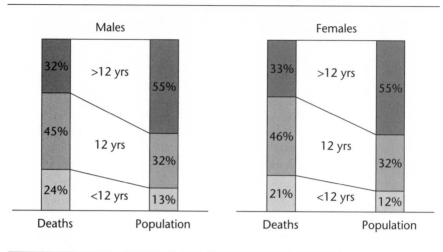

Source: Miniño et al. 2002.

TABLE 6.1.   COMMONLY USED DISPROPORTIONALITY FUNCTIONS.

Index Name	Disproportionality Function
Squared coefficient of variation (CV^2)	$(r_j - 1)^2$
Gini index (G)	Individual-level data: $\lvert r_i - r_j \rvert /2$
	Grouped data: $r_j(q_j - Q_j)$, where q_j is the proportion of the total population in groups less healthy than group j, and Q_j is the proportion of the total population in groups healthier than group j (i.e., $p_j + q_j + Q_j = 1$)
Relative concentration index (RCI)	Same as for G, but groups are ranked by social group position instead of by health, so that q_j is the proportion of the total population in groups less advantaged than group j, and Q_j is the proportion of the total population in groups more advantaged than group j (i.e., $p_j + q_j + Q_j = 1$)
Theil index (T)	$r_j \ln(r_j)$
Mean logarithmic deviation (MLD)	$\ln(1/r_j) = -\ln(r_j)$
Variance of log-health ($VarLog$)	$[\ln r_j - E(\ln r_j)]^2$

Note: Adapted from Firebaugh (2003).

Entropy Indices

One class of disproportionality measures that are popular among economists are measures of general entropy, developed by Henri Theil (1967). The following example is for measuring the inequality in body mass index (BMI). Theil's index is calculated (with grouped data) by summing the product of each group's BMI share of the population's total BMI and the natural log of each group's BMI share. Measures of entropy may also be used to measure total inequality, such that for individual-level data, total inequality in BMI measured by Theil's index can be written as

$$T = \sum_{i=1}^{N} p_i r_i \ln(r_i), \tag{11}$$

where p_i is an individual's population share (which in the case of individual data will be $1/n$, so that $\Sigma\, p_i = 1$) and r_i is the ratio of the individual's BMI to the population average BMI (that is, $r_i = y_i / \overline{Y}$); however, T can also be used to measure social group inequality. When the population of individuals is arranged into J groups, Theil showed that equation (11) is the exact sum of two parts: between-group inequality and a weighted average of within-group inequality:

$$T = \sum_{j=1}^{J} p_j r_j \ln(r_j) + \sum_{j=1}^{J} p_j r_j T_j, \tag{12}$$

where T_j is the inequality in BMI *within* group j. The within-group component (the second term on the right side of equation [12]) is weighted by group j's share of the total BMI, because $p_j \times r_j = y_j$ (where y_j is the *share* of total BMI) when the denominator for r_j is mean BMI for the total population. The ability of entropy-based measures of inequality to decompose total inequality into between-group and within-group components is referred to as additive decomposability (Sen and Foster 1997). More important, the previous decomposition example also makes it clear that it is possible to calculate between-group inequality in BMI—the primary quantity of interest with respect to social inequalities in health—in the absence of data on each individual. The only data needed are the group proportions and the ratio of the group's BMI to the population average BMI; however, between-group inequality may increase because total inequality is increasing (that is, both between-group and within-group inequality are increasing simultaneously). The primary advantage of using additively decomposable inequality measures is that it allows one to determine not just whether between-group inequality is increasing but whether the share of total inequality that is due to inequality between groups is increasing or decreasing. Although this measure has very attractive qualities, the between-group and within-group decomposition requires continuous outcome data measurable in individuals, so it is not clear whether this can be applied to many relevant non-continuous health outcomes (for example, incidence, mortality, or health behaviors). But even for non-continuous outcomes, entropy indices can easily be used to calculate between-group inequalities in the absence of individual-level data.

Measuring between-group inequality in BMI using equation (11) makes clear that changes in the value of inequality over time are a function of two quantities: changing group proportions (p_j) and changing social group BMI ratios (r_j). This is important because, in the case of obesity for example, differentiating between these two components of change has different public health implications for the obesity epidemic and may be the result of very different social policies. If we find that inequality is increasing but that the main reason for the observed change is that the share of the population among groups at the tails of the BMI distribution has increased, it simply demonstrates that the inequality increase is primarily due to the movement into and out-of different social groups—not to differentially increasing rates of BMI within subgroups of a social group. If we find, however, that population shares have remained relatively constant over time but BMI inequality has increased because BMI ratios are increasing, this implicates differential sources of BMI change among particular groups—which may then become the target of public health intervention.

Atkinson's Measure

Atkinson's index actually is not a single index of inequality but depends on specifying the relative sensitivity of the index to different parts of the distribution. One way of writing Atkinson's index is:

$$A = 1 - \left[\sum_{j=1}^{J} p_j r_j^{1-\varepsilon} \right]^{1/[1-\varepsilon]}, \quad \varepsilon > 0, \tag{13}$$

where p_j and r_j are again, respectively, the share of population and the health ratio (relative to the total population rate) as defined previously. Clearly, when one uses this index, the extent of inequality hinges on specifying the parameter ε, which indicates the degree of aversion to inequality. Larger values of ε indicate stronger aversion to inequality, which may also be interpreted as placing increased weight on the least healthy groups. For example, if we are particularly concerned about improving the health of least-healthy individuals we could make the measure of inequality more sensitive to changes in the bottom of the health distribution.

Gini Coefficient

The Gini summarizes social group differences in, for example, BMI for the entire population and can be thought of as a measure of association between each social group's share of population, ranked by their health, and their share of health. Its formula for individual data is given earlier in this chapter for the IID in equation (2)

FIGURE 6.10. GRAPHICAL REPRESENTATION OF THE GINI COEFFICIENT OF HEALTH INEQUALITY.

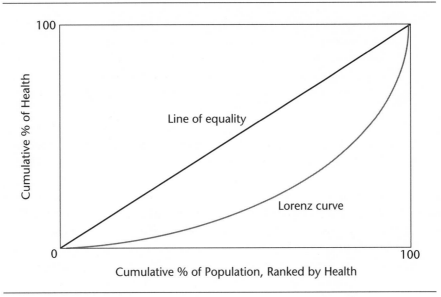

when $\alpha = 2$ and $\beta = 1$. The formula for grouped data can be obtained by applying the general formula for measures of disproportionality in equation (10) and substituting the disproportionality function for the Gini using grouped data in Table 6.1. Formally, the Gini coefficient is the ratio of the area between the line of equality in Figure 6.10 and the Lorenz curve to the total area of the triangle beneath the line of equality (Sen and Foster 1997). Because the Gini coefficient is a function of the disproportionality between shares of population and shares of health, one can see from Figure 6.10 that health inequality increases as the Lorenz curve moves further away from the line of equality (that is, as the disproportionality between shares of population and shares of health increases).

Concentration Index

The Concentration Index is another measure of economic inequality that has been adapted to measure health inequality (Kakwani et al. 1997). It is calculated similarly to the Gini index, but it results from a bivariate distribution of health and social group ranking. In the same way that the Gini coefficient is derived from the Lorenz curve, the Concentration Index is similarly derived from a Health Concentration curve, where the population is first ordered by social group status (rather than by health status, as for the Gini) and the cumulative percent of the population is then plotted against their share of total ill-health. When the y-axis is the share of ill-health, this results in the Relative Concentration Index (RCI); however, an Absolute Concentration Index (ACI) may also be derived by plotting the cumulative share of the population against the cumulative amount of ill-health (that is, the cumulative contribution of each subgroup to the mean level of health in the population). Figure 6.11 shows relative and absolute concentration curves for current smoking among U.S. females of different education groups in 1965 and 2003.

Note the similarity between the relative Concentration curve on the top in Figure 6.11 and the Lorenz curve drawn in Figure 6.10 to illustrate the Gini coefficient. The two curves, and thus, the Gini coefficient and the RCI are calculated similarly, the only difference being the ordering of the social groups. In the case of the Gini, the social groups are ordered by their health status (lowest to highest), regardless of their social group ranking, whereas for the RCI the social groups are ordered by their ranking in terms of years of education, regardless of their health status. It is important to note that, because the RCI incorporates information on *both* health and social group status, the Concentration curve may lie either above or below the line of equality. Thus, the top graph of Figure 6.11 shows that in 1965 smoking was disproportionately concentrated among those with higher education but in 2003 smoking was concentrated among those with less education. The general formula for the RCI for grouped data is given by Kakwani et al. (1997) as:

$$RCI = \frac{2}{\mu} \left[\sum_{j=1}^{J} p_j \mu_j R_j \right] - 1 \tag{14}$$

where p_j is the group's population share, μ_j is the group's mean health, and R_j is the relative rank of the jth socioeconomic group, which is defined as:

$$R_j = \sum_{j=1}^{J} p_\gamma - \frac{1}{2} p_j \tag{15}$$

where p_γ is the cumulative share of the population up to and including group j and p_j is the share of the population in group j; R_j indicates the cumulative share of the population up to the midpoint of each group interval, as in the categorization of the Slope and Relative Indexes of Inequality previously mentioned. In fact, the RCI has a specific mathematical relationship with the RII:

$$RCI = 2 \, \text{var}(R) RII, \tag{16}$$

where R is the relative rank variable identified in equation (15). Thus, the SII/RII and the ACI/RCI will produce the same rank ordering of health inequality over

FIGURE 6.11.   RELATIVE AND ABSOLUTE HEALTH CONCENTRATION CURVES FOR CURRENT SMOKING AMONG FEMALE EDUCATION GROUPS, 1965 AND 2003.

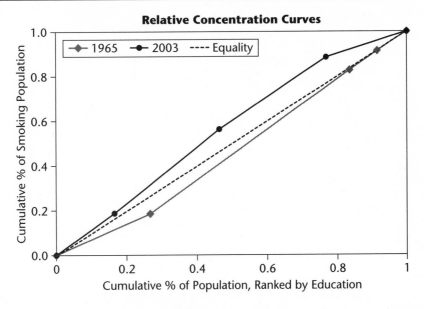

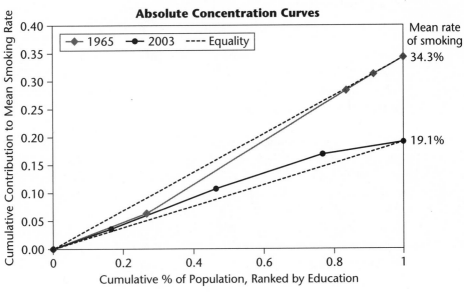

Source: Authors' calculation of the 1965 and 2003 NHIS.

TABLE 6.2.   EDUCATIONAL INEQUALITY IN CURRENT SMOKING AMONG FEMALES, 1965 AND 2003.

Education	Smoking Prevalence	Population Share	Relative Rank	RCI
1965				
<12 years	23.8%	0.267	0.133	0.008
12 years	38.7%	0.568	0.551	0.121
13–15 years	37.1%	0.079	0.875	0.026
16+ years	35.0%	0.086	0.957	0.029
Total	34.3%	1.0		0.184
		Relative Concentration Index →		**0.074**
		Absolute Concentration Index →		**0.025**
2003				
<12 years	21.7%	0.165	0.083	0.003
12 years	24.0%	0.299	0.315	0.023
13–15 years	20.2%	0.304	0.616	0.038
16+ years	9.5%	0.232	0.884	0.020
Total	19.1%	1.0		0.083
		Relative Concentration Index →		**−0.132**
		Absolute Concentration Index →		**−0.025**

Note: Authors' calculations of the 1965 and 2003 NHIS.

time but will differ in scale. The absolute version of the concentration index (ACI) is calculated by multiplying the RCI by the mean rate of the health variable:

$$ACI = \mu RCI, \tag{17}$$

where μ is the mean level of health in the population. Table 6.2 shows a simple example of how the RCI and ACI are calculated using equations (14) and (17) with grouped data using rates of current smoking in 1965 and 2003 among education groups for U.S. females.

One of the advantages of the Concentration Index is that it "reflects the socioeconomic dimension to inequalities in health" (Wagstaff et al. 1991, p. 548). That is, a downward health gradient (such that health worsens with increasing social group rank) results in a positive RCI, whereas an upward health gradient results in a negative RCI. For example, the data in Table 6.2 show that in 1965, when rates of smoking tended to be higher among the better-educated women, the RCI was 0.074, whereas in 2003, when rates of smoking were highest among the less educated, the RCI was −0.132. This sensitivity to the direction of the health gradient is not a property of other disproportionality measures like the Gini coefficient and the Index of Dissimilarity, because they do not depend on the strict ordering of social groups.

This is undoubtedly a particular advantage of the Concentration Index, but as with all inequality measures, it may also be seen as a disadvantage. Because of its sensitivity to *gradients* in health, the Concentration Index may not register any inequality when health is not ranked directly by social group. So when a social group ranked in the middle of a hierarchy bears a disproportionate burden of ill-health, the index may well register minimal inequality. This is not just a theoretical limitation for the RCI. For instance, age-adjusted rates of breast cancer death (per 100,000) in the United States in 1998 were 20.0 among those with less than a high school education, 28.4 among those with a high school education, and 22.0 among those with at least some college education (United States Department of Health and Human Services 2000). If the respective shares of the population in each of the education groups were approximately 38.8 percent, 20 percent, and 41.2 percent, the RCI would be virtually 0, indicating no educational mortality inequality, yet those with a high school education will contribute roughly 40.3 percent of breast cancer deaths. A reasonable case could be made that a disproportionate burden of breast cancer falls on the high school-educated (using this categorization of education), but the RCI would not reveal this pattern. And this pattern of the worst health among those in the middle social group is not simply an artifact of breast cancer as an unusual cause-of-death. This pattern is also seen for colorectal, prostate, and melanoma mortality as well.

We use the breast cancer example not necessarily to suggest that the Concentration Index is a poor index for measuring social group inequalities in health but rather to emphasize that all inequality measures have advantages and disadvantages that one should consider when selecting and interpreting an inequality index, and no summary inequality measure should be used as a substitute for detailed inspection of the health status indicators for each social group via tables and graphs.

Recommendations

Monitoring progress toward the elimination of inequalities in health involves a number of ethical, conceptual, and methodological issues that must be given careful consideration in order to answer the question of which measure or measures we should employ to monitor progress toward the elimination of health inequalities between social groups. One possibly useful way to approach the measurement of health inequality is to consider a sequence of methodological steps.

First, closely inspect the underlying subgroup specific health outcomes (rate or prevalence, and so forth), either via tabular or graphical inspection. This is likely to reveal important population health patterns, highlight the situation of specific sub-groups of interest, and lend an understanding of any underlying heterogeneity that a summary measure of health inequality may not emphasize.

Next, consider the relevant question that is to be answered. If one is interested in the health inequality between two particular groups, for example the trend in the inequality between black and white males in lung cancer mortality, then the use of a pairwise comparison of absolute and relative trends is all that is needed.

If one is interested in monitoring the health inequality trend across the entire range of subgroups within a social group category, for example across all education groups rather than a comparison of, say, the least and most educated groups— or if the social group category has many subgroups, such as the fifty U.S. states—then summary measures of health inequality are warranted. The first decision involved in choosing a summary measure is dictated by whether or not the social group in question has a natural ordering.

Ordered Social Groups

If the social group does have a natural ordering, as with education and income groups, then we recommend using the Absolute Concentration Index (ACI) or the Slope Index of Inequality (SII) as a measure of absolute health inequality and the Relative Concentration Index (RCI) or the Relative Index of Inequality (RII) as a measure of relative inequality. The major reasons for choosing these particular measures are that they: account for changes in the underlying population distributions in the social groups over time and use information across the entire range of social groups; are flexible enough to allow for incorporating different levels of aversion to inequality; and are sensitive to the direction of the social gradient in health.

Whereas this last criterion is what mainly distinguishes these measures from other summary measures of inequality, such as the Gini coefficient or the Index of Dissimilarity, we would also reemphasize that if the social groups in the middle of the distribution (for example, those with a high school education as opposed to those with less or more education) experience a disproportionate burden of ill-health, our selected measures may indicate no inequality exists when in fact it could be argued otherwise. But of course, if the sequence laid out in the previous paragraphs is adhered to, then a simple and careful inspection of the basic sub-group data should reveal this.

This is part of the "cost" of using summary measures of inequality, but in this case a comparison of the RCI or RII with another measure of disproportionality that is not strictly sensitive to health gradients, like the Gini coefficient or Theil index, may reveal important information about the social distribution of health. Lastly, because the ACI and RCI are mathematically related to the SII/RII, they will always result in the same rank ordering of health distributions. That being said, one additional desirable feature of the ACI/RCI is the ability to graph its associated health concentration curve, which may aid in interpretation for policy makers. Although the ability of any summary measure of health inequality to communicate important information about inequality trends to health policymakers may be limited, the ACI/RCI may serve this purpose better than the SII/RII.

Unordered Social Groups

Our recommendations for health inequality measures for ordered groups restate the recommendations of earlier reviews of health inequality measures (Kunst and Mackenbach 1995; Wagstaff et al. 1991). Groups with a natural ordering, however, represent only a small number of the social groups across which we want to eliminate health inequalities. Therefore, we need also to think about inequality measures that can be applied to unordered social groups, such as race and ethnicity or geography. Again, we would emphasize choosing a summary measure of health inequality only when one is interested in monitoring the extent of inequality across more than two or three social groups. For comparisons of two specific groups there is no substitute for simple pairwise measures of absolute and relative inequality.

If comparisons across multiple unordered groups are needed, then we recommend the between-group variance (BGV) as a summary of absolute inequality and the general entropy class of measures developed by Henri Theil as summary measures of relative inequality (more specifically, the Theil index and the Mean Log Deviation). An important reason for choosing the between-group variance and the entropy-based measures is that they are inequality measures that can be perfectly decomposed into between-social group and within-social group components, given a continuous health outcome. This cannot be said for other measures, such as the Gini coefficient and Atkinson's measure (Cowell and Jenkins 1995; Shorrocks 1980). The ability of the variance and the entropy class of inequality measures to decompose inequality is important because it allows one to look at any number of cross-classified social groups, whether ordered or not. For example, race and income, or gender and education can be jointly examined to assess the trend in inequality between certain dimensions of society. In addition, the entropy-based measures can also be decomposed to investigate the relative effects of changing social group distributions versus changing health distributions. This is important because both of these aspects of the population are constantly changing over time. Understanding the relative impact of health changes versus compositional changes in social groups is important for understanding the prospects for intervening to eliminate health inequalities.

Conclusions

These recommendations for measures of health inequality derive from our consideration of a number of ethical, conceptual, and pragmatic issues. The measurement strategies we recommend reflect what we think are desirable characteristics of the statistics because of the way they capture important dimensions of health inequality. In doing so we have explicitly chosen to adopt a population health perspective toward monitoring health inequalities. Thus we recommend measures that emphasize: (1) the use of the total population as the reference group for measuring health inequality, (2) weighting social groups according to the number of individuals they represent, and (3) absolute as well as relative inequalities. In this way we can account for changing demographic structures over time and the population health burden of inequalities in health.

In this chapter we reviewed a number of existing measures of health inequality, and one might reasonably ask whether new measures of health inequality are needed. Although we would welcome additional research into new measures of health inequality, particularly with respect to measuring inequality among social groups with no inherent ranking, it seems unlikely that any single measure of inequality will be able to capture all of the dimensions of a concept so fraught with ambiguity (Temkin 1993). Perhaps more beneficial would be empirical comparisons of a range of existing measures of health inequality with an eye toward understanding the conditions under which the selected measures agree or disagree in practice. This would be particularly helpful for comparisons of health inequality across different social group categories, different health outcomes, and over time. Such research would likely reinforce the links between statistical measurement and ethical considerations, both of which are instrumental to reducing and ultimately eliminating social inequalities in health.

References

Asada, Y. & Hedemann, T. (2002). A problem with the individual approach in the WHO health inequality measurement. *International Journal of Equity Health* [serial online] [cited 2003], *1*, [5 p]. Available at http://www.equityhealthj.com/content/pdf/1475-9276-1-2.pdf

Bach, P. B., Cramer, L. D., Warren, J. L., & Begg, C. B. (1999). Racial differences in the treatment of early-stage lung cancer. *N Engl J Med, 341,* 1198–1205.

Berkman, L. F., & Kawachi, I. (2000). *Social epidemiology.* New York: Oxford University Press.

Braveman, P., & Gruskin, S. (2003). Defining equity in health. *Journal of Epidemiology and Community Health, 57,* 254–258.

Braveman, P., Krieger, N., Lynch, J. (2000). Health inequalities and social inequalities in health. *Bulletin of the World Health Organization, 78,* 232–234.

Braveman, P., Starfield, B., Geiger, H. J., & Murray, C.J.L. (2001). World health report 2000: How it removes equity from the agenda for public health monitoring and policy commentary: Comprehensive approaches are needed for full understanding. *BMJ, 323,* 678–681.

Breen, N., Wagener, D. K., Brown, M. L., Davis, W. W., & Ballard-Barbash, R. (2001). Progress in cancer screening over a decade: Results of cancer screening from the 1987, 1992, and 1998 national health interview surveys. *Journal of the National Cancer Institute, 93,* 1704–1713.

Brookmeyer, R., & Stroup, D. F. (Eds.). (2004). *Monitoring the health of populations.* New York: Oxford University Press.

Carter-Pokras, O., & Baquet, C. (2002). What is a "health disparity?" *Public Health Reports, 117,* 426–434.

Cowell, F. A., & Jenkins, S. P. (1995). How much inequality can we explain? A methodology and an application to the United States. *The Economic Journal, 105,* 421–430.

Ebrahim, S. (2002). Addressing health inequalities. *The Lancet, 360,* 1691.

Firebaugh, G. (1999). Empirics of world income inequality. *American Journal of Sociology, 104,* 1597–1630.

Firebaugh, G. (2003). *The new geography of global income inequality.* Cambridge, MA: Harvard University Press.

Gakidou, E., & King, G. (2002). Measuring total health inequality: Adding individual variation to group-level differences. *International Journal of Equity Health, 1,* 3.

Gakidou, E. E., Murray, C. J., & Frenk, J. (2000). Defining and measuring health inequality: An approach based on the distribution of health expectancy. *Bulletin of the World Health Organization, 78,* 42–54.

Hobbs, F., & Stoops, N. (2002). *Demographic trends in the 20th century. Census 2000 special reports, Series CENSR-4.* Washington, DC: United States Government Printing Office, United States Census Bureau.

Houweling, T.A.J., Kunst, A. E., & Mackenbach, J. P. (2001). World health report 2000: Inequality index and socioeconomic inequalities in mortality. *Lancet, 357,* 1671–1672.

Illsley, R., & Le Grand, J. (1986). The measurement of inequality in health. In A. Williams (Ed.), *Health and economics* (pp. 12–36). London: Macmillan Press.

Kakwani, N., Wagstaff, A., & Vandoorslaer, E. (1997). Socioeconomic inequalities in health: Measurement, computation, and statistical inference. *Journal of Econometrics, 77,* 87–103.

Keppel, K. G., Pearcy, J. N., & Klein, R. J. (2004). *Measuring progress in healthy people 2010* (Healthy People 2000 Statistical Notes, no. 25). Hyattsville, MD: National Center for Health Statistics.

Kunst, A. E., & Mackenbach, J. (1994). International variation in the size of mortality differences associated with occupational status. *International Journal of Epidemiology, 23,* 742–750.

Kunst, A. E., & Mackenbach, J. P. (1995). *Measuring socioeconomic inequalities in health.* Copenhagen: World Health Organization, Regional Office for Europe.

LaVeist, T. A. (2002). Measuring disparities in healtcare quality and utilization. In E. K. Swift (Ed.), *Guidance for the national healthcare disparities report* (pp. 75–98). Washington, DC: National Academy Press.

Liberatos, P., Link, B. G., & Kelsey, J. L. (1988). The measurement of social-class in epidemiology. *Epidemiologic Review, 10,* 87–121.

Mackenbach, J. P., & Kunst, A. E. (1997). Measuring the magnitude of socio-economic inequalities in health: An overview of available measures illustrated with two examples from Europe. *Social Sciences & Med, 44,* 757–771.

Mackenbach, J. P., Cavelaars, A. E. J. M., & Kunst, A. E. (1997). Socioeconomic inequalities in morbidity and mortality in Western Europe—reply. *The Lancet, 350,* 517–518.

Miniño, A. M., Arias, E., Kochanek, K. D., Murphy, S. L., & Smith, B. L. (2002). Deaths: Final data for 2000. *National vital statistics reports, 50,* 15, Hyattsville, MD: National Center for Health Statistics.

Murray, C. J., Gakidou, E. E., & Frenk, J. (1999). Health inequalities and social group differences: What should we measure? *Bulletin of the World Health Organization, 77,* 537–543.

Navarro, V. (2001). World health report 2000: Responses to Murray and Frenk. *The Lancet, 357,* 1701–1702.

Oliver, A., Healey, A., & Le Grand, J. (2002). Addressing health inequalities. *The Lancet, 360,* 565–567.

Pamuk, E. R. (1988). Social-class inequality in infant mortality in England and Wales from 1921 to 1980. *European Journal of Population, 4,* 1–21.

Pearcy, J. N., & Keppel, K. G. (2002). A summary measure of health disparity. *Public Health Report, 117,* 273–280.

Preston, S. H., Haines, M. R., & Pamuk, E. (1981). Effects of industrialization and urbanization on mortality in developed countries. In International Union for the Scientific Study of Population, *International population conference, Manila, 1981: Solicited papers* (Vol. 2. pp. 233–254). Liege, Belgium: Ordina Editions.

Reardon, S. F., & Firebaugh, G. (2002). Measures of multigroup segregation. *Sociological Methodology, 32,* 33–67.

Regidor, E. (2004a). Measures of health inequalities: Part 1. *Journal of Epidemiology and Community Health, 58,* 858–861.

Regidor, E. (2004b). Measures of health inequalities: Part 2. *Journal of Epidemiology and Community Health, 58,* 900–903.

Ries, L.A.G., Eisner, M. P., Kosary, C. L., et al. (Eds.). (2003). *SEER cancer statistics review, 1975–2000.* Bethesda, MD: National Cancer Institute. Available at: http://seer.cancer.gov/csr/1975_2000/

Rothman, K. J., & Greenland, S. (1998). *Modern Epidemiology,* (2nd ed.). Philadelphia: Lippencott-Raven Publishers.

Sen, A. (2002). Why health equity? *Health Economics, 11,* 659–666.

Sen, A. K. (1992). *Inequality reexamined.* Cambridge, MA: Harvard University Press.

Sen, A. K., & Foster, J. E. (1997). *On economic inequality* (Expanded ed.). Oxford: Clarendon Press.

Shorrocks, A. F. (1980). The class of additively decomposable inequality measures. *Econometrica, 48,* 613–626.

Spasoff, R. A. (1999). *Epidemiologic methods for health policy.* New York: Oxford University Press.

Szklo, M., & Nieto, F. J. (2000). *Epidemiology: Beyond the basics.* Gaithersburg, MD: Aspen.

Temkin, L. S. (1993). *Inequality.* New York: Oxford University Press.

Theil, H. (1967). *Economics and information theory.* Amsterdam: North-Holland.

United States Department of Health and Human Services. (2000). *Healthy people 2010: Understanding and improving health.* Washington, DC: United States Department of Health and Human Services.

Vågerö, D., & Erikson, R. (1997). Socioeconomic inequalities in morbidity and mortality in Western Europe. *The Lancet, 350,* 516.

Wagstaff, A. (2002). Inequality aversion, health inequalities and health achievement. *Journal of Health Economics, 21,* 627–641.

Wagstaff, A., & Van Doorslaer, E. (2004). Overall versus socioeconomic health inequality: A measurement framework and two empirical illustrations. *Health Economics, 13,* 297–301.

Wagstaff, A., Paci, P., & van Doorslaer, E. (1991). On the measurement of inequalities in health. *Social Sciences & Medicine, 33,* 545–557.

Walter, S. D. (2000). Choice of effect measure for epidemiological data. *Journal of Clinical Epidemiology, 53,* 931–939.

Whitehead, M. (1992). The concepts and principles of equity and health. *International Journal of Health Services, 22,* 429–445.

Wolfson, M., & Rowe, G. (2001). On measuring inequalities in health. *Bulletin of the World Health Organization, 79,* 553–560.

CHAPTER SEVEN

A CONCEPTUAL FRAMEWORK FOR MEASURING SEGREGATION AND ITS ASSOCIATION WITH POPULATION OUTCOMES

Sean F. Reardon

One of the central sets of questions in both epidemiological and sociological research concerns the patterns of association between where individuals live and their health and social outcomes. Interest in such "neighborhood effects" research has grown dramatically in recent decades, owing in part to theoretical and methodological advances that have helped illuminate the associations among neighborhood characteristics and individual outcomes. An important subset of such research is particularly concerned with whether aggregate differences in health and social outcomes among population subgroups (especially groups defined by race, ethnicity, or socioeconomic characteristics) are attributable to—or at least associated with—patterns of racial, ethnic, or socioeconomic residential segregation. In short, this research investigates whether racial, ethnic, and socioeconomic differences in health and social outcomes are due to the fact that different subgroups live in different social, physical, and institutional environments. More bluntly, it asks, "Does segregation contribute to racial or ethnic inequalities?"

To ask whether segregation is associated with subgroup differences in health or social outcomes requires first, a clear definition of what we mean by "segregation"; second, a strategy for measuring segregation; and third, a methodology for inferring descriptive and causal associations between measured segregation and patterns of subgroup differences. The chapter is organized into three sections, in which these three requirements are discussed in turn. The first section reviews definitions of "segregation," pointing out the different ways that the term is used and suggesting a general framework for conceptualizing segregation. The second section briefly reviews the methodological literature on the measurement of segregation, describing several of the most useful segregation measures. The third section discusses analytic strategies for estimating the association between segregation and individual and subgroup outcome patterns.

What is Segregation?

What does it mean to say a neighborhood or city is segregated? Consider the following three uses of the term "segregated":

> Chicago is a segregated city.
>
> Most black children live in segregated neighborhoods.
>
> Some housing projects were deliberately segregated.

In the first sentence, "segregated" is an adjective describing the uneven distribution of (racial) groups across the city. In this case, segregation is seen as a *characteristic of a region* and describes the extent to which population subgroups are (un)evenly distributed throughout that region. By this usage, a city with 90 percent black residents would not be segregated, so long as those black residents were evenly distributed throughout the city. Conversely, a city with equal proportions of white, black, and Latino residents but where each of the three groups occupied distinct areas of the city would be highly segregated.

In the second sentence, "segregated" is an adjective describing individual neighborhoods. In this case, segregation is a *characteristic of a local neighborhood* and is used essentially as shorthand to describe the (racial) composition of that particular neighborhood—so a neighborhood is segregated if it has a high proportion of minority residents. By this usage, a 90-percent black neighborhood might be described as highly segregated, even if all other neighborhoods in the city were also 90-percent black. This leads to a possible contradiction between the first and second uses of the term—a city where every neighborhood was 90-percent black would be completely unsegregated by the first definition, but each neighborhood would be highly segregated by the second definition. The contradiction occurs because the second usage describes local racial composition, whereas the first describes regional unevenness.

In the third sentence, "segregated" is a verb describing deliberate action on the part of some legislative, judicial, or administrative body to ensure that members of different (racial) groups live in different neighborhoods. In this case, the term "segregated" is used to indicate not only racial differences in housing patterns but also the presence of some active policy mechanism that produced these differences. In the case of legislative—explicit segregation policies, as with school segregation laws in the South prior to 1954—the use of "segregate" as an active verb is relatively transparent, because both the agent (state and local governments) and the mechanisms (Jim Crow segregation laws) are apparent. In the case of current housing patterns, however, the causes of racial unevenness in residential location are less clear. Thus, the use of "segregated" in this sense depends on some inference about the causes of residential patterns.

Although each of these three usages is meaningful within some contexts, this chapter will generally use the term "segregation" in only the first sense. By this definition, a region is segregated to the extent to which individuals of different groups live in different neighborhoods within the region. The term segregation does not apply to individual neighborhoods but only to larger regions. In describing individual neighborhoods, then, it will be more useful to describe the (racial or socioeconomic) *composition* of the neighborhood; the term is more precise and better disentangles local composition from regional demographics. Moreover, to say that a region is segregated in this sense is merely to describe the existing patterns of racial or socioeconomic residential patterns; no assumption about the cause of these patterns should be inferred.

Why Does Segregation Matter?

The conceptual distinctions among the uses of the term segregation arise, in part, because of different implicit theories about why and how segregation patterns might matter for health and social outcomes. To see this, consider why it might matter where people live.

In part, it matters where people live because residential location influences individuals' proximity to important resources and shapes the possibilities for intergroup contact. From a social inequality perspective, segregation matters because it may be—and generally is—related to the differential proximity of groups to important resources. Such resources may be both institutional (for example, schools, health clinics and hospitals, child care facilities, and labor markets and employment opportunities) and social (for example, access to social networks and other forms of social capital). In addition, segregation matters because it may be related to the differential proximity of groups to a variety of potential hazards, including environmental hazards (for example, poor air or water quality, substandard housing, exposure to lead) and social hazards such as exposure to crime and violence (Acevedo-Garcia 2001; Acevedo-Garcia et al. 2003; Downey 2003; Lopez 2002; Massey and Denton 1993; see for example, Wilson 1987).

From the social inequality perspective, it might not matter if different population groups were residentially separated from one another, so long as both groups had equal proximity to all social resources and hazards. In a society where all social goods (including institutional, social, and environmental resources) were evenly distributed throughout residential space, where one lived would be, in principle, unrelated to one's access to these social goods. In this case, segregation might not matter for health or social outcomes.

From a social interaction perspective, in contrast, segregation matters because it affects the potential for intergroup contact among members of different social groups. And if intergroup contact leads to better social relations among groups and if groups have, on average, different levels of social resources (wealth and access to social networks and social and cultural capital), then proximity to other groups would provide greater potential for the distribution of social resources through intergroup contact. From this perspective, segregation might matter even if institutional and environmental goods were evenly distributed throughout social space, because some social groups might have greater access to forms of capital that provide advantages for health and social outcomes.

Conceptual and Methodological Issues in the Measurement of Segregation

To measure the segregation of a region, several methodological and conceptual issues must be addressed. First, because segregation indicates the extent to which individuals of different groups live in different neighborhoods, we must clarify the meaning of "neighborhood"; to do this, we must make some determination about the proximity of residential locations to one another within a region. Second, we must decide on a conceptual definition of segregation—Massey and Denton (1988) describe five different *dimensions* of segregation, which they term *evenness*, *exposure*, *clustering*, *concentration*, and *centralization*; strategies for measuring segregation will depend on which of these aspects of segregation we are particularly interested in. Third, we must define the population dimension along which we wish to measure segregation—measuring segregation among two or more distinct, unordered groups requires a different set of measurement tools than does measuring segregation along some ordered or continuous dimension, such as educational attainment or family income. Moreover, even if we are interested in measuring segregation among some set of distinct, categorical groups (for example, race or ethnic groups), measuring segregation among more than two population subgroups requires different measures than if we are measuring segregation between only two groups.

Spatial and Aspatial Measures of Segregation

Segregation can be thought of as the extent to which individuals of different groups occupy or experience different social environments. A measure of segregation, then, implicitly requires that we define the social environment of each individual. Most traditional measures of segregation implicitly define an individual's social environment as equivalent to some organizational or areal unit (for example, a school or census tract), without regard for the patterning of these units in social space. Such measures—termed *aspatial* measures—typically treat all individuals in a given census tract, for example, as occupying the same social environment, the composition of which is independent of the makeup of nearby tracts.

Aspatial segregation measures have often been criticized in the residential segregation context for their failure to account for the spatial patterning of census tracts (Grannis 2002; Massey and Denton 1988; Morrill 1991; Wong 1993, 2002). In particular, aspatial measures are criticized for their sensitivity to the "checkerboard problem" (Morrill 1991; White 1983) and the "modifiable areal unit problem" (Openshaw and Taylor 1979; Wong 1997). Each of these can be seen as critiques of the definition of the social environment implicit in the traditional segregation measures.

The "checkerboard problem" stems from the fact that aspatial segregation measures ignore the spatial proximity of neighborhoods and focus instead only on the racial composition of neighborhoods. To visualize the problem, imagine a checkerboard where each square represents an exclusively black or exclusively white neighborhood (Figure 7.1). If all the black squares were moved to one side of the board and all white squares to the other, we would expect a measure of segregation to register this change as an increase in segregation, because not only would each neighborhood be racially homogeneous but most neighborhoods

FIGURE 7.1. THE CHECKERBOARD PROBLEM.

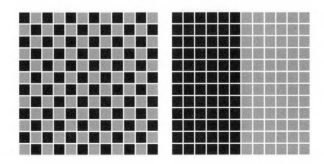

would now be surrounded by similarly homogeneous neighborhoods. Aspatial measures of segregation, however, do not distinguish between the first and second patterns, because in each case the racial compositions of individual neighborhoods are the same (White 1983).

The "modifiable areal unit problem" (MAUP) arises in residential segregation measurement because residential population data are typically collected, aggregated, and reported for spatial units (such as census tracts) that have no necessary correspondence with meaningful social or spatial divisions. This data collection scheme implicitly assumes that individuals living near one another (perhaps even across the street from one another) but in separate spatial units are more distant from one another than are two individuals living relatively far from one another but within the same spatial unit. As a result—unless spatial subarea boundaries correspond to meaningful social boundaries—all measures of spatial and aspatial segregation that rely on population counts aggregated within subareas are sensitive to the definitions of the boundaries of these spatial subareas. Figure 7.2 illustrates two aspects of the MAUP: aggregation effects, which result in differences in measured segregation if different-sized subareas are used to compute it; and zoning effects, which result in differences in measured segregation if the subarea boundaries are shifted, even if the number and size of the subareas remain fixed (Openshaw and Taylor 1979; Wong 1997, 1999).

In some cases it is possible to define organizational units (for example, schools) that meaningfully delimit social interactions and among which spatial proximity is irrelevant (that is, schools meaningfully bound students' "school environments"); in such cases, aspatial measures of segregation are perfectly appropriate. In other cases, as when measuring residential segregation, the checkerboard problem and MAUP pose conceptual difficulties to the measurement of segregation. Reardon and O'Sullivan (2004), however, argue that the "checkerboard problem"

FIGURE 7.2.   THE MODIFIABLE AREAL UNIT PROBLEM.

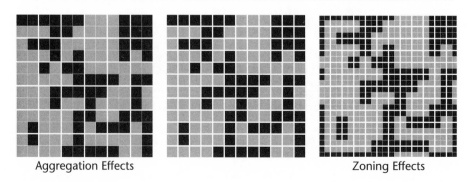

Aggregation Effects   Zoning Effects

and the MAUP are both measurement error artifacts resulting from a reliance on subarea (for example, tract) boundaries in the computation of segregation measurement. In principle, segregation measures that use information on the exact locations of individuals and their proximities to one another in residential space would eliminate the "checkerboard problem" and MAUP issues entirely from the measurement of residential segregation. Measures that explicitly account for the spatial patterning of residential locations—so-called *spatial* measures of segregation—are discussed later in this chapter.

The Dimensions of Segregation

The reliance on census tract or other administrative boundaries for the computation of segregation measures has led to some conceptual confusion in the segregation measurement literature. In an oft-cited article, Massey and Denton (1988) describe five conceptually distinct "dimensions" of residential segregation that they term *evenness, exposure, clustering, centralization,* and *concentration.* In their formulation, evenness and exposure are aspatial dimensions (because they ignore the spatial patterning of census tracts and so are subject to the checkerboard problem), whereas clustering, concentration, and centralization are explicitly spatial dimensions of segregation and require information on the locations and areas of census tracts to compute.

Reardon and O'Sullivan (2004), however, argue that, like the "checkerboard problem" and the MAUP, the distinction between aspatial "evenness" and spatial "clustering" is an artifact of the reliance on spatial subareas (for example, census tracts) at some chosen geographical scale of aggregation. Evenness, in Massey and Denton's formulation, refers to the degree to which members of different groups are overrepresented and underrepresented in different subareas relative to their overall proportions in the population. Clustering refers to the proximity of subareas with similar group proportions to one another; however, evenness at one level of aggregation (say, census tracts) is clearly strongly related to clustering at a lower level of aggregation (block groups), because tracts where a minority group is overrepresented will tend to be "clusters" of block groups where the minority population is overrepresented. Unless subarea boundaries correspond to meaningful social boundaries, the distinction between "evenness" and "clustering" is arbitrary.

As a result of this insight, Reardon and O'Sullivan (2004) suggest an alternative to the Massey and Denton (1988) dimensions of residential segregation, arguing instead for two primary conceptual dimensions to spatial residential segregation—a *spatial exposure-isolation dimension* and a *spatial evenness-clustering dimension.* The *spatial exposure-isolation dimension* indicates the extent that members of one group encounter members of another or their own group in their local spatial environments. The *spatial evenness-clustering dimension* indicates the extent to which groups are similarly distributed in residential space. Spatial exposure-isolation, like aspatial exposure, is a measure of the typical environment experienced by individuals; it depends in part on the overall racial composition of the population in the region under investigation. Spatial evenness-clustering, in contrast, is independent of the population composition. In this framework, Massey and Denton's evenness and clustering dimensions are collapsed into a single dimension. Their exposure dimension remains intact but is now conceptualized as explicitly spatial. Their centralization and concentration dimensions can be seen as specific subcategories of spatial evenness-clustering.

Measuring Segregation Among Different Population Dimensions

Because sociologists initially developed and used segregation indices primarily to study a particular set of social concerns—black or white school and residential segregation during the civil rights era from the 1950s through the 1970s and occupational sex segregation during the 1970s—most segregation indices are designed to measure segregation between two discrete population groups. But the world is not dichotomous, of course. Social classifications and such markers as race, ethnicity, religion, political affiliation, and occupation encompass multiple distinct categories. Moreover, as U.S. society becomes increasingly racially diverse, two-group measures of racial and ethnic segregation are increasingly inadequate for describing complex patterns of racial segregation and integration.

In addition, given the theoretical importance of income segregation and inequality in sociology, epidemiology, geography, economics, and public policy, measures of income segregation are particularly important. Unless household income is dichotomized, however, traditional categorical measures of segregation are not useful for describing segregation along an income dimension. Thus, in defining and measuring segregation, it is important to choose indices that appropriately measure segregation along the population dimension of interest.

Although most traditional measures of segregation measure between two discrete groups, some have been developed to measure segregation among multiple groups (Reardon and Firebaugh 2002) and along a continuous dimension, such as income (Jargowsky 1996; Jargowsky and Kim 2004). Such measures are described later in this chapter.

Measures of Residential Segregation

A large number of indices of residential segregation have been proposed, evaluated, and used in the social science research on segregation and its consequences. To the casual reader, the literature on segregation measurement offers a sometimes bewildering array of proposed indices and an equally extensive literature criticizing these indices (for reviews and evaluations of many such indices, see James and Taeuber 1985; Massey and Denton 1988; Reardon and Firebaugh 2002; Reardon and O'Sullivan 2004; Zoloth 1976). The following section briefly describes the most useful and most commonly-used (not always the same ones) segregation indices, with particular attention to the circumstances under which each might be used.

As noted earlier, in choosing a segregation index, several considerations are important. First, the choice of index will depend on the dimension of segregation to be measured (for example, exposure, evenness). Second, the choice of index will depend on the definition of the population dimension among which segregation is to be measured. This dimension may be defined by a binary variable (for example, white or nonwhite, male or female), a multigroup categorical variable (white or black or Hispanic or Asian or other), or a continuous variable (income).[1] Third, the choice of a measure will depend on a definition of subareas among which population groups are distributed (for example, census tracts, schools) and the extent to which it is important to account for the spatial or social proximity of these subareas to one another. The following section describes segregation measures used to measure exposure and evenness. Among those that measure evenness, the section describe two-group, multigroup, and continuous-variable measures of segregation. Finally, the measures that can take into account the spatial or social patterning of population distributions are described.

Notation

Throughout this chapter the following notation is used: consider a spatial region R populated by M mutually-exclusive population subgroups (for example, racial groups), indexed by m. Let p index points within the region R; and let r index subareas of the region R (for example, census tracts). Let τ denote population density and π denote population proportion. Thus we have

$$t_r \;\;= \text{population count of subarea } r$$

$$t_{rm} = \text{population count of group } m \text{ in subarea } r \text{ (note that } \textstyle\sum_m t_{rm} = t_r)$$

$$\tau_p \;\;= \text{population density at point } p$$

$$\tau_{pm} = \text{population density of group } m \text{ at point } p$$

$$T \;\;= \text{total population in } R \text{ (note that } \textstyle\sum_{r \in R} t_r = T \text{ and } \int_{p \in R} \tau_p \, dp = T)$$

$$\pi_m = \text{proportion in group } m \text{ of total population (for example, proportion black)}$$

$$\pi_{rm} = \text{proportion in group } m \text{ in subarea } r \text{ (defined as } \pi_{rm} = t_{rm}/r_r)$$

[1]One could also imagine wanting to measure segregation among a set of ordered population groups, such as those defined by educational attainment (those without a high school diploma, those with a high school diploma but without a college degree, those with a bachelor's degree but no advance degree, and those with an advanced degree), but no segregation measures have been developed to measure segregation among such ordered categorical groups.

In addition, a super-positioned tilde ($\sim$) indicates that a parameter describes the spatial environment of a given point rather than the point itself (for example, $\tilde{\pi}_{pm}$ denotes the proportion in group m in the local environment of point p).

Measures of "Exposure"

Exposure-based indices of segregation measure the average exposure of members of one group (group m) to another group (group n), where "exposure" is understood as the proportion of group n in the local environment of a member of group m. A region is highly segregated—from the exposure perspective—if members of group m, on average, inhabit local environments containing few members of group n. In the aspatial case, where each individual's local environment is defined by the subarea (for example, census tract) inhabited, the exposure index (Bell 1954; Lieberson and Carter 1982a, 1982b) for the exposure of group m to group n (denoted $_mP_n^*$) is formally defined as

$$_mP_n^* = \sum_{r \in R} \frac{t_{rm}}{T_m} \pi_m . \tag{1}$$

In concrete terms, $_mP_n^*$ is simply the average proportion of group n in the subareas of members of group m. Note that the P^* index is not symmetric—the exposure of group m to group n is not, in general, equal to the exposure of group n to group m.

More generally, exposure-based measures might be thought of as measuring the average exposure of a population (or subpopulation) to some environmental characteristic. If X_r measures some characteristic of a local environment r (air quality, percentage of low-income residents, toxic waste facilities, and so forth), then the average exposure of members of group m to X will be given by

$$_mP_X^* = \sum_{r \in R} \frac{t_{rm}}{T_m} X_r . \tag{2}$$

Equation (1) is simply a special case of equation (2), where the proportion of group n is the environmental characteristic of interest. In concrete terms, $_mP_X^*$ measures the average value of characteristic X across the subareas of members of group m.

Reardon and O'Sullivan (2004) suggest a spatial version of equation (2), the spatial exposure index, which indicates the average exposure of members of group m to some aspect X of their local environment (for details, see Reardon and O'Sullivan 2004):

$$_m\tilde{P}_X^* = \int_{p \in R} \frac{\tau_{pm}}{T_m} \tilde{X}_p \, dp. \tag{3}$$

Because an exposure index measures some characteristic of the average environment of a group, it is dependent on the overall prevalence of that characteristic in the region of interest. As the black proportion of the population grows, for example, then the exposure of whites to blacks may increase even if the spatial distribution of the black and white populations across a region remains the same.

Measures of "Evenness"

In contrast to exposure measures, "evenness" measures of segregation measure the extent to which population groups are evenly distributed (relative to one another or to some environmental characteristic) across a region. A region is highly segregated—from the evenness perspective—if members of group m are distributed very differently throughout a region than are members of group n. In this case, members of group m will inhabit local environments where group n is disproportionately underrepresented relative to its share of the regional population. Evenness measures, unlike exposure measures, are not sensitive to the overall proportions of groups in the population but rather measure the extent to which groups are differentially distributed throughout a region, regardless of their overall share of the population. Thus a region can, for example, exhibit high exposure of group m to n while also being characterized by perfect evenness—if group n makes up a large share of the population and groups m and n are identically distributed throughout the region.

There are a number of segregation measures designed to measure "evenness." Most commonly used is the dissimilarity index (denoted D), though D has been criticized for possessing a number of mathematical properties that are inconsistent with intuitive notions of segregation (James and Taeuber 1985; Reardon and Firebaugh 2002; Winship 1978). In particular, D does not appropriately register changes in the population distribution that should, in principle, change segregation levels—if, for example, a black family moves from a neighborhood that is disproportionately black to a less-black neighborhood, D does not necessarily indicate that the latter configuration of households is less segregated than the former.

Other useful measures of evenness are the information theory index (H), the Gini index (G), and the variance ratio index (V).[2] More detail on the definitions, interpretations, and properties of these indices can be found in James and

---

[2]The variance ratio index has gone by many names in the literature–the segregation index (S) (James 1986; Zoloth 1976), the correlation ratio (CR or $eta2$) (Duncan and Duncan 1955; Massey and Denton 1988; Stearns and Logan 1986), the proportional reduction in error (Grannis 1998), the revised index of isolation (Bell 1954), the adjusted group isolation index (White 1986), the gap-based measure of segregation (Clotfelter 1999), the normalized exposure index (Reardon and Yun 2002), $r(ij)$ (Coleman et al 1982), and the variance ratio index (V) (James and Taeuber 1985). These different names arise because the index can be derived and interpreted in a variety of ways. For simplicity's sake, the chapter follows James and Taeuber and refers to this index as the variance ratio index (V).

Taeuber (1985), Massey and Denton (1988), Reardon and Firebaugh (2002), White (1986), and Zoloth (1976).

The dissimilarity index. Formally, the dissimilarity index (Taeuber and Taeuber 1965) can be written

$$D = \sum_{r \in R} \frac{t_r |\pi_{rm} - \pi_m|}{2T\pi_m(1 - \pi_m)}, \tag{4}$$

The dissimilarity index can be interpreted as the percentage of all individuals who would have to transfer among units to equalize the group proportions across units divided by the percentage that would have to transfer if the system started in a state of complete segregation.

The Gini index. The Gini segregation index (James and Taeuber 1985) is

$$G = \sum_{r \in R} \sum_{s \in R} \frac{t_r t_s |\pi_{rm} - \pi_{sm}|}{2T^2\pi_m(1 - \pi_m)}, \tag{5}$$

where π_m, π_{rm}, and π_{sm} are the proportions of group m in the population and in subareas r and s, respectively (the index is symmetric with respect to the two groups, so it does not matter whether we use group m or n in the calculation). The Gini index can be interpreted as the sum of the weighted average absolute difference in group proportions between all possible pairs of subareas divided by the maximum possible value of this sum (obtained if the system were in a state of complete segregation). Note that the Gini segregation index is related to, but distinct from, the more familiar Gini index of inequality, which is a common measure of income inequality (see for example, Schwartz and Winship 1980). Like the dissimilarity index, the Gini index of segregation exhibits several undesirable properties (James and Taeuber 1985; Reardon and Firebaugh 2002), though perhaps the primary reason it has been less commonly used is that it is computationally more demanding to calculate than D and other indices.

The variance ratio index. The variance ratio index (James and Taeuber 1985) is defined as

$$V = \sum_{r \in R} \frac{t_r(\pi_{rm} - \pi_m)^2}{T\pi_m(1 - \pi_m)}, \tag{6}$$

where π_m and π_{rm} are the group m proportions in the total population and in subarea r, respectively (again, the index is symmetric with respect to groups m and n, so it does not matter which group is used in the calculation). The variance ratio index can be interpreted as the proportion of the variance in group membership that is accounted for by between-subarea differences in group proportions.[3]

The information theory index. The information theory index (also called the Theil index, after its originator) measures the variation in diversity across subareas, where the diversity of a population is defined as the entropy (E) of the population:

$$E = \sum_{m=1}^{M} \pi_m \ln \frac{1}{\pi_m}, \tag{7}$$

where there are $M \geqslant 2$ groups in the population.[4] The entropy takes on a value of 0 if and only if the population is made up of a single group and has its maximum if each of the M groups are equally represented in the population. The information theory index (Theil 1972; Theil and Finezza 1971) is then defined as

$$H = \sum_{r \in R} \frac{t_r(E - E_r)}{TE}, \tag{8}$$

where E_r is the entropy in subarea r. Note that H—unlike D, G, and V—is implicitly defined as a measure of segregation among multiple population groups, because the entropy is defined for any $M \geqslant 2$.

These are not the only measures of "evenness" that have been proposed and used in research on segregation, but they are the most commonly used. In each case, the index has a minimum value of 0—obtained if and only if each subarea has the same group composition—and a maximum value of 1—obtained if and only if each subarea is comprised of a single group.

Measures of Multigroup Segregation

The dichotomous indices of segregation that measure evenness (D, G, and V) each have multigroup analogs (Reardon and Firebaugh 2002), whereas H is implicitly

---

[3]Note that V can also be defined in terms of the ratio of the exposure of group m to group n to the proportion of group n in the population:

$$V = 1 - \frac{_mP_n^*}{\pi_n}$$

Thus, V can be interpreted as a "normalized" exposure index or as a measure of the relative gap between the actual exposure of group m to n and the exposure that would be experienced if the two groups were both evenly distributed through a region.

[4]Note that we define:

$$0 \cdot \ln(1/0) = \lim_{\pi \to 0}[\pi \cdot \ln(1/\pi)] = 0$$

Note also that E can be defined with logarithms to any base; we use the natural logarithm for simplicity here.

defined as a multigroup measure (Theil 1972; Theil and Finezza 1971). Each of these multigroup measures of evenness describes the extent to which $M \geq 2$ population groups are similarly distributed among subareas. Reardon and Firebaugh (2002) provide an extensive review of these multigroup indices and their mathematical properties, concluding that the information theory index (H) is the most flexible and conceptually appropriate multigroup measure of evenness.

The choice of whether to use a two-group or multigroup index of segregation depends on the specific question of interest. In a region where the population is composed of three groups (white non-Hispanic, black non-Hispanic, and Hispanic, for example), we may be interested in the segregation between two specific groups (for example, how segregated are white from black residents?); or we may be interested in the segregation among all three groups (for example, how segregated are white, black, and Hispanic residents from one another?). In the first case, any of the two-group indices would be appropriate; in the second case, a multigroup index is required.

Measures of Income Segregation

Segregation indices to measure income segregation (or, more generally, segregation along any continuous variable) have only recently been developed. The most useful measure of income segregation is the Neighborhood Sorting Index (NSI), which measures the proportion of income variation that lies between subareas (Jargowsky 1996, 1997). If X_i is a measure of income for person i, then the NSI is defined as

$$NSI = \sqrt{\frac{\sum_{r \in R} t_r (\overline{X}_r - \overline{\overline{X}})^2}{\sum_i (\overline{X}_i - \overline{\overline{X}})^2}},$$ (9)

where $\overline{X}_r$ is the mean income in subarea r and $\overline{\overline{X}}$ is the mean income in the region. The NSI can be interpreted as the ratio of the standard deviation of subarea mean incomes (weighted by subarea population) to the standard deviation of income in the regional population.

Measures of Spatial Segregation

All of the segregation indices described thus far are aspatial—meaning that they treat each census tract as an isolated neighborhood and do not account for the spatial patterning of tracts. Although such indices have been commonly used in many studies of residential segregation, they suffer from the checkerboard problem and MAUP issues, as previously described. A class of spatial racial and ethnic segregation indices developed in recent decades, however, is designed to better account for spatial patterns of residential locations (Frank 2003; Grannis 2002; see, for example, Morgan 1983a, 1983b; Morrill 1991; O'Sullivan and Wong 2004; Reardon and O'Sullivan 2004; White 1983; Wong 1993, 1998, 1999; Wu and Sui 2001). Although there are many such spatial indices, Reardon and O'Sullivan (2004) show that most fail to meet a set of criteria that ensure they adequately address MAUP issues and match theoretically meaningful conceptions of segregation.

One reason for relying on explicitly spatial measures of segregation is to reduce MAUP-induced measurement error. Measurement error is typically only a minor concern in cross-sectional analyses of segregation, as the error typically constitutes only a small portion of the variance in segregation levels across regions. In analyzing *changes* in segregation levels, however, measurement error is an important concern, because measurement error constitutes a greater portion of the variance of changes than of cross-sectional levels. This point is largely overlooked in research on changes in segregation, although it has important implications for research on the causes and consequences of segregation changes. Moreover, studying changes in segregation levels is more likely to reveal important relationships between segregation, social policy, and social outcomes—it enables researchers to understand how social policy affects patterns of residential change and helps to isolate the relationship between exogenous changes in segregation patterns and changes in average child and family outcomes as an effective way to determine if reducing segregation levels would improve children's and families' life chances. For both of these types of research questions, statistical models of change (for example, fixed-effects models) will provide less biased estimates of causal relationships among policies, segregation levels, and outcomes. Because spatial segregation measures are arguably less susceptible to MAUP-induced measurement error, they are preferred in such analyses, though they have been relatively little used in research on changes in segregation.

Reardon and O'Sullivan (2004) propose a conceptually straightforward and general approach to measuring two-group and multigroup segregation in a way that accounts for spatial patterns. They suggest that a segregation index should measure the extent to which the local environments of individuals differ in their racial or socioeconomic composition (or, more generally, in any population or environmental trait), where each individual inhabits a "local environment" whose population is made up of the spatially-weighted average of the populations (or other characteristics) at each point in the region of interest. Typically, the population at nearby locations will contribute more to the local environment of an individual than will more distant locations (a "distance-decay" effect). Given a particular spatial weighting function and data on the residential location of households, it is straightforward to compute the spatially-weighted racial (or socioeconomic) composition of the local environment of each location (or person) in the study region. Given this, spatial exposure is measured by computing the average composition of the local environments of members of each group. Spatial evenness is measured by examining how similar, on average, the racial (or socioeconomic) compositions of all individuals' local environments are to the overall composition of the study region. If each person's local environment is relatively similar in composition to the overall population, there is little spatial unevenness; conversely, if there is considerable deviation from the overall composition, there is high spatial segregation (unevenness).

For example, to compute a spatial version of the information theory index, Reardon and O'Sullivan first define the spatially-weighted entropy at each point p as

$$\widetilde{E}_p = -\sum_{m=1}^{M} (\widetilde{\pi}_{pm}) \log_M(\widetilde{\pi}_{pm}) \tag{10}$$

This is the entropy of the local environment of point p. It is analogous to the entropy of an individual tract, E_r, used in the computation of the aspatial segregation index H (if we define the local environment of p to be tract r, then $\widetilde{E}_p = E_r$), except that $\widetilde{E}_p$ may incorporate (proximity-weighted) information on the racial composition at all points in R, not just the racial composition of the tract where p is located. The spatial information theory segregation index, $\widetilde{H}$, is then defined as

$$\widetilde{H} = 1 - \frac{1}{TE} \int_{p \in R} \tau_p \widetilde{E}_p \, dp \tag{11}$$

where T is the total population and E is the overall regional entropy as in equation (8). The spatial information theory index $\widetilde{H}$ is the spatial analog to the usual information theory index H, a measure of how much less diverse, on average, individuals' local environments are than those of the total population of region R.

Jargowsky and Kim (2004) have recently proposed a spatial index of income segregation, based on the *NSI*. This index, the Generalized *NSI*, takes into account the spatial patterning of census tracts in measuring income segregation.

Choosing Appropriate Segregation Indices

In any given study, the choice of a segregation index depends on: (1) the dimension (exposure or evenness) of segregation of interest; (2) the population dimension of interest (which may be indicated by a binary variable, such as gender, a multigroup categorical variable, such as race, or a continuous variable, such as income); and (3) the extent to which it is important to account for the spatial proximity of locations. Table 7.1 summarizes the previously described indices with regard to these three aspects. In addition, Table 7.1 indicates whether each index is decomposable in two different ways (Reardon and Firebaugh 2002; Reardon and O'Sullivan 2004; Reardon et al. 2000). Here, organizational decomposability indicates that an index can be decomposed into components of

TABLE 7.1. PROPERTIES OF SEGREGATION MEASURES.

	P*	D	G	V	H	NSI
Dimension						
Exposure	✓					
Evenness		✓	✓	✓	✓	✓
Variable Types						
2-Group	✓	✓	✓	✓	✓	
Multigroup		✓	✓	✓	✓	
Continuous						✓
Spatial						
Aspatial	✓	✓	✓	✓	✓	✓
Spatial	✓	✓		✓	✓	✓
Decomposability						
Organizational	✓			✓	✓	✓
Grouping					✓	

segregation attributable to between- and within-subregion segregation (for example, into segregation between a city and suburbs and within cities and suburbs separately); grouping decomposability indicates that a multigroup index can be decomposed into components of segregation attributable to segregation between and within different clusters of population subgroups (for example, into segregation between white and minority families and segregation among different minority subgroups).

If a measure of exposure is required, then a version of the P^* exposure index must be used; both spatial and aspatial versions are available. There are more indices that measure evenness for two-group and multigroup population dimensions, each of which (except the Gini index) have both spatial and aspatial versions. Reardon and Firebaugh (2002) and Reardon and O'Sullivan (2004), however, note that the information theory index (H) and the variance ratio index (V) have more attractive mathematical properties than the others, in part because they are decomposable and in part because they register changes in segregation more appropriately in response to household mobility. Finally, if segregation is to be measured along some continuous population dimension—such as income—then the Neighborhood Sorting Index (NSI) is available in both spatial and aspatial versions.

Computing Segregation Indices

The formulae for computing aspatial segregation indices generally require summing (or double-summing, in the case of the Gini index) over all subareas in a region. Most software packages do not have built-in routines for computing these indices, though the formulae are relatively easily programmed and require only data on population subgroup counts for each tract or subarea.[5] The spatial measures of segregation, however, are more complicated to compute and typically require geographic information systems (GIS) software and data on the spatial patterning of census tracts.

The Association of Segregation with Population Outcomes

One of the primary reasons for measuring segregation is to assess the association between segregation patterns and group differences in some health or social outcome. In education, for example, we are interested in knowing whether racial segregation among schools is associated with racial achievement gaps. Likewise, in public health, we are interested in whether racial or socioeconomic segregation is associated with racial or socioeconomic differences in disease rates or mortality.

This final section gives a brief introduction to methods of assessing the association between segregation and health and social outcomes. The section begin by considering three simple models for the ways that segregation may be associated with some social outcome Y (for example, asthma). First, suppose that residents of neighborhoods with higher proportions of black residents have higher rates of asthma, regardless of their individual race (this might happen, for example, if air quality were negatively correlated with the proportion of black residents in a neighborhood and if air quality affects black and white residents similarly). Formally, this would imply that

$$Corr(Y_{ir}, \overline{G}_r) \,|\, G_{ir} \neq 0, \tag{12}$$

where G indicates racial group membership, and r indexes neighborhoods. In this first model, neighborhood racial composition is associated with asthma, resulting in an observed racial difference in asthma rates across a region, even if there is no difference in asthma rates between black and white residents living in the same neighborhoods.

A second model would suggest that the segregation level of a region might be associated with average outcomes of all groups within a region. It might not be farfetched to imagine that mortality rates are higher for all racial groups in more segregated cities, if segregation leads to increased stress, conflict, and violence among groups. If this were true, we would expect to observe

$$Corr(\overline{Y}_j, S_j) \neq 0, \tag{13}$$

---

[5]In the Stata statistical software package, the command *seg* (installed by typing "ssc install seg" from within Stata) will compute each of the aspatial measures of exposure and evenness described here (Reardon 2002; Stata Corporation 2003).

where j indexes regions and S_j is a measure of segregation in region j. In this model, segregation is associated with mean outcomes for all racial groups equally.

More likely, perhaps segregation is associated with unequal outcomes among segregated groups. Returning to the asthma example, if air quality were correlated with neighborhood racial composition, then we would expect to observe larger racial differences in asthma rates in more segregated regions, because the racial differences in average exposure to poor air quality will be larger in more segregated regions. Formally, if m and n indicate distinct groups in region j, we would expect to observe

$$Corr(\overline{Y}_{mj} - \overline{Y}_{nj}, S_j) \neq 0. \tag{14}$$

Such a model implicitly assumes that either group m or n tends to benefit more, on average, from segregation patterns.

Hypotheses of these types can be tested with regression techniques. Shown first are models with individual-level data that also show that one can estimate these with only group-specific aggregate data on an outcome Y. To test model 1, suppose one collects data on some outcome of interest for a sample of members of groups $G = 0$ and $G = 1$ in some region. One can estimate the average difference in outcomes between the groups by fitting the simple regression model

$$Y_i = \delta_0 + \delta_1 G_i + \varepsilon_i. \tag{15}$$

From this model, one obtains $\hat{\delta}_1$, an estimate of the difference in the average value of Y between the two groups. If we let r index neighborhoods (often operationalized as census tracts or blocks but not necessarily) and define $\overline{G}_r$ as the average value of G in neighborhood r (this will be the proportion of the population in neighborhood r who are members of the group indicated by G), we can then estimate the following regression model:

$$Y_{ri} = \beta_0 + \beta_1 G_{ri} + \beta_2 \overline{G}_r + \varepsilon_{ri}. \tag{16}$$

Fitting this model yields $\hat{\beta}_1$, an estimate of the within-neighborhood association between G and Y, and $\hat{\beta}_2$, an estimate of the between-neighborhood association between $\overline{G}$ and Y after controlling for individuals' group membership (β_2 is often termed the neighborhood compositional effect of group membership, though the term "effect" here should be understood as describing as association, not a causal process). Note that β_2 is the parameter of interest in model 1, as it describes the association between neighborhood racial composition and Y, holding individual race constant. A useful relationship between equations (15) and (16) is that

$$\delta_1 = \beta_1 + \beta_2 V, \tag{17}$$

where V is the variance ratio index segregation measure between the two groups defined by the dichotomous variable G (see equation 6). This result allows us to decompose the average difference in outcomes into a within-neighborhood component (β_1) and a between-neighborhood component (the product of the association between neighborhood composition and the outcome [β_2] and the level of segregation in the region [V]).

If the within-neighborhood effect is zero, this means that there is, on average, no difference in outcomes between members of different groups residing in the same neighborhoods, and so the total difference in outcomes between groups is associated with neighborhood segregation. If the between-neighborhood effect is zero, in contrast, then segregation cannot be responsible for the difference between groups (assuming the model specified is correct), regardless of how high segregation levels are. Conversely, if segregation levels are very low, then even a strong association between neighborhood composition and the outcome will not produce a large outcome gap.

Next consider models 2 and 3. In these models, we are interested in how segregation is associated with the observed outcomes (on some variable Y) of two groups (denoted by $G = 0$ and $G = 1$). If we have data on a number of regions (indexed by j) and we measure segregation with some segregation index S, we can write a multilevel linear model (Raudenbush and Bryk 2002) describing the association between Y, G, and S:

$$Y_{ij} = \beta_{0j} + \beta_{0j}(G_{ij} - \overline{G_j}) + \varepsilon_{ij}$$

where:

$$\beta_{0j} = \gamma_{00} + \gamma_{01}(S_j - \overline{S}) + u_{0j}$$
$$\beta_{1j} = \gamma_{10} + \gamma_{11}(S_j - \overline{S}) + u_{1j}. \tag{18}$$

In this model, γ_{00} indicates the average outcome Y in a region with an average level of segregation S; likewise, γ_{10} indicates the average within-region between-group difference in outcomes Y in a region with an average level of segregation S. The coefficient γ_{01} indicates the association between segregation levels and the average value of Y; the coefficient γ_{11} indicates the association between segregation levels and the within-region between-group difference in average values of Y.

Note that we do not need individual-level data to estimate this model. If we average equation (18) over all individuals within each region j, we obtain

$$\overline{Y}_j = \gamma_{00} + \gamma_{01}(S_j - \overline{S}) + u_{0j}. \tag{19}$$

We can estimate γ_{00} and γ_{01} directly from aggregated data on Y and measured levels of segregation S. The parameter γ_{01} is the parameter of interest in model 2, as it describes the association of regional segregation with Y for all individuals.

Likewise, if we average equation (18) over all individuals of groups $G = 1$ and $G = 0$ separately within each region j, we obtain

$$\overline{Y}_{1j} = \gamma_{00} + \gamma_{01}(S_j - \overline{S}) + (\gamma_{10} + \gamma_{11}(S_j - \overline{S}) + u_{1j})(1 - \overline{G_j}) + u_{0j} \tag{20}$$

and

$$\bar{Y}_{0j} = \gamma_{00} + \gamma_{01}(S_j - \bar{S}) - (\gamma_{10} + \gamma_{11}(S_j - \bar{S}) + u_{1j})\bar{G}_j + u_{0j}. \quad (21)$$

Subtracting (21) from (20), we obtain the between-group gap on Y in region j (denoted by (δ_{1j})):

$$\delta_{1j} = \bar{Y}_1 - \bar{Y}_{0j} \quad (22)$$
$$= \gamma_{10} + \gamma_{11}(S_j - \bar{S}) + u_{1j}$$

Thus, we can estimate γ_{10} and γ_{11} directly from the observed within-region average between-group differences in Y and measured levels of segregation S. In model 3, γ_{11} is the parameter of interest, as it describes the association between segregation and the size of the between-group difference in Y.

If segregation S is measured with the variance ratio index V, then from equations (22) and (17), we have

$$\delta_{1j} = \gamma_{10} + \gamma_{11}(V_j - \bar{V}) + u_{1j}$$
$$= [\gamma_{10} - \gamma_{11}\bar{V} + u_{1j}] + \gamma_{11}V_j. \quad (23)$$
$$= \beta_{1j} + \beta_{2j}V_j$$

This implies

$$\beta_{2j} = \gamma_{11}$$
$$\beta_{1j} = \gamma_{10} - \gamma_{11}\bar{V} + u_{1j}. \quad (24)$$
$$= \delta_{1j} - \gamma_{11}V_j$$

Thus, we can estimate β_{1j} and β_{2j} in equation (17) for each region j from aggregated data alone, so long as we have data from multiple regions (and we assume model [18] is correct). With only a measure of the between-group gap in Y for each region and the computed variance ratio index for each region, we can estimate the average within-neighborhood gap for each region and the association between neighborhood composition and Y, net of group membership.

Finally, note that we can add to any of these models a vector of variables representing mechanisms through which segregation may be related to the outcomes. In the asthma model, for example, we might add measures of air quality to equations (16) and (22); if the inclusion of this variable reduced the coefficient γ_{11} to 0, this would suggest that the association between segregation and asthma was explained by between-neighborhood differences in air quality. It is important to note, however, that the inclusion of potential mediator or confounder variables, or both, is not necessarily straightforward in contextual effect models, owing to selection mechanisms, endogeneity, and cross-level interactions (for more discussion of the complexities in making causal inferences from contextual effect models, see Morgenstern 1995; Oakes 2004).

Summary

In this chapter, three central issues involved in answering the question of whether segregation is associated with subgroup differences in health or social outcomes were addressed. Careful analyses of segregation and health and social outcomes require, first, a clear conceptualization of what is meant by "segregation." Theory and prior research are typically useful for determining which conceptual definition of segregation is most appropriate in a given context. Second, segregation research requires a measure or measures of segregation appropriate to the conceptual framework and hypothesized mechanisms. This chapter has briefly reviewed this literature; the interested researcher, however, should consult some of the articles cited here for further detail. Finally, the chapter described some simple statistical models for inferring descriptive associations between measured segregation and individual and subgroup outcome patterns. The models described in this section are intended as outlines only. In particular, models of the sort described here may be appropriate for estimating patterns of association between segregation and outcomes, but they do not necessarily produce unbiased estimates of *causal* associations between segregation and observed health and social outcomes. As in all statistical analyses, the old caveat applies: correlation does not imply causation. In fact, designing studies and analytic strategies for inferring the effects of segregation on health and social outcomes is an area of research where much work remains to be done, both methodologically and substantively. This is a rapidly developing field where social epidemiologists might make important contributions.

References

Acevedo-Garcia, D. (2001). Zip code-level risk factors for tuberculosis: Neighborhood environment and residential segregation in New Jersey, 1985–1992. *American Journal of Public Health, 91,* 734–741.

Acevedo-Garcia, D., Lochner, K. A., Osypuk, T. L., & Subramanian, S. V. (2003). Future directions in residential segregation and health research: A multilevel approach. *American Journal of Public Health, 93,* 215–220.

Bell, W. (1954). A probability model for the measurement of ecological segregation. *Social Forces, 43,* 357–364.

Clotfelter, C. T. (1999). Public school segregation in metropolitan areas. *Land Economics, 75,* 487–504.

Coleman, J., Hoffer, T., & Kilgore, S. (1982). Achievement and segregation in secondary schools: A further look at public and private school differences. *Sociology of Education, 55,* 162–182.

Downey, L. (2003). Spatial measurement, geography, and urban racial inequality. *Social Forces, 81,* 937–952.

Duncan, O. D., & Duncan, B. (1955). A methodological analysis of segregation indexes. *American Sociological Review, 20*(2), 210–217.

Frank, A. I. (2003). Using measures of spatial autocorrelation to describe socio-economic and racial residential patterns in U.S. urban areas. In D. Kidner, G. Higgs, & S. White (Eds.), *Socio-economic applications of geographic information science, Innovations in GIS* (pp. 147–162). London: Taylor & Francis.

Grannis, R. (1998). The importance of trivial streets: Residential streets and residential segregation. *American Journal of Sociology, 103*(6), 1530–1564.

Grannis, R. (2002). Discussion: Segregation indices and their functional inputs. *Sociological Methodology, 32*, 69–84.

James, D. R., & Taeuber, K. E. (1985). Measures of segregation. *Sociological Methodology, 14*, 1–32.

James, F. J. (1986). A new generalized "exposure-based" segregation index. *Sociological Methods and Research, 14*(3), 301–316.

Jargowsky, P. A. (1996). Take the money and run: Economic segregation in U.S. metropolitan areas. *American Sociological Review, 61*, 984–998.

Jargowsky, P. A. (1997). *Poverty and place: Ghettos, barrios, and the American city.* New York: Russell Sage Foundation.

Jargowsky, P. A., & Kim, J. (2004). *A measure of spatial segregation: The generalized Neighborhood Sorting Index.* Richardson: University of Texas at Dallas.

Lieberson, S., & Carter, D. K. (1982a). A model for inferring the voluntary and involuntary causes of residential segregation. *Demography, 19*, 511–526.

Lieberson, S., & Carter, D. K. (1982b). Temporal changes and urban differences in residential segregation: A reconsideration. *American Journal of Sociology, 88*, 296–310.

Lopez, R. (2002). Segregation and black-white differences in exposure to air toxics in 1990. *Environmental Health Perspectives, 110*, 289–295.

Massey, D. S., & Denton, N. A. (1988). The dimensions of residential segregation. *Social Forces, 67*, 281–315.

Massey, D. S., & Denton, N. A. (1993). *American apartheid: Segregation and the making of the underclass.* Cambridge, MA: Harvard University Press.

Morgan, B. S. (1983a). An alternate approach to the development of a distance-based measure of racial segregation. *American Journal of Sociology, 88*, 1237–1249.

Morgan, B. S. (1983b). A distance-decay interaction index to measure residential segregation. *Area, 15*, 211–216.

Morgenstern, H. (1995). Ecologic studies in epidemiology: Concepts, principles, and methods. *Annual Review of Public Health, 16*, 61–81.

Morrill, R. L. (1991). On the measure of spatial segregation. *Geography Research Forum, 11*, 25–36.

O'Sullivan, D., & Wong, D. W. S. (2004). *A density surface-based approach to measuring spatial segregation.* Paper presented at the Annual Meeting of the Association of American Geographers, Philadelphia, PA (March 14–19).

Oakes, J. M. (2004). The (mis)estimation of neighborhood effects: Causal inference for a practicable social epidemiology. *Social Science & Medicine, 58*, 1929–1952.

Openshaw, S., & Taylor, P. (1979). A million or so correlation coefficients: Three experiments on the modifiable area unit problem. In N. Wrigley (Ed.), *Statistical applications in the spatial sciences* (pp. 127–144). London: Pion.

Raudenbush, S. W., & Bryk, A. S. (2002). *Hierarchical linear models: Applications and data analysis methods.* Thousand Oaks, CA: Sage Publications.

Reardon, S. F. (2002). SEG: Stata module for computing multiple-group diversity and segregation indices. Available at http://ideas.repec.org/c/boc/bocode/s375001.html.

Reardon, S. F., & Firebaugh, G. (2002). Measures of multi-group segregation. *Sociological Methodology, 32,* 33–67.

Reardon, S. F., & O'Sullivan D. (2004). Measures of spatial segregation. *Sociological Methodology, 34,* 121–162.

Reardon, S. F., & Yun, J. T. (2002). *Private school racial enrollments and segregation.* Cambridge, MA: Civil Rights Project, Harvard University.

Reardon, S. F., Yun, J. T., & Eitle, T. M. (2000). The changing structure of school segregation: Measurement and evidence of multi-racial metropolitan area school segregation, 1989–1995. *Demography, 37,* 351–364.

Schwartz, J., & Winship, C. (1980). The welfare approach to measuring inequality. *Sociological Methodology, 9,* 1–36.

Stata Corporation. (2003). *Stata.* College Station, TX: Author.

Stearns, L. B., & Logan, J. R. (1986). Measuring trends in segregation: Three dimensions, three measures. *Urban Affairs Quarterly, 22*(1), 124–150.

Taeuber, K. E., & Taeuber, A. F. (1965). *Negroes in cities: Residential segregation and neighborhood change.* Chicago: Aldine Publishing Co.

Theil, H. (1972). *Statistical decomposition analysis* (Vol. 14). Amsterdam: North-Holland Publishing Company.

Theil, H., & Finezza, A. J. (1971). A note on the measurement of racial integration of schools by means of informational concepts. *Journal of Mathematical Sociology, 1,* 187–194.

White, M. J. (1983). The measurement of spatial segregation. *American Journal of Sociology, 88,* 1008–1018.

White, M. J. (1986). Segregation and diversity measures in population distribution. *Population Index, 52,* 198–221.

Wilson, W. J. (1987). *The truly disadvantaged: The inner city, the underclass, and public policy.* Chicago: University of Chicago Press.

Winship, C. (1978). The desirability of using the index of dissimilarity or any adjustment of it for measuring segregation: Reply to Falk, Cortese, and Cohen. *Social Forces, 57,* 717–720.

Wong, D. S. (1993). Spatial indices of segregation. *Urban Studies, 30,* 559–572.

Wong, D.W.S. (1997). Spatial dependency of segregation indices. *The Canadian Geographer, 41,* 128–136.

Wong, D.W.S. (1998). Measuring multiethnic spatial segregation. *Urban Geography, 19,* 77–87.

Wong, D.W.S. (1999). Geostatistics as measures of spatial segregation. *Urban Geography, 20,* 635–647.

Wong, D.W.S. (2002). Spatial measures of segregation and GIS. *Urban Geography, 23,* 85–92.

Wu, X. B., & Sui, D. Z. (2001). An initial exploration of a lacunarity-based segregation measure. *Environment and Planning B: Planning and Design, 28,* 433–446.

Zoloth, B. S. (1976). Alternative measures of school segregation. *Land Economics, 52,* 278–298.

CHAPTER EIGHT

MEASURES OF RESIDENTIAL COMMUNITY CONTEXTS

Patricia O'Campo and Margaret O'Brien Caughy

This chapter concerns approaches that are used to characterize communities or neighborhoods within public health research. Research on the influence of community context or residential neighborhoods has increased exponentially in the last decade of the twentieth century (Diez-Roux 2000; Duncan et al. 1998; Kawachi and Berkman 2003; O'Campo 2003; Sampson et al. 2002). Because this research has primarily focused upon urban environments, we will not address non-urban research on neighborhoods except to say that more research is needed on how neighborhood is conceptualized and how it influences the health of suburban and rural residents.

The literature distinguishes between *neighborhood*, which usually refers to a geographically bounded area, and *community*, which often identifies a group of individuals concerned with a common issue (for example, school issues, crime control, or urban development). Communities can also have a geographic component (for example, communities concerned with a local school issue), so there is some overlap between the two terms. Even this simplistic description of neighborhood, however, fails to capture the challenges related to ensuring the identification of appropriate geographic boundaries of relevance to residents within neighborhoods or boundaries appropriate for particular health issues. Nevertheless, neighborhoods are thought to possess physical characteristics, social and economic resources (or lack of), and an element of social interaction (positive, negative, or neutral) between residents. It is the measurement of these components of neighborhood that we devote our attention to in this chapter.

Because of the convenience of using data readily available by census units—census tract, census block groups—census designations are often used in the United States and Canada as a proxy for geographically based neighborhoods. Although it is clear that residents do not normally consider specific census boundaries to describe the borders of their neighborhoods, emerging research suggests that census units—census block groups and census tracts—are reasonable proxies for neighborhoods (Bond-Huie 2001; Krieger et al. 2003a, 2003b; O'Campo 2003; Ross et al. 2004). Although there is much concern about the issue of the appropriate unit of analysis or best geographic designation in the literature on "neighborhoods," it is unlikely that a single answer will, or needs, to emerge. The tradeoffs of using smaller versus larger geographic units of analysis, however, are noted extensively in the literature (for example, Duncan et al. 1998; Raudenbush and Sampson 1999) and should be considered when designing a neighborhood study.

Measurement Strategies for Residential Neighborhoods

To effectively examine effects of neighborhoods on individual outcomes, careful attention is required as to how characteristics of neighborhoods are operationalized. A variety of approaches have been used in the neighborhood literature, each with its own strengths and weaknesses. We will loosely organize existing sources of neighborhood measures as either *subjective measures* (based upon individuals' reported perceptions) or so-called *objective measures*. The most common source of objective data used to operationalize neighborhood characteristics is the census. *Census data* have been used to provide indicators of socioeconomic position of the neighborhood (poverty rate, unemployment rate, average household income, and so forth), population stability (for example, proportion of residents who have moved in the last five years), as well as race or ethnic composition. Some researchers have employed census data as single indicators (Brooks-Gunn et al. 1993; Diez-Roux et al. 1997; O'Campo et al. 1997; Ross 2000), whereas others have used indices that combine information from multiple census variables (Beyers et al. 2003; Caughy et al. 2003; Malmstrom et al. 1999). Regardless of the specific census variables used or whether they are combined into indices or not, the researcher interested in neighborhood effects should be guided by theory in identifying the best use of census data. Rajaratnam et al. (2005) conducted a comprehensive review of the maternal and child health literature between January 1999 and

March 2004 and identified 32 research articles that included measurement of neighborhood characteristics. Census data, particularly data regarding economic characteristics, were by far the most frequent data used to characterize neighborhoods; however, few of the articles reviewed by Burke et al. (2005) used health-specific theories to explicate why certain census indicators were used.

There are aspects of census data that have not been capitalized upon in the extant neighborhood research literature. Few researchers have used historical census data to capture the manner in which neighborhoods may have changed over time. For example, data from the 1970, 1980, 1990, and 2000 census regarding poverty rates could be used to identify neighborhoods that have experienced significant declines, improvements, or change in recent decades. Relying on cross-sectional data of neighborhoods masks the fact that neighborhoods are dynamic, and the change experienced in a neighborhood over time may be as important as or more important than its status at a single point in time. Another aspect of census data that has not been exploited is the variability within neighborhoods. Most operational measures of neighborhoods using census data have relied on measures of central tendency, such as average household income. Income inequality theorists suggest that disparities in economic resources between individuals may be an important explanatory factor for understanding social inequalities in health outcomes. Likewise, inequalities within neighborhoods may be important because they may undermine social cohesion and collective efficacy, neighborhood social processes that have been suggested as important mediators of neighborhood effects (Sampson 1991, 1992).

Although census data are the most frequently exploited of the objective sources of neighborhood data, they are not the only sources. Administrative data sources such as crime data, liquor license data, tax parcel data, and city data on housing violations are all examples of sources of objective data that may be useful in operationalizing neighborhood context. Just as with census data, however, the investigator's theory regarding how neighborhoods affect individuals should guide the selection of measures to use and how they should be formulated (Rajaratnam et al. 2005). For example, crime data can be used in a variety of different formats. Should one include all crimes or only "serious" crimes such as murder or rape? Should crimes against property (burglary, auto theft, and so forth) be considered separately from crimes against people? Should the crime variable be calculated to represent number of crimes per capita or number of crimes per square mile? The driving force behind these decisions should be the investigator's theory regarding *how* crime is related to individual health and well-being. For example, one may hypothesize that the negative effects of crime are mediated by the stress created by living in crime-ridden areas; however, there is empirical evidence that individual perceptions of crime may be inconsistent with actual crime rates. Taylor (2001) reports that Baltimore residents perceived that crime was increasing during a period of time when rates were actually falling. His conclusion was that these perceptions were driven more by discrepancies between the city of Baltimore and the surrounding metropolitan area than by the actual crime rates themselves. If a researcher is interested in stress-related reactions to neighborhood crime, focusing on discrepancies between area crime rates and surrounding areas may be a more fruitful approach.

Observational Measures of Neighborhoods

Another objective measure of neighborhoods that has been used less frequently is *systematic observation of the neighborhood context.* Observational methods used have ranged from making videotapes while driving through the neighborhood and coding them at a later time (Raudenbush and Sampson 1999) to shorter "windshield" assessments (so called because the neighborhood is observed and coded while driving through; Laraia et al., unpublished manuscript under review) or checklists that are coded while walking through the neighborhood on foot (Caughy et al. 2001). Observations allow one to characterize neighborhoods in terms of factors that are not captured in routine data sources such as the census. Most frequently, neighborhood observations have been used to collect data regarding physical incivilities, such as trash, graffiti, or boarded-up homes. In addition, some researchers have used observations to collect data on social incivilities such as drug dealing or other illegal activity, levels of social interaction, or resources in the neighborhood, such as facilities for child play. Although collecting observational data provides an opportunity for characterizing neighborhoods in a much richer way as compared to that provided by routine data sets, the collection and analysis of these data provide their own unique set of challenges. The timing of data collection should be considered, especially with regard to observing social interaction and other human behavior. Qualitative data have extensively documented that patterns of activity in neighborhoods often vary significantly across the day, both in terms of volume of activity as well as the characteristics of the individuals out and about in the neighborhood (Burton and Price-Spratlen 1999). Neighborhood activity level is also affected by time of year, with outdoor activity more likely when weather permits. The relevance of these neighborhood characteristics to the particular research question should be paramount in determining the timing of data collection. For example, if the objective is to observe social interactions of children in the neighborhood, scheduling observations during weekday school hours would be problematic. Likewise, if observing illegal drug activity is a high priority for the researcher, scheduling observations during morning hours would likely give a skewed view of such activity in the neighborhood. One option is to standardize observation times across the neighborhoods being observed to avoid confounding the neighborhood measures with time of assessment. Other researchers have used time of day as a covariate in analyses using observational data to address this issue (Raudenbush and Sampson 1999).

Data reduction of neighborhood observational data provides another set of challenges. Different approaches have been used by different researchers, which have complicated the comparison of findings across studies. Some researchers have used complex analytic models to estimate the probability of different latent constructs at a larger geographic unit, such as a census block group (Caughy et al. 2001; Raudenbush and Sampson 1999). Other researchers have created simple summary measures for the block on which the respondent lives. For example, Kohen et al. (2002) rated the traffic; garbage and litter; people loitering, arguing, or intoxicated; and the general condition of buildings for an area 500 feet in either direction from the respondents' homes. Differing levels of aggregation of observational data may have differing implications, depending upon the health or well-being outcome under examination. For example, the physical characteristics of the immediate block may be most relevant when studying the activities of daily living of elderly individuals who have limited mobility in the neighborhood, whereas, the physical and social characteristics of a broader geographic area might be important for studying the delinquent behavior of adolescents.

Additional research is needed to explore how observational measures of neighborhoods perform in a variety of settings, both urban and rural. To date, the use of such measures has been almost wholly limited to urban areas, primarily in cities in the northeast. Virtually no application of these observational measures in rural areas has been conducted. In addition, few studies have used the same measures, limiting our ability to compare findings across investigations. Laraia et al. compared application of the same tool in an urban area in the south with the tool reported by Caughy et al. (2001) and found very different neighborhood environments than those in Baltimore (Laraia et al., unpublished manuscript under review).

Measures on Perceptions of Neighborhoods

Subjective measures of the neighborhood environment have been extensively used in research on neighborhood effects. In most cases, neighborhood residents are asked to report their perceptions of their neighborhood or their neighbors with regard to a variety of dimensions, such as physical and social disorder in the community, degree of connectedness between community residents, and perceptions regarding the degree to which community members are willing to act collectively on behalf of the community as a whole. Robert Sampson, a sociologist at the University of Chicago, has written extensively regarding neighborhood social processes, focusing most explicitly on what Sampson et al. (1997) have coined *collective efficacy* (see also Sampson 1991). Sampson (1991, p. 10) has defined collective efficacy as the "linkages of mutual trust and the shared willingness to intervene for the common good" of the community and as comprising two components: *social cohesion,* or the sense of connectedness, and *informal social control,* the willingness to intervene in community problems. Sampson et al. have developed a neighborhood perceptions measure in their work with the Project for Human Development in Chicago Neighborhoods (Earls 1999). In addition, neighborhood perceptions measures have been reported by Buckner (1988), Coulton et al. (1996), and McGuire (1997). Although specific items and constructs differ across the individual measures, most of them attempt to tap into some aspect of social cohesion and informal social control, and some go further by tapping into physical and social disorder, patterns of social interaction and mutual exchange, community involvement, and use of and satisfaction with community resources.

Perceptions of neighborhood climate and social processes represent data that cannot be obtained in any way other than by interviewing individuals who live in the neighborhood. Certain analytic issues, however, must be kept in mind when relying upon perceptions data as a way of measuring neighborhood context. First, each respondent can be viewed as an imperfect "informant" about the neighborhood in which he lives. Raudenbush et al. (1991) has described the analytic issues of dealing with such data collected to assess characteristics of schools as well as neighborhoods (Raudenbush and Sampson 1999). The accuracy of a neighborhood informant is affected by his length of residence in the neighborhood as well as such personal characteristics as psychological well-being, among other things. Individuals who moved to a neighborhood recently would have a different length of experience in the neighborhood and therefore present different perceptions of neighborhood social processes. Depending on length of residence, they may not have had a chance to develop social networks in the community. Individuals who are psychologically depressed may have perceptions that are skewed as a function of their own mental health status.

Care must be taken when using neighborhood perceptions data to create neighborhood-level variables. One approach that is frequently used is to aggregate the individual responses of neighborhood residents to create a neighborhood-level average for each variable or construct. The problem with this approach is that it does not account for the measurement error inherent in each individual's response as a function of length of residence in the neighborhood, psychological status, or other individual factors. One approach to address this issue includes incorporating individual-level variables into the analysis that the investigator believes influence perceptions of the neighborhood, such as a measure of the individual's psychological status. Another method is to use random effects analytic approaches (Bryk and Raudenbush 1992; Goldstein 1995; Muthen and Muthen 1998) that separate the variance in neighborhood perceptions between neighborhoods from the variance in neighborhood perceptions between individuals in the same neighborhood.

The researcher should also consider carefully how the perceptions variables are operationalized when they are included in the analysis. The form of the variable should be dictated by the theory that the researcher has regarding the nature of the relationship between the neighborhood variable and the outcome of interest. For example, using a variable in continuous form assumes that the relationship with the outcome is linear as well as similar along the entire continuum of the neighborhood variable. In contrast, perhaps the true form of the relationship is a "threshold" effect. That is, any relationship between the conditions in the neighborhood and health outcomes is only observed at certain extreme levels, either low or high. For example, social cohesion is a characteristic of neighborhoods that is often considered to be protective of good health and positive outcomes (Cattell 2001; Franzini et al. 2005; Ross 2000). It may be, however, that the protective effects of neighborhood cohesion for a particular health problem are only seen once a certain threshold is achieved, with levels above that being inconsequential. If, in this situation, the neighborhood variable is incorporated in the analysis as a continuum rather than a binary variable to capture the threshold effect, any association between the neighborhood social processes and that health problem will be missed. In our own work, we have found that very low levels of psychological sense of community (a construct similar to social cohesion) was predictive of child mental health outcomes, whereas the continuous form of the measure was unrelated (Caughy et al. 2003).

Another issue regarding neighborhood perceptions data is the agreement, or lack thereof, with objective measures that tap the same neighborhood characteristics. For example, one can ask residents about the degree of physical disorder in the neighborhood such as graffiti or trash or about the degree of social disorder such as disorderly groups of adults or teens. In contrast, one can make direct observations of these conditions by walking through the neighborhood, as previously described. Agreement between individual perception of neighborhood conditions and objective observations of neighborhood conditions may be quite low. To illustrate this, we use data from two studies conducted in Baltimore, Maryland: a study of 307 preschoolers and their families living in fifty-seven different census block groups, and a study of 405 elementary school-age children and their families living in ninety-one different census block groups. Data collection methods and measures were similar between the two studies. During a visit to the home, the primary caregiver of the participating child answered a number of questions about the physical and social conditions of the neighborhood, using the Neighborhood Environment for Children Rating Scales (NECRS) (Coulton et al. 1996). The "physical/social disorder" scale of the NECRS included fifteen items reflecting frequency of such neighborhood problems as trash, graffiti, abandoned cars, drug dealers, gangs, and loitering. Objective assessments of neighborhoods by trained observers were conducted in a similar manner with a checklist adapted from the work of Ralph Taylor (Perkins et al. 1992; Taylor et al. 1984) and the Project for Human Development in Chicago Neighborhoods (National Opinion Research Center 1996) The data collection tool and methodology is described in detail in Caughy et al. (2001); in brief, two observers rated each face block on a forty-five- to fifty-item checklist that included ratings of the amount of graffiti and trash, the condition of buildings, the condition of grounds and undeveloped spaces, indications of block uniformity and territoriality, type of street, neighborhood resources, and presence and activities of people. In the preschoolers study, ratings were conducted for every face block in each of the fifty-seven block groups in the study, for a total of 1,135 streets observed. For the elementary school study, ratings were conducted for the face block on which the participating child lived plus a cluster of up to six streets surrounding this street, for a total of 1,290 streets observed.

For each study, a summary indicator of physical disorder was created from the observational data that included the amount of graffiti and trash and the condition of buildings and grounds. For the preschoolers study, this indicator was created as a summary measure from every face block in the entire census block group. For the elementary school study, two indicators were created: one that was a summary measure for the street on which the target child lived, and one that was a summary measure for the cluster of streets surrounding the child (including the street on which the child lived). Higher scores on these summary measures indicated higher rates of graffiti and trash and a greater density of abandoned or boarded up buildings and poorly kept spaces. To compare physical disorder as objectively assessed by our observers with the perceptions of physical disorder of our participants, we used data of participants' reports of their neighborhood physical disorder. We then ranked and categorized both participants' reports of their neighborhood perceptions as well as the measure of physical disorder based on our observations into quartiles. We used a weighted Kappa statistic to quantify the degree of agreement between perceptions and observed measures of physical disorder. For the preschoolers study, with observed physical disorder summarized at the block group level, Kappa was .49. This indicates that there was very little agreement between the quartile of physical disorder as perceived by the participant with that observed by trained data collectors. Among those individuals whose physical disorder was observed to be in the lowest quartile of all block groups observed, approximately 22 percent of the reported perceptions of physical disorder in their neighborhood fell into the highest quartile. Of those observed to be in the highest quartile of all block groups observed, approximately 10 percent of the perceptions of their neighborhoods fell into the lowest quartile of physical disorder.

One possible reason for this low level of agreement could be the degree of heterogeneity within a block group. If physical disorder varies widely from one part of a block group to another, then a summary measure estimated for the block group may not agree with how an individual perceives the neighborhood immediately surrounding his or her home. As described previously, the observed measures of physical disorder in the second sample from Baltimore were summarized at a smaller geographic area—one summary measure for a cluster of six or seven streets surrounding the participant's house and another summary measure for the face block on which the participant lived. The level of agreement between perceived disorder and observed disorder did not improve when the geographic area was smaller. For the cluster of six or seven streets, the level of agreement between perceived and observed disorder was .34. For the individual block on which the participant lived, the level of agreement between perceived and observed physical disorder was .25.

The obvious lack of agreement between objective measures of neighborhood context and residents' perceptions of those same neighborhood characteristics forces the researcher to critically consider the mechanisms underlying neighborhood effects on individual well-being. If neighborhoods affect health, there must be a mechanism whereby conditions of the neighborhood—conditions that by definition are external to the individual—are translated into differences in physiological or psychological processes (or both) that are internal to individual residents. Whether neighborhood effects are derived from physical exposure to risk factors (such as environmental pollutants or conditions that increase risk of injury) or effects of neighborhood stress in compromising individual psychological well-being or both, different mechanisms have different implications for understanding and dealing with the discrepancy between observed and perceived neighborhood characteristics. In cases in which psychological effects are believed to mediate neighborhood effects on individual health and well-being, how individuals perceive the conditions of their neighborhood may be more important than an objective assessment of those conditions by an outsider. The characteristics that predict differences in perceptions of neighborhood context among individuals living in the same neighborhood need to be systematically investigated. Furthermore, researchers need to expand their conceptualization regarding how neighborhoods affect individual health outcomes. Roosa et al. (2003) have proposed a "transactional" model of neighborhood influences. According to this model, individuals are not passive recipients of neighborhood influences, nor is the direction of influence solely from neighborhoods to individuals. Rather, residents are "active cognizers and constructors of their environments" and their responses to the neighborhood environment are a function of that transactional process. The lack of congruity between objective neighborhood assessments and perceptions of the neighborhood environment by its residents is a concrete example of how individuals actively evaluate and cope with the neighborhood environment in which they live.

Bringing in the Community Perspective

The literature concerning neighborhood effects on individual health has almost exclusively been conducted without input from those who reside in these community settings. As noted earlier, these multilevel neighborhood studies have often lacked a strong conceptual foundation linking neighborhood characteristics to individual-level risks and outcomes. Although social epidemiologists have consulted the social sciences—criminology, social geography, community psychology, sociology—as a source of theory and conceptual information about neighborhood processes, the processes identified are often most relevant to non-health outcomes, such as delinquency, school drop-out, and teen pregnancy (see for example, Crane 1991; Sampson et al. 1999; Taylor 2001; Taylor et al. 1984). Social epidemiologists should begin, however, to develop frameworks and testable hypotheses regarding the pathways of neighborhood environments to individual well-being that are specific to processes that affect health. There has been recent recognition of the importance of "lay knowledge" in facilitating a greater understanding about the importance and meaning of "place" (Burke et al. 2005; O'Campo et al. 2005). Popay et al. (2003) note that lay knowledge about the "meanings people attach to their experience of places and how this shapes social action . . ." may provide the "missing link in our understanding of the causes of inequalities in health."

The community perspective can provide complimentary knowledge to that generated by researchers, as neighborhood residents possess "lived experience" of their environments. The case of research on neighborhood effects on intimate partner violence (IPV) provides a good example. Published studies on neighborhood effects and the risk of IPV consistently report that low neighborhood socioeconomic position is associated with higher risk of partner violence (Cunradi et al. 2000; Grisso et al. 1999), and recent studies have examined additional neighborhood characteristics such as high levels of collective efficacy serving as protective factors against partner violence (Browning 2002) and high levels of neighborhood mobility increasing the risk of partner violence (Grisso et al. 1999).

Yet, taken together, the breadth of neighborhood characteristics that have been examined in relation to IPV is narrow and cannot begin to contribute to a comprehensive understanding of how neighborhoods affect the risk of partner violence, a characteristic that is shared with the more general literature on neighborhoods and health (O'Campo 2003).

To gain the perspective of residents on neighborhood factors and IPV, a study was undertaken with participant-driven methods of concept mapping to obtain data on how characteristics of neighborhoods are related to IPV (O'Campo et al. 2005). Briefly, the concept mapping research involved over seven hours of discussion with participants about neighborhoods and IPV (Burke et al. 2005).

Whereas the published literature has examined four neighborhood characteristics, participants listed over fifty neighborhood characteristics that were important for IPV. Many of the characteristics were related to each other and, upon statistical analyses with multidimensional scaling and hierarchical cluster analyses, yielded seven clusters of the neighborhood items that were related to perpetration, severity, and cessation of violence (see Figure 8.1). The dots on the figure are the fifty or so items within each of the seven clusters. Those items and clusters

FIGURE 8.1.   CLUSTER MAP FROM CONCEPT MAPPING OF URBAN NEIGHBORHOOD FACTORS AND INTIMATE PARTNER VIOLENCE.

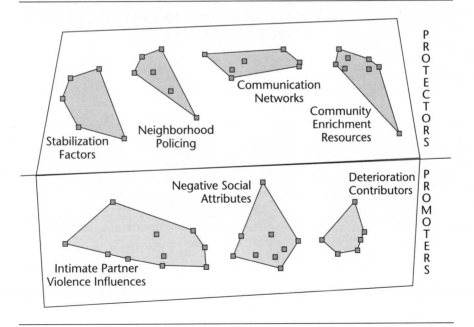

closer together in Figure 8.1 are more closely related to each other. For example, the two clusters "communication networks" and "community enrichment resources" are more closely related to one another than the two clusters of "communication networks" and "deterioration contributors," as indicated by the distance between the clusters.

Participants identified items as being "promoters" of as well as "protectors" from IPV. Participants also rated the importance of these items and clusters of items for IPV perpetration, severity, and cessation. Results show that those factors important for perpetration of IPV are similar to those important for severity but were not the same factors that were critical for cessation of IPV (O'Campo et al. 2005).

Finally, in small discussion groups, the participants created figures that represented the pathways by which these clusters of items were related to IPV (see Figures 8.2 and 8.3). Some diagrams represented straightforward "chain" relationships between items, such as for "Stabilization Factor" items and their relationship to IPV cessation (Figure 8.2), whereas some groups perceived more complex relationships between items (Figure 8.3). As shown in Figure 8.3, neighborhoods with many "families with young children" positively influenced neighborhood "cultural norms" that, in turn, created more people in the neighborhood who "intervened" and, ultimately, results in less IPV. The

FIGURE 8.2. NEIGHBORHOOD STABILIZATION FACTORS AND IPV CESSATION.

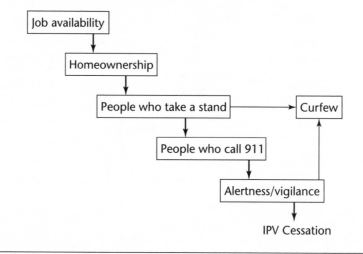

FIGURE 8.3.   NEIGHBORHOOD MONITORING CLUSTER AND IPV.

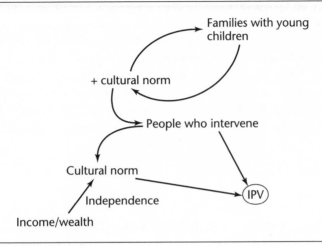

participants who drew the diagram intentionally used curved arrows to suggest that the relationships between the factors were not direct but dynamic, complex, and potentially influenced by other factors (not identified in the diagram). In this diagram, "income and wealth" also influence neighborhood norms.

This type of research with community residents may yield a missing perspective on neighborhood influences from those with lived experiences. This research can identify gaps in current research on community. In this case, numerous neighborhood characteristics were identified by community residents that researchers have, to date, not yet examined. Moreover, the information about the perceived pathways from neighborhoods to IPV contributes to the design of testable hypotheses about neighborhoods and individuals.

Future Directions on Measuring Neighborhood Environments

Given the recency of adoption within public health of multilevel modeling of residential neighborhoods on health outcomes, major methodological gains have been made in a short period of time. Hopefully, the methodological advancements will continue to improve our understanding of whether and how residential neighborhoods affect health. Social epidemiologists should move beyond their overreliance on census data as the primary and sole source for characterizing neighborhoods. Moreover, more research should focus upon developing relevant health-specific theories. Use of such theories should be the primary driving force in determining neighborhood characteristics and how to operationalize them in studies of multilevel models. To ensure that such studies ultimately contribute to intervention and policy design, this body of research must begin to tease apart the mechanisms of neighborhood effects. Finally, the community perspective has been virtually excluded from neighborhood research up to this point. Incorporating the community perspective in social epidemiology's theories and hypotheses regarding neighborhoods is essential for developing effective and viable community-level interventions.

References

Beyers, J. M., Bates, J. E., Pettit, G. S., & Dodge, K. A. (2003). Neighborhood structure, parenting processes, and the development of youths' externalizing behaviors: A multilevel analysis. *American Journal of Community Psychology, 31,* 35–53.

Bond-Huie, S. (2001). The concept of neighborhood in health and mortality research. *Sociological Spectrum, 21,* 341–358.

Brooks-Gunn, J., Duncan, G. J., Klebanov, P. K., & Sealand, N. (1993). Do neighborhoods influence child and adolescent development? *American Journal Sociology, 99,* 353–395.

Browning, C. (2002). The span of collective efficacy: Extending social disorganization theory to partner violence. *Journal of Marriage and Family, 64,* 833–850.

Bryk, A. S. & Raudenbush, S. W. (1992). *Hierarchical linear models: Application and data analysis methods.* Newbury Park, CA: Sage Publications.

Buckner, J. C. (1988). The development of an instrument to measure neighborhood cohesion. *American Journal of Community Psychology, 16,* 771–790.

Burke, J., O'Campo, P., Peak, G., Gielen, A., McDonnell, K., & Trochim, W. (2005). Concept mapping as a participatory public health research tool: Application to neighborhoods and intimate partner violence. *Qualitative Health Research, 10,* 1392–1410.

Burton, L. M., & Price-Spratlen, T. (1999). Through the eyes of children: An ethnographic perspective on neighborhoods and child development. In A. S. Masten (Ed.), *Cultural processes in child development. The Minnesota Symposia on Child Psychology* (pp. 77–96). Mahwah, NJ: Lawrence Erlbaum Associates, Inc.

Cattell, V. (2001). Poor people, poor places, and poor health: The mediating role of social networks and social capital. *Social Science & Medicine, 52,* 1501–1516.

Caughy, M.O.B., O'Campo, P., & Patterson, J. (2001). A brief observational measure for urban neighborhoods. *Health & Place, 7,* 225–236.

Caughy, M.O.B., O'Campo, P. J., & Muntaner, C. (2003). When being alone might be better: Neighborhood poverty, social capital, and child mental health. *Social Science & Medicine, 57,* 227–237.

Coulton, C. J., Korbin, J. E., & Su, M. (1996). Measuring neighborhood context for young children in an urban area. *American Journal of Community Psychology, 24,* 5–33.

Crane, J. (1991). Effects of neighborhoods on dropping out of school and teenage childbearing. In C. Jencks & P. E. Peterson (Eds.), *The Urban Underclass* (pp. 299–321). Washington, DC: The Brookings Institute.

Cunradi, C. B., Caetano, R., Clark, C., & Schafer, J. (2000). Neighborhood poverty as a predictor of intimate partner violence among White, Black, and Hispanic couples in the United States: A multilevel analysis. *Annals of Epidemiology, 10,* 297–308.

Diez-Roux, A. (2000). Multilevel analysis in public health research. *Annual Review of Public Health, 21,* 171–192.

Diez-Roux, A. V., Nieto, F. J., Muntaner, C., Tyroler H. A., Comstock, G. W., Shahar, E., et al. (1997). Neighborhood environments and coronary heart disease: A multilevel analysis. *American Journal of Epidemiology, 146,* 48–63.

Duncan, C., Jones, K., & Moon, G. (1998). Context, composition and heterogenity: Using multilevel models in health research. *Social Science & Medicine, 46,* 97–117.

Earls, F. (1999). *Project on human development in Chicago neighborhoods: Community survey.* Boston, MA: Harvard Medical School.

Franzini, L., Caughy, M. O., Spears, W., & Fernandez Esquer, M. E. (2005). Neighborhood economic conditions, social processes, and self-rated health: A multilevel latent variables model. *Social Science & Medicine, 61*(6), 1135–1150.

Goldstein, H. (1995). *Multilevel statistical models.* New York: Halstead Press.

Grisso, J., Schwarz, D. F., Hirschinger, N., Sammel, M., Brensinger, C., Santanna, J., et al. (1999). Violent injuries among women in an urban area. *New England Journal of Medicine, 341,* 1899–1905.

Kawachi, I., & Berkman, L. (2003). *Neighborhoods and health.* New York: Oxford.

Kohen, D. E., Brooks-Gunn, J., Leventhal, T., & Hertzmann, C. (2002). Neighborhood income and physical and social disorder in Canada: Associations with young children's competencies. *Child Development, 73,* 1844–1860.

Krieger, N., Chen, J. T., Waterman, P. D., Rehkopf, D. H., & Subramanian, S. V. (2003a). Race/ethnicity, gender, and monitoring socioeconomic gradients in health: A comparison of area-based socioeconomic measures—the public health disparities geocoding project. *American Journal of Public Health, 93,* 1655–1671.

Krieger, N., Chen, J. T., Waterman, P. D., Soobader, M. J., Subramanian, S. V., & Carson, R. (2003b). Choosing area based socioeconomic measures to monitor social inequalities in low birth weight and childhood lead poisoning: The Public Health Disparities Geocoding Project (US). *Journal of Epidemiology and Community Health, 57,* 186–199.

Laraia, B. A., Messer, L., Kaufman, J. S., Dole, N., Caughy, M., O'Campo, P., et al. (under review). *Direct observation of neighborhood attributes in an urban area of the U.S. South.*

Malmstrom, M., Sundquist, J., & Johansson, S. E. (1999). Neighborhood environment and self-reported health status: a multilevel analysis. *American Journal of Public Health, 89,* 1181–1186.

McGuire, J. B. (1997). The reliability and validity of a questionnaire describing neighborhood characteristics relevant to families and young children living in urban areas. *Journal of Community Psychology, 25,* 551–566.

Messer, L., Kaufman, J., Laraia, B., Eyster, J., Holzman, C., Culhane, J., et al. (under review). *The development of a standardized neighborhood deprivation index.*

Muthen, L. L., & Muthen, B. O. (1998). *MPlus: The comprehensive modeling program for applied researchers. User's guide.* Los Angeles: Muthen and Muthen.

National Opinion Research Center (1996). Project for Human Development in Chicago Neighborhoods; Harvard Project 4709. *SSO (Systematic Social Observation) Coding Manual,* June.

O'Campo, P. (2003). Invited commentary: Advancing theory and methods for multilevel models of residential neighborhoods and health. *American Journal of Epidemiology, 157,* 9–13.

O'Campo, P., Burke, J., Peak, G. L., McDonnell, K. A., & Gielen, A. C. (2005). Uncovering neighbourhood influences on intimate partner violence using concept mapping. *Journal of Epidemiology and Community Health, 59,* 603–8.

O'Campo, P., Xue, X., Wang, M., & Caughy, M. O. (1997). Neighborhood risk factors for low birthweight in Baltimore: A multilevel analysis. *American Journal of Public Health, 87,* 1113–1118.

Perkins, D. D., Meeks, J. W., & Taylor, R. B. (1992). The physical environment of street blocks and resident perceptions of crime and disorder: Implications for theory and measurement. *Journal of Environmental Psychology, 12,* 21–34.

Popay, J., Williams, G., Thomas, C., & Gatrell, A. (2003). Theorizing inequalities in health: The place of lay knowledge. In R. Hofrichter (Ed.), *Health and social justice: Politics, ideology, and inequity in the distribution of disease* (pp. 385–409). San Francisco: Jossey-Bass.

Rajaratnam, J., Burke, J., & O'Campo, P. (2005). Maternal & child health and neighborhood context: The selection and construction of area-level variables. *Health & Place.*

Rajaratnam, J., Burke, J., & O'Campo, P. (in press). Maternal & Child Health and Neighborhood Context: The Selection and Construction of Area-Level Variables. *Health & Place.*

Raudenbush, S. W., Rowan, B., & Kang, S. J. (1991). A multilevel, multivariate model for studying school climate with estimation via the EM algorithm and application to U.S. high school data. *Journal of Educational Statistics, 16,* 295–330.

Raudenbush, S. W., & Sampson, R. J. (1999). Ecometrics: Toward a science of assessing ecological settings, with application to the systematic social observation of neighborhoods. *Sociological Methodology, 29,* 1–41.

Roosa, M. W., Jones, S., Tein, J.-Y., & Cree, W. (2003). Prevention science and neighborhood influences on low-income children's development: Theoretical and methodological issues. *American Journal of Community Psychology, 31,* 55–72.

Ross, C. E. (2000). Walking, exercising, and smoking: Does neighborhood matter? *Social Science & Medicine, 51,* 265–274.

Ross, N. A., Tremblay, S. S., & Graham, K. (2004). Neighbourhood influences on health in Montreal, Canada. *Social Science & Medicine, 59,* 1485–1494.

Sampson, R. J. (1991). Linking the micro and macrolevel dimensions of community social organization. *Social Forces, 70,* 43–64.

Sampson, R. J. (1992). Family management and child development: Insights from social disorganization theory. In J. McCord (Ed.), *Facts, frameworks, and forecasts. Advances in criminological theory* (pp. 63–93). New Brunswick, NJ: Transaction Publishers.

Sampson, R. J., Morenoff, J. D., & Gannon-Rowley, T. (2002). Assessing "neighborhood effects": Social processes and new directions in research. *Annual Review of Sociology, 28,* 443–478.

Sampson, R. J., Morenoff, J. D., & Raudenbush, S. W. (1999). Assessing neighborhood-level theories of crime: Social mechanisms and spatial dynamics. In *Neighborhood effects.* Chicago: Joint Center for Poverty Research, Northwestern University/University of Chicago.

Sampson, R. J., Raudenbush, S. W., & Earls, F. (1997). Neighborhoods and violent crime: A multilevel study of collective efficacy. *Science, 277,* 918–924.

Taylor, R. B. (2001). *Breaking away from broken windows: Baltimore neighborhoods and the nationwide fight against crime, grime, fear, and decline.* Boulder, CO: Westview Press.

Taylor, R. B., Gottfredson, S. D., & Brower, S. (1984). Block crime and fear: Defensible space, and territorial functioning. *Journal of Research in Crime and Delinquency, 21,* 303–331.

CHAPTER NINE

USING CENSUS DATA TO APPROXIMATE NEIGHBORHOOD EFFECTS

Lynne C. Messer and Jay S. Kaufman

Despite the development of innovative neighborhood data collection methods, such as systematic social observation (Caughy et al. 2001; Sampson and Raudenbush 1999), and the use of novel administrative data sources, including delinquent tax records, homelessness shelter use, reports of housing violations (O'Campo et al. 2000), and crime reports (Messer et al. 2006; Morenoff 2003; O'Campo et al. 1997), the U.S. Census remains a rich and convenient data source for characterizing neighborhood environments and exposures in the United States. For researchers who wish to learn how societal structures influence health and disease outcomes, sociodemographic census data are useful because they can offer insight into aspects of community stratification, opportunity structures, and social conditions (Berkman and Macintyre 1997; Krieger et al. 1997; Link and Phelan 1996; Singh 2003). Given the data's ready availability for researchers and extensive geographic coverage, understanding how to employ census data in research on neighborhood or area effects on health is an important tool for social epidemiology.

Drawing on literature from geography, social epidemiology, and sociology, this chapter will offer an introduction to census geography and describe the various ways that the U.S. Census divides physical space. This is followed by an overview of the various types of available census data with special emphasis on information collected in the decennial census that can be used to characterize neighborhoods. Next, the chapter provides a brief description of the ways in which census data have been used previously in association with health outcomes and will offer a worked example of using census data to estimate neighborhood influences on adverse birth outcomes. Significant racial disparity exists for all birth outcomes, despite considerable research and various interventions. Birth outcomes were chosen to illustrate the use of census data to approximate neighborhood effects because neighborhood-level factors may contribute to these persistent racial disparities and this topic is an active area of research in perinatal epidemiology. The chapter concludes with a discussion of the strengths and limitations of using census data to approximate neighborhood effects.

Neighborhood Defined

Neighborhood is a term used to refer to a person's immediate residential environment, which has been hypothesized to have both material and social characteristics related to health (Diez-Roux 2001) and has been operationalized in various ways. The word "neighborhood" most often connotes a physical or geographic space but has also been used to represent a community of shared identity or conceptual entity or the place where one spends the bulk of one's day (for instance, the work or school environment). Each operationalization of neighborhood is accompanied by a different measurement approach (see, for example, an extensive review of this topic by Sampson et al. 2002). Because using census data to estimate neighborhood effects requires defining neighborhoods with administrative boundaries, the remainder of this chapter will assume neighborhoods represent geographic units.

Census Geography

At the national level, census data branch into two systems of aggregation: 1) the region and state system, and 2) the metropolitan and urban system (Figure 9.1, adapted from a U.S. Census Bureau figure). The United States is divided into four census regions, Northeast, Midwest, South, and West, each containing two or three divisions. For instance, the South region is composed of three divisions, the South Atlantic, East South Central, and West South Central. Divisions are divided into states. The South Atlantic division includes the states of Delaware, Florida, Georgia, Maryland, North Carolina, South Carolina, Virginia, West Virginia, and the District of Columbia (United States Census Bureau 1994). States are further divided into counties, the primary legal subdivision in most states, which are further divided into census tracts. Census tracts are small, relatively permanent statistical subdivisions of counties containing 4,000 residents on average (generally ranging from 1,500 to 8,000) (United States Census Bureau 2000a). Tract

FIGURE 9.1.   HIERARCHY OF CENSUS GEOGRAPHIC ENTITIES.

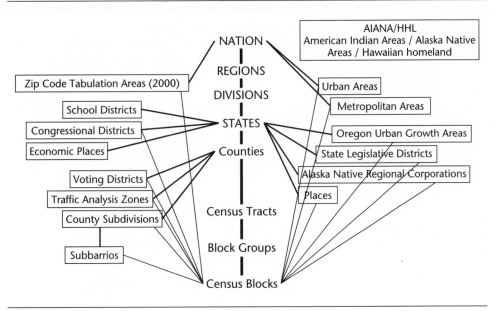

boundaries are delineated by a local committee of census data users for the purpose of representing data and are designed to be relatively homogeneous units with respect to sociodemographic characteristics and living conditions (United States Census Bureau 2000a). Areas experiencing rapid population growth or decline may become heterogeneous during the decennial census period. Tract boundaries usually follow visible features (for example, roads or rivers) but may follow governmental unit boundaries and other non-visible features. Census tracts reduce to block groups, which are the smallest geographic units for which the Census Bureau tabulates sample data. Census block groups are nested within census tracts and generally contain between 600 and 3,000 people, with an optimal size of 1,500 (United States Census Bureau 2000a). Block groups are further subdivided into census blocks, which are the smallest geographic units for which the Census Bureau tabulates 100-percent data. Many blocks correspond to individual city blocks bounded by streets, but blocks—especially in rural areas—may include many square miles and may have some boundaries that are not streets (United States Census Bureau 2000a).

Another dimension along which epidemiologists and the U.S. Census Bureau classify neighborhoods is the degree to which they are urban or rural. Population density is one common basis for making rural–urban distinctions and one that is available at every level of aggregation for which a population size and area can be defined. One drawback of this simple metric is that population may be unevenly clumped within the area; for example, densely populated urban areas within large and mostly rural counties commonly occur in the western states. Alternatively, the U.S. Census includes a binary urban–rural indicator that is based on an algorithm that is respecified for each decennial census. The year 2000 definition used population density of interrelated geographic units, along with a new designation of "urban clusters," which have a smaller total population than urbanized areas (Hall et al., forthcoming, Hart et al. 2005).

An alternate scale at the county level is Bluestone's Classification system, which categorizes counties into six levels of urbanization. This definition does not consider adjacency but considers population density and percent of population that is urbanized according to the census definition. Another designation made at the county level or at the level of groups of counties is that of "Metropolitan Areas" (MAs), which defines urban areas by considering economic integration and population size by county. In 2000, these MA designations were changed to "Core-Based Statistical Areas" (CBSAs), which include both "Metropolitan Statistical Areas" (MeSAs) (for urban clusters of at least 50,000), and "Micropolitan Statistical Areas" (MiSAs) (for urban clusters of 10,000–49,999). Economic and social interdependence is recognized by annexing counties adjacent to MeSAs or MiSAs, if a specified proportion of the population works in the county considered central to the CBSA. And MeSAs and MiSAs may also be combined, if geographically contiguous, into "Combined Statistical Areas" (Hall et al., forthcoming; Hart et al. 2005).

When rural areas are specifically of interest, "Urban Influence Codes" (UICs) make finer distinctions of rurality than the previously described measures. UICs are county-level classifications developed by the U.S. Department of Agriculture that consider adjacency to other areas, including both geographic contiguity and also the percent of population commuting. Similarly, "Rural-Urban Continuum Codes" (RUCCs) are comparable ordinal-categorical measures at the county level but take into account adjacency to a larger economy while ignoring the size of the adjacent MA. Even finer distinctions can be made with "Rural-Urban Commuting Area Codes" (RUCACs), which are similar to UICs and RUCCs but which make additional distinctions based on the type of community to which commuting primarily flows (Hall et al., forthcoming; Hart et al. 2005).

Types of Census Data

The U.S. government orchestrates or participates in multiple censuses, including the Census for countries around the world, the Census of Governments, the Census of Agriculture (sponsored by the U.S. Department of Agriculture), and the Economic Census, which is produced by the U.S. Census Bureau every five years. When census data is used in epidemiologic research, however, it is usually the decennial data obtained from the Census of Population and Housing that is considered.

Since 1790, the census has been taken every ten years, as required by the U.S. Constitution (Rosenthal 2000). The year 2000 census resulted in a 67-percent national response rate from U.S. households, which mailed back either the short form or long form of the Census instrument (United States Census Bureau 2000a). The short form queries the type of household and the number of people included as well as the name and phone number of household head and the sex and race of up to twelve people in the household. The long form also asks about age, education, language, citizenship, residential stability, disabilities, military status, employment, sources of income and employer, household type and condition, and expenses. These questions are asked for up to six people living in a household. In 2003, the American Community Survey is scheduled to become a national survey; its ongoing design is intended to replace the long form and reduce the decennial census to a handful of questions (Rosenthal 2000).

Individual and household responses to the census may be aggregated to multiple geographic units (blocks, block groups, tracts, and so forth) to produce proportions of various characteristics, including percent of total population over age sixty-five, percent black non-Hispanic (NH) race, percent unemployed, median household income, percent receiving public assistance, percent living in the same house since 1995, and so forth. The population characteristics are generally available as percents of individuals, families, or households within the given unit of aggregation, and these data are released to the public through four U.S. Census Bureau Summary files. Summary files 1 and 2 comprise 100 percent data collected from all people and housing units. Summary file 1 provides population characteristics, including age, sex, race, ethnic origin, household relationship, and home rental status; Summary file 2 provides similar characteristic information iterated for multiple detailed racial and ethnic groups. Summary files 3 and 4 contain the sample data that were collected with the long form from one of six families and weighted to represent the total population. Summary file 3 provides detailed population and housing data (place of birth, education, employment status, income, housing value, age of structure, and so forth), whereas Summary file 4 provides this information for 336 racial, ethnic, and ancestry categories. Summary file information related to special populations (for example, American Indian and Alaskan Natives or Congressional Districts) is also available. Not all census data is aggregated to areal units (Ruggles et al. 2004), but these data contain poor geographic measures to protect respondent confidentiality. The directory of population and housing census variables available at the various levels of aggregation is readily accessible from American Fact Finder [http://factfinder.census.gov/home/].

Overview of Research Assessing Census-Defined Neighborhood Deprivation and Health

The body of research in epidemiology, sociology, and community psychology assessing census-defined neighborhood sociodemographic environments and health is substantial, and an exhaustive review of these literatures is beyond the scope of this chapter. Rather, this chapter will provide an overview of various epidemiologic studies conducted over the last five years that have used census data to estimate neighborhood effects on health behaviors, intermediates, and outcomes. Living in a disadvantaged neighborhood, defined as such with census indicators of deprivation, has been associated with such health behaviors as gambling (Welte et al. 2004) and perinatal substance use (Finch et al. 1999). It has also been associated with health intermediates, including late stage cancer diagnoses (Barry and Breen 2005; Klassen et al. 2004), pediatric injury (Shenassa et al. 2004), partner violence (Cunradi et al. 2000), and poor self-rated health among Mexican Americans (Patel et al. 2003). Furthermore, living in deprived neighborhood environments has been associated with excess mortality (Robbins and Webb 2004), AIDS incidence (Zierler et al. 2000), violent injuries to women (Grisso et al. 1999), cardiovascular disease mortality (Borrell et al. 2004), homicide risk (Gjelsvik et al. 2004), and breast cancer incidence (Yost et al. 2001). Neighborhood disadvantage has also been associated with perinatal outcomes (Buka et al. 2003; Kogan 1995; Kramer 1987; Krieger et al. 2003; O'Campo et al 1997; Parker et al. 1994; Pearl et al. 2001; Rauh et al. 2001; Roberts 1997; Wilcox et al. 1995). Income distribution, constructed with census variables, has been associated with fatal drug overdose (Galea et al. 2003), lower self-rated health (Blakely et al. 2002), and cardiovascular disease (Cooper 2001) but has also been observed to be unassociated with population or individual health after covariate adjustment (Mellor and Milyo 2003).

Neighborhood deprivation effects differ by urban and rural status (Barnett et al. 2002) and respondent age or life stage (Robert and Li 2001). The effect of deprived neighborhoods on health is mediated by individual deprivation status, and living in a deprived neighborhood appears to have the most negative health effects on poor individuals (Stafford and Marmot 2003), but adjustment for individual status often does not eliminate the effect of area disadvantage on health behaviors, intermediates, or outcomes.

Approaches to Analysis with Census Data

Area deprivation is multidimensional, composed of poverty, housing, employment, education, racial composition, and occupational domains. Despite its multidimensionality, single variable constructs are commonly used to approximate the deprivation environment. For instance, poverty is the socioeconomic construct employed most frequently in epidemiologic research, and its various forms include proportion of individuals or households below the federal poverty level, percent on public assistance, and percent of female-headed households with dependent children. If one is interested in testing a specific hypothesis about the association of poverty or education with a specific health outcome, the use of a single census item is clearly appropriate. If, however, one is interested in the broader issues of neighborhood deprivation, an index including multiple domains of disadvantage, which more accurately reflects the multidimensional character of community socioeconomic position (Singh 2003; Singh and Siahpush 2002; Singh et al. 2002), may be more appropriate.

Research in the United Kingdom represents an important model for approaching area-level assessment with local census data. There, established area-level indices such as the Townsend Material Deprivation Score and the Carstairs Deprivation Index are widely used, which allows for the comparison of deprivation effects across a variety of geographic regions. The Townsend Material Deprivation Score (Townsend et al. 1988), an area-level index composed of unemployment, overcrowding, and ownership of a car or a home, is the most widely used deprivation index and tends to be favored by health authorities. It has been applied in many studies, for example, to assess the effect of area deprivation on height, weight, and body mass index in two birth cohorts (Wright and Parker 2004). The Carstairs Deprivation Index, developed to study health outcomes in Scotland, is similar to the Townsend Index but replaces non-home ownership with a low social class variable (Carstairs and Morris 1989, 1991). It has been used to assess area-level deprivation and birth weight (Dolk et al. 2001) as well as a variety of other health outcomes. Other frequently employed indices include the Jarman Underprivileged Area Score 8 (Jarman 1983, 1984), the Department of the Environment's All Area Social Index, Scottish Development Department Index, Forrest and Gorden's Matdep (material deprivation) and Socdep (social deprivation) (Forrest and Gordon 1993), and the Department of the Environment's Index of Local Conditions (Department of Environment 1994). Because these indices are used regularly in the United Kingdom, their application and interpretation have become widely understood.

Research in the United States has thus far taken a less uniform approach when using census data to asses "neighborhood effects." As mentioned previously, the most common approach involves using single census variables, such as percent poverty, to represent the spectrum of deprivation for an area. Other research has combined multiple census variables, representing either one or multiple deprivation domains, using factor analysis (FA) or principal components analysis (PCA) methods. Principal components analysis and FA are data reduction techniques that assess underlying data structure by condensing a large number of variables into a smaller number of components or factors. The goal of PCA is to extract maximum variance from a data set by analyzing the total available variance. In contrast, FA seeks to uncover underlying factor structure by analyzing only the shared variance (or "communalities"). Researchers interested in a unique theoretical solution uncontaminated by error variability generally use FA, whereas those seeking an empirical data summary employ PCA (Statistica 2003; Tabachnick and Fidell 1996), but both methods take a similar data reduction approach. Both FA (Bell et al. 1998; James and Mustard 2004; Singh 2003; Wang and Luo 2005) and PCA (Buka et al. 2003; Ewing et al. 2003; Mares et al. 2005; Martens et al. 2002; Salmond et al. 1998; Singh et al. 2002; Stafford et al. 2005; Yost et al. 2001) have been widely used in health research to reduce census data.

Regardless of the data reduction approach employed, it is clearly advantageous for those who use census data, either with or without other sources of neighborhood data, to select a broad array of neighborhood characteristics rather than to focus on one or two variables. By broadly characterizing neighborhoods, researchers run less risk of misestimating neighborhood effects (Sampson et al. 2002).

Worked Example: Low Birth Weight and Neighborhood Deprivation

With census data from four sociodemographically diverse areas, this section will 1) outline a neighborhood deprivation index development process undertaken for use in perinatal and reproductive epidemiologic research and 2) demonstrate its utility in differentiating areas with adverse outcomes from those with normal birth outcomes across different geographies.

Methods

The Multilevel Modeling of Disparities Explaining Preterm Delivery (MODE-PTD) project is a collaborative partnership of four universities and their government health department partners, with the purpose of identifying policy-relevant contextual factors associated with infant and child health disparities to better inform state Maternal and Child Health officials of modifiable environmental factors for policy development and program planning.

Project Areas. Four university-health department partnerships representing eight study areas, including three urban centers (Philadelphia, Pennsylvania; Baltimore City, Maryland; and sixteen combined cities in Michigan), three racially heterogeneous Maryland counties near Washington, D.C., and two urban counties in

North Carolina participated in the deprivation index development process. Hereafter, each of these eight study areas will be referred to as a study "site."

Data Sources. Birth outcome and maternal characteristics were obtained from birth certificates for selected years between 1995 and 2001 (Table 9.1). Year 2000 Census of Population and Housing Data from the U.S. Census Bureau (2000)(70) representing the eight study sites were used to develop the deprivation index.

Unit of Analysis. *Neighborhood* is used here to refer to a person's immediate residential environment, which is hypothesized to have both material and social characteristics related to health (Diez-Roux 2001). Census tract data were chosen to maximize the precision and stability of area adverse birth outcome rates and still ensure a rough approximation of each woman's immediate physical neighborhood. Previous research has indicated that the largest statistical effect of economic disadvantage on low birth weight, among other outcomes, is observed at the block group and census tract levels. But effects of lesser magnitude at larger levels of aggregation, such as zip codes or counties (Krieger et al. 2003) are also evident.

Data Reduction Method. The MODE-PTD team postulated a domain or factor structure underlying many of the census variables used to estimate area-level disadvantage. Rather than reproduce this structure with FA, the team sought to produce a single summary index containing variables from multiple domains that could be used to empirically estimate "neighborhood deprivation." For this reason, PCA was chosen for index construction.

Variable Selection. Socioeconomic variables at the neighborhood level represent aspects of community stratification, opportunity structures, and social conditions (Berkman and Macintyre 1997; Krieger et al. 1997; Link and Phelan 1996; Singh 2003). The investigators first created a comprehensive, broadly conceptualized list of census variables to represent social class and stratification from seven broad deprivation domains: poverty, housing, employment, occupation, worker class, education, and racial heterogeneity. Variables were eliminated from inclusion in the PCA analysis if they showed limited variability across strata of adverse birth outcomes, were too redundant, or were gender-specific. Fifteen variables, including three housing, six income and poverty, two employment, one occupation, one worker class, one education, and one racial distribution, were retained for possible inclusion in the deprivation index.

Component Extraction and Interpretation. Although it is possible to form as many independent linear combinations as there are variables, the first principal

TABLE 9.1. MATERNAL CHARACTERISTICS IN THE ≥ TWENTY-YEAR-OLD NON-HISPANIC WHITE AND NON-HISPANIC BLACK VITAL RECORDS COHORT BY AREA.

Maternal Attributes n (%)	Baltimore, MD 1995–2001	Baltimore County, MD 1995–2001	Montgomery County, MD 1995–2001	Prince Geo. County, MD 1995–2001	MI-16 Cities 1995, 1998–1999	Durham County, NC 1999–2001	Wake County, NC 1999–2001	Philadelphia, PA 1999–2000
Total Births	41490	46578	52976	52335	69924	8200	24297	26593
PTB	5791 (14.0)	3816 (8.2)	3649 (6.9)	5180 (9.9)	7743 (11.1)	961 (11.7)	2022 (8.3)	2837 (10.7)
LBW	5100 (12.3)	2871 (6.2)	2689 (5.1)	4384 (8.4)	6848 (9.8)	737 (9.0)	1448 (5.7)	2412 (9.1)
NH Black	28723 (69.2)	11423 (24.5)	12520 (23.6)	38252 (75.0)	42210 (60.4)	4552 (53.3)	6536 (25.8)	15577 (58.6)
Age								
20–24	15011 (36.2)	88335 (19.0)	5128 (9.7)	11788 (22.5)	26365 (37.7)	1817 (23.7)	3865 (16.1)	8845 (33.3)
25–29	11829 (28.5)	14133 (30.3)	11880 (22.4)	15384 (29.4)	22522 (32.2)	2303 (30.1)	6849 (28.6)	7855 (29.5)
30–34	9106 (21.9)	15103 (32.4)	20482 (38.7)	15480 (29.6)	13879 (19.9)	2285 (29.8)	8402 (35.0)	6129 (23.0)
35+	5544 (13.4)	8507 (18.3)	15486 (29.3)	9683 (18.5)	7159 (10.2)	1260 (16.4)	4867 (20.3)	3764 (14.2)
Education								
<12 yrs	9300 (22.4)	2741 (5.9)	1501 (2.8)	2427 (4.6)	15084 (21.6)	812 (10.2)	1166 (4.8)	3939 (14.8)
=12 yrs	16712 (40.3)	14005 (30.1)	8180 (15.4)	17565 (33.6)	26471 (37.9)	1829 (23.1)	4615 (18.8)	11247 (42.3)
>12 yrs	15478 (37.3)	29832 (64.1)	43295 (81.7)	32343 (61.8)	28369 (40.6)	5292 (66.7)	18770 (76.5)	11407 (42.9)

Note: LBW = low birth weight (infant born weighing <2,500 grams); NH = non-Hispanic; PTB = preterm birth (birth at <37 weeks gestational age and <3,888 grams).

component is the unique linear combination that accounts for the largest possible proportion of the total variability in the component measures (Tabachnick and Fidell 1996). Of the fifteen variables considered for index inclusion, ten variables from four domains (poverty, housing, employment, and education) were included in the index because their loadings clustered between 0.2 and 0.4 and they made conceptual sense as constituting "deprivation," whereas the remaining five loaded at substantially lower levels (Table 9.2).

Index Construction. Item loadings from the first component were used to weight the contribution of each item to the summary score for neighborhood deprivation for each census tract. Each variable in the deprivation index is standardized with a mean of 0 and variance of 1, resulting in a weighted summed index with a median of −0.50, a mean of 0.00, and a standard deviation of 2.61. A deprivation index was created for the combined eight-site study sample, which accounted for 68 percent of the total all-site variance. The second component added only 7–10 percent to the explained variance and so was not used.

Variable and Study Population Definitions. Vital record birth outcome data were obtained from each site's state or city department of vital statistics for selected years between 1995 and 2001. Low birth weight, a crude birth outcome indicator of impaired fetal growth, shortened gestation, or both impaired growth and short gestation, was defined as birth at less than 2,500 grams. Less than 1 percent of records were missing birth weight data. Data analyses were restricted to singleton births, because multiple gestations often result in low birth weight even in otherwise normally progressing pregnancies. Analyses were further restricted to NH white and NH black births, owing to the limited number of births from other ethnic groups. Births for women under age twenty were excluded, because data were not available for all sites.

Statistical Analysis. Data reduction and PCA were performed with the Stata software package. Proportions of low birth weight deliveries were estimated for each quartile of the deprivation score with tabular analyses. The authors employed deprivation quartiles (with three indicator variables) to allow the dose response relations to take any arbitrary functional form and thus avoid linearity assumptions. Risk differences, 95 percent Confidence Intervals, and P-for-trend statistics were estimated. All analyses were race-stratified.

Results

Tracts were of varying population, ranging from a mean of 3,009 for Michigan 16-cities to 5,979 in Wake County, North Carolina (Table 9.3). The largest variation among sites was evident in the census socioeconomic descriptors. On

TABLE 9.2. SITE-SPECIFIC AND ALL-SITE FIRST PRINCIPAL COMPONENT SCORE LOADINGS FOR EACH MODE-PTD SITE.

Deprivation Index Variables	Baltimore, MD 200 Tracts	Baltimore Co., MD 204 Tracts	Montgomery Co., MD 177 Tracts	Prince Geo. Co., MD 183 Tracts	MI-16 Cities 607 Tracts	Durham Co., NC 53 Tracts	Wake Co., NC 105 Tracts	Philadelphia, PA 381 Tracts	All-Site 1908 Tracts
% Poverty	0.35	0.33	0.39	0.36	0.37	0.32	0.35	0.37	0.36
% FHHH	0.31	0.24	0.31	0.28	0.30	0.36	0.34	0.32	0.31
% < $30K	0.36	0.42	0.40	0.38	0.35	0.35	0.35	0.36	0.35
% Pub asst	0.33	0.31	0.28	0.26	0.33	0.34	0.33	0.34	0.33
% No car	0.36	0.34	0.35	0.36	0.30	0.35	0.30	0.33	0.31
% No phone	0.31	0.29	0.22	0.30	0.32	0.35	0.32	0.29	0.30
Costs > 50%	0.26	0.25	0.30	0.31	0.30	0.15	0.29	0.27	0.28
Med HH value	−0.24	−0.30	−0.24	−0.27	−0.24	−0.31	−0.23	−0.18	−0.26
% Unemp	0.32	0.33	0.31	0.32	0.32	0.22	0.31	0.34	0.33
% No HS ed	0.31	0.31	0.32	0.30	0.32	0.35	0.33	0.32	0.32
% Variance[a]	68.9%	49.4%	53.9%	58.0%	62.0%	55.9%	68.6%	65.4%	68.0%

Notes: % Poverty = percent of individuals with income in 1999 below the poverty level; % FHHH = percent of families with female-headed household with dependent children; % < $30K = percent of households with income less than $30,000; % Pub asst = percent households with public assistance income; % No car = percent households with no vehicle; % No phone = percent households with no telephone; Costs > 50% = households with rent or selected monthly owner costs exceeding 50% of income; Med HH value = median value of owner occupied unit; % Unemp = percent males and females unemployed; % No HS = percent males and females with no high school education.

[a]Percent total variance explained

TABLE 9.3. MEAN (SD) OF SOCIODEMOGRAPHIC DATA OF EACH MODE-PTD SITE, YEAR 2000 U.S. CENSUS DATA.

Variable Mean (SD)	Baltimore, MD 200 Tracts	Baltimore Co., MD 204 Tracts	Montgomery Co., MD 177 Tracts	Prince Geo. Co., MD 183 Tracts	MI-16 Cities 607 Tracts	Durham Co., NC 53 Tracts	Wake Co., NC 105 Tracts	Philadelphia, PA 381 Tracts
Tract pop[a]	3256 (1434)	3698 (1771)	4934 (1906)	4380 (1699)	3009 (1546)	4213 (2175)	5979 (3375)	3854 (2416)
% Poverty	24.5 (13.7)	7.1 (8.9)	5.4 (3.8)	7.9 (6.0)	24.9 (13.8)	17.4 (16.6)	9.8 (9.6)	22.1 (15.5)
% FHHH	14.5 (8.85)	6.3 (4.8)	5.4 (3.4)	11.1 (6.5)	25.2 (13.2)	17.4 (15.0)	11.0 (8.6)	19.0 (13.1)
% < $30K	51.3 (15.9)	27.1 (13.9)	14.6 (9.2)	21.8 (11.7)	50.5 (16.5)	40.4 (23.1)	26.2 (15.0)	47.0 (19.4)
% Pub asst	8.2 (6.0)	1.7 (1.9)	1.3 (1.2)	2.0 (1.8)	10.2 (6.9)	3.6 (5.1)	1.9 (2.6)	8.8 (8.6)
% No car	10.2 (6.6)	3.2 (2.6)	1.9 (1.6)	2.7 (1.8)	20.0 (14.1)	5.4 (5.7)	2.6 (4.4)	34.8 (20.2)
% No phone	1.1 (1.6)	0.2 (0.4)	0.1 (0.2)	0.2 (0.4)	6.8 (5.6)	2.6 (3.3)	1.5 (2.3)	2.7 (3.6)
Costs > 50%	17.8 (6.3)	10.2 (8.3)	9.3 (3.8)	11.1 (4.4)	16.8 (7.4)	16.0 (15.2)	10.3 (5.1)	17.1 (8.8)
Med HH Value ($)	70441 (44918)	137150 (65835)	250451 (126954)	140940 (34148)	66822 (45374)	109898 (51775)	167339 (65721)	72519 (70156)
% Unemp	12.4 (8.0)	4.5 (4.0)	3.2 (2.0)	5.8 (3.6)	12.5 (8.1)	7.2 (8.9)	4.5 (5.4)	11.1 (7.8)
% No HS	33.8 (13.3)	17.1 (11.4)	9.9 (8.3)	16.2 (9.9)	28.2 (13.7)	20.1 (14.4)	12.0 (9.8)	28.1 (15.0)
% White NH[a]	31.9 (33.3)	75.6 (25.9)	61.0 (20.2)	24.4 (22.7)	32.6 (32.8)	44.3 (30.2)	67.1 (23.8)	42.6 (36.6)

Notes: % White NH = percent white non-Hispanic; other abbreviations as in Table 9.2.

[a]Tract population not included in deprivation index.

average, Montgomery County, Maryland, had the wealthiest tracts according to the census characteristics: 14.6 percent of the population had income less than $30,000 compared with 51.3 percent of Baltimore city residents. The three most urban sites—Baltimore City, Philadelphia, and Michigan 16 cities—were characterized as the "most deprived," based on these sociodemographic indicators. The Michigan 16-city site appeared to be the poorest according to poverty-related indicators including, among others, percent poverty (24.9 percent) and percent of female-headed households with dependent children (25.2 percent). Philadelphia had the largest percentage of households with no vehicle (34.8 percent). Prince George's County, Maryland, had the lowest percentage of white NH population (24.4 percent) compared with Baltimore City, Maryland, with the highest proportion (75.6 percent) in these data. Thus, these eight urban and suburban regions demonstrated considerable socio-demographic variability.

Figure 9.2 graphically demonstrates the significant socioeconomic heterogeneity in the distribution of the all-site deprivation scores across the eight sites. Philadelphia had the largest range in deprivation scores, from −5.8 to 10.4, followed by Michigan-16 cities. Particularly noteworthy is Montgomery County, with deprivation index values ranging from −5.4 to −0.5. The majority of tracts in

FIGURE 9.2.   BOX PLOT OF ALL-SITE DEPRIVATION INDEX BY MODE-PTD SITE.

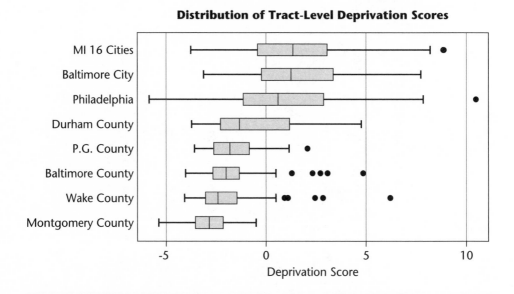

Distribution of Tract-Level Deprivation Scores

Durham, Prince George's, Wake, and Baltimore counties were at the affluent end of the all-site deprivation continuum, compared with the three most densely urban sites (Michigan 16-cities, Baltimore City, and Philadelphia), which had a greater representation of tracts at the more deprived end of the range.

Three important patterns emerged from the site-specific and all-site first principal component score loadings (Table 9.2). The first was the consistency *within each site* of variable loadings that comprised the first principal component, with values ranging from 0.2 to 0.4. These results suggest that each component contributed similarly to the empirical "neighborhood deprivation" summary score. Second, the component loadings were quite consistent *across the sites;* for instance, poverty loadings ranged from 0.3 to 0.4, despite significant geographic and sociodemographic variability. The consistency of the loadings across sites suggested these variables function similarly across geography, despite meaningful heterogeneity in demographics and economic status. Unemployment, for instance, made as important a contribution to deprivation in Philadelphia as it did in Durham County. The third important pattern emerging from these analyses was the consistency of the principal component loadings on the all-site deprivation score. The all-site weights were of similar magnitude to the site-specific weights. The all-site deprivation index represented a weighted average of the component variables from diverse geographic and socioeconomic sites, the loadings for which could be therefore reasonably applied to census variables from a variety of dissimilar areas to produce a comparable deprivation index.

A substantial number of births occurred during the study years at the eight sites (Table 9.1). The proportions of these births that were classified as having a low birth weight ranged from 5.1 percent to 12.3 percent. Baltimore City had the highest, whereas Montgomery County had the lowest proportions of adverse birth outcomes. The proportion of NH black women delivering singleton births varied across the sites, from 75 percent in Prince George's County to 25 percent in Baltimore County. Michigan had the fewest births to women ≥35 years of age (10.2 percent), whereas Montgomery County had the most (29.3 percent). Maternal education varied by site. Uniformly, the fewest singleton mothers obtained <12 years and the most obtained >12 years, but the relative percentages differed geographically. In Baltimore City, 22.4 percent of women received <12 years of education compared with 2.8 percent in Montgomery County. In Wake County, 76.5 percent of women had >12 years of schooling compared with 40.6 percent in Michigan.

Among white NH women, there was a gradient in the relationship between deprivation and birth outcomes: larger percentages of low birth weights (Table 9.4) occurred at higher levels of deprivation. For instance, Montgomery

TABLE 9.4. PERCENTAGE OF WHITE NON-HISPANIC LOW BIRTH WEIGHT (LBW; TOTAL NUMBER OF BIRTHS) AND Q4–Q1, Q3–Q1 RISK DIFFERENCES (RD; 95% CONFIDENCE INTERVALS [CI]) IN THE ≥ TWENTY-YEAR-OLD COHORT IN EACH QUARTILE (Q) OF DEPRIVATION BY MODE-PTD GEOGRAPHIC AREA.

All-Site Deprivation Index Quartiles	Baltimore, MD 1995–2001	Baltimore County, MD 1995–2001	Montgomery County, MD 1995–2001	Prince Geo. County, MD 1995–2001	MI - 16 Cities 1995, 1998–1999	Durham County, NC 1999–2001	Wake County, NC 1999–2001	Philadelphia, PA 1999–2000
Q1: −5.85–2.12	3.3 (1467)	4.0 (18797)	3.7 (34447)	4.1 (9305)	3.9 (4583)	4.1 (2559)	3.6 (14,962)	2.6 (734)
Q2: −2.12–0.50	4.7 (4414)	5.1 (13719)	4.3 (5829)	5.1 (3291)	4.8 (6695)	4.2 (1000)	4.9 (3074)	4.3 (5,732)
Q3: −0.50–1.97	7.4 (5063)	6.7 (2406)	5.0 (180)	5.2 (481)	5.8 (12129)	6.3 (192)	7.1 (239)	5.1 (3,238)
Q4: 1.98–10.45	9.8 (1823)	6.9 (231)	a	b	7.6 (4307)	b	b	7.3 (1,312)
P for trend	P < 0.001	P < 0.001	P = 0.023	P = 0.013	P < 0.001	P = 0.331	P < 0.001	P < 0.001
Q3–Q1 RD	4.1	2.7	1.3	1.1	1.9	2.2	3.5	2.5
95% CI	(2.9, 5.3)	(1.7, 3.7)	(−1.9, 4.5)	(−0.9, 3.1)	(1.2, 2.6)	(−1.3, 5.7)	(0.2, 6.8)	(1.1, 3.9)
Q4–Q1 RD	6.5	2.9	a	b	3.7	b	b	4.7
95% CI	(4.9, 8.1)	(−0.4, 6.2)			(2.7, 4.7)			(2.9, 6.5)
Percent LBW	6.4	4.7	3.8	4.4	5.5	4.3	3.9	4.8
(# LBW/Total)	(812/12767)	(1640/35153)	(1534/40456)	(574/13083)	(1526/27714)	(165/3826)	(712/18301)	(528/11016)

[a] no tracts fell into this deprivation quartile; [b] data not shown; fewer than 100 births in deprivation quartile.

County, the most affluent of the sites, had low birth weight percentages that ranged from 3.7 percent to 5.0 percent in the first to third quartiles of deprivation (no Montgomery County tracts fell into the fourth quartile of all-site deprivation). In more deprived areas, these rates were similar; for example, the low birth weight percentages in the Michigan-16 cities site increased from 3.9 percent to 5.8 percent. Risk differences were estimated for the contrasts of low birth weight proportions for women living in quartiles four or three compared with those living in the lowest quartile of deprivation. Across the sociodemographically diverse sites, the relationship between adverse birth outcomes and neighborhood deprivation appeared consistent among white NH women.

The relationship between deprivation and low birth weight for black NH women was less clear (Table 9.5). Whereas the low birth weight percentages in the highest quartile of deprivation were consistently large, high risk of low birth weight throughout the continuum was apparent. For instance, Philadelphia ranged from 8.1 percent to 13.5 percent low birth weight in the first compared with fourth quartile. The relationship between deprivation and adverse birth outcomes among black NH women in these data was not as consistent with the hypothesized pattern of monotonically increasing risk.

Summary of Findings

Literature posits that the Weberian dimensions of class, status, and party (or power), contemporarily operationalized as occupation, education, and income, are differentially distributed and may influence opportunities for health and well-being (Liberatos et al. 1988). In the absence of direct measures of "status" and related concepts, research in epidemiology has struggled with how best to approximate these constructs at individual and area levels. By finding consistent loadings on the first principal component both within site and across each of the eight sites, this work provides insight into the relative importance of each of the components to the concept of "deprivation," despite significant sociodemographic and economic heterogeneity across the geographic units. The index was further able to differentiate between areas of higher and lower low birth weight risks for white and, to a lesser extent, for black NH women, confirming previous findings on the association of deprivation and adverse birth outcomes (Buka et al. 2003; Kogan 1995; Kramer 1987; O'Campo et al 1997; Parker et al. 1994; Pearl et al. 2001; Rauh et al. 2001; Roberts 1997; Wilcox et al. 1995). Ongoing work considers the relative utility of the deprivation index compared with single-variable associations with adverse birth outcomes.

TABLE 9.5. PERCENTAGE OF BLACK NON-HISPANIC LOW BIRTH WEIGHT (LBW; TOTAL NUMBER OF BIRTHS) AND Q3–Q1, Q4–Q1 RISK DIFFERENCES (RD; 95% CONFIDENCE INTERVALS [CI]) IN THE ≥ TWENTY-YEAR-OLD COHORT IN EACH QUARTILE (Q) OF DEPRIVATION BY MODE-PTD GEOGRAPHIC AREA.

All-Site Deprivation Index Quartiles	Baltimore, MD 1995–2001	Baltimore County, MD 1995–2001	Montgomery County, MD 1995–2001	Prince Geo. County, MD 1995–2001	MI-16 Cities 1995, 1998–1999	Durham County, NC 1999–2001	Wake County, NC 1999–2001	Philadelphia, PA 1999–2000
Q1: −5.85–2.12	a	9.8 (2639)	9.1 (6331)	8.8 (14675)	10.9 (697)	12.5 (861)	9.2 (2686)	8.1 (160)
Q2: −2.12–0.50	12.3 (2930)	11.1 (6540)	9.3 (5799)	10.0 (16193)	10.9 (3727)	12.0 (1494)	11.2 (1960)	9.8 (1,721)
Q3: −0.50–1.97	13.7 (10774)	10.5 (2009)	9.7 (390)	10.7 (8072)	12.0 (15961)	13.5 (974)	12.3 (1055)	10.4 (4,733)
Q4: 1.98–10.45	16.3 (14938)	14.8 (236)	b	11.2 (312)	13.5 (21825)	14.7 (1045)	14.2 (522)	13.5 (8,963)
P for trend	P < 0.001	P = 0.077	P = 0.696	P < 0.001	P < 0.001	P = 0.069	P < 0.001	P < 0.001
Q3–Q1 RD	a	0.7	0.6	1.9	1.1	1.0	3.1	2.3
95% CI	a	(−1.1, 2.5)	(−2.4, 3.6)	(1.1, 2.7)	(−1.3, 3.5)	(−2.1, 4.1)	(0.8, 5.4)	(−2.0, 6.6)
Q4–Q1 RD	a	5.0	b	2.4	2.6	2.2	5.0	5.4
95% CI		(0.3, 9.7)		(−1.1, 5.9)	(0.2, 5.0)	(−0.9, 5.3)	(1.8, 8.2)	(1.1, 9.7)
Percent LBW	14.9	10.8	9.2	9.7	12.6	13.1	10.8	12.1
(# LBW/Total)	(4288/28723)	(1231/11424)	(1155/12520)	(3810/39252)	(5322/42210)	(572/4374)	(671/6223)	(1884/15577)

[a] data not shown; fewer than 100 births in deprivation quartile; [b] no tracts fell into this deprivation quartile.

Limitations of Using Census Data to Estimate Deprivation

Using census data to approximate neighborhood-level exposures can be problematic in several ways. Using geographically defined data in the absence of solid theory or proposed mechanisms can result in the modifiable areal unit problem (MAUP). The MAUP arises from the imposition of artificial units of spatial reporting on continuous geographical phenomenon, resulting in the generation of artificial spatial patterns (Heywood 1998). Area-level data must be contained within recognized boundaries to be useful. For instance, knowing that a specific household is below the poverty line is less useful for population research than knowing the proportion of households within a given geographic space that are under the poverty line. Socioeconomic and epidemiologic analyses select and use artificial boundaries regularly, but it is precisely this practice that generates the MAUP (Oliver 2001).

The MAUP describes two effects that influence statistical and epidemiological results: scale and aggregation effects. The scale effect produces different statistical results by altering the denominator within the same dataset (Armhein 1995). For instance, imagine the nine boxes in Figure 9.3 as indicating the preterm birth percentages for each block group and those in Figure 9.4 indicating the preterm

FIGURE 9.3. BLOCK GROUP PRETERM BIRTH PROPORTIONS.

10	15	15
6	10	15
6	6	10
Mean = 10.33; N = 9		

FIGURE 9.4. CENSUS TRACT PRETERM BIRTH PROPORTIONS.

7.33	10.33	13.33
Mean = 10.33; N = 3		

birth proportions for the census tracts. The block groups with high preterm birth are clustered and separated from block groups characterized by lower rates of preterm birth. In this example, although the overall mean remains the same, much of the variability in the preterm birth proportions is obscured by the tract-level grouping.

The aggregation or zoning effect arises from variability in the way units can be grouped at a given scale (Armhein 1995). For instance, using the same preterm birth proportions from Figure 9.3, differences in adverse birth outcome rates can be observed by grouping outcomes by postal zip code (Figure 9.6) compared with grouping them by metropolitan statistical areas (MSA) (Figure 9.5), despite the same number of adverse birth events being used in the calculation of both numerators.

Although generally viewed as a problem, the multiple levels for which census data are available can also be seen as substantive opportunity for exploring the relationships between scales using multilevel modeling methods (Subramanian et al. 2001). Because different exposure effects will be observed at various units of aggregation, it is important to choose the unit of geographic aggregation that best corresponds to the proposed exposure level. For instance, assessing the mortality prevention effect of motorcycle helmet laws will be most appropriately done at the state level, where the laws are made and implementation is enforced, whereas

FIGURE 9.5.   MSA PRETERM BIRTH PROPORTIONS.

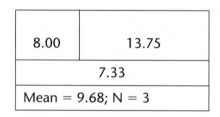

FIGURE 9.6.   ZIP CODE PRETERM BIRTH PROPORTIONS.

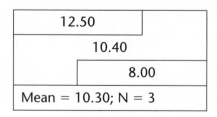

school performance and lead paint exposure research can conceivably be conducted at a smaller level of aggregation.

Other limitations to using decennial census data include their inability to capture the rapidly changing nature of geographic areas in transition. Census data are collected every ten years, but neighborhood environments can change over a very short period of time. These changes will not be reflected in research using census data, but use of the American Community Survey may reduce this limitation. Because census data are produced by aggregating individual level responses, they are not reflective of contextual features of neighborhoods. Increasingly, research suggests that important neighborhood characteristics exist, such as the presence of resources, the nature of social interactions, the quality of shared space, and the investments in infrastructure and community life, that can not be assessed with aggregated individual level data (Cummins et al. 2005; Yen and Syme 1999). Furthermore, census variables and their definitions have changed over time, and their specific meaning can vary by state or region. This temporal and geographic variability reduces researcher's ability to compare data from multiple censuses.

Census variables are often highly correlated with each other. Making inferences based on the inclusion of one census variable in a model, for example finding an "employment effect," while not simultaneously considering the remaining constellation of factors that contribute to the neighborhood sociodemographic environment risks producing incomplete or inappropriate conclusions. Moreover, the highly correlated nature of census data may often result in findings that are not easily translated into policy recommendations.

Research using census data to approximate neighborhood effects is inherently limited in its ability to address causality or mechanistic hypotheses (Macintyre et al. 2002). Several pathways through which deprived environments may affect health have been suggested in the literature and include: increased stress, allostatic load, and weathering (Fremont and Bird 2000; Geronimus 1992; Geronimus et al. 1996; McEwen 2000; Taylor et al. 1997); decreased social relations or collective efficacy (Berkman 1995; Fullilove et al. 1998; Sampson 2003; Sampson and Raudenbush 1999; Sampson et al. 2002); decreased physical activity (Cohen et al. 2003; Ross and Mirowsky 2001); and resource limitation. Nonetheless, these mechanisms have been explored minimally to date. Innovative research strategies including systematic social observation (Caughy et al. 2001; Cohen et al. 2000; Laraia et al., "Direct observation of neighborhood attributes in an urban area of the US south," *International Journal of Health Geographics* [in press]) and qualitative work (Burke et al. 2005) promise to shed new light on the mechanisms through which neighborhood environments influence health intermediates and outcomes.

Although there can be no consensus about the definition of neighborhoods in any general sense, census information is often used as a convenient means to delineate a geographically defined neighborhood. In some regions, block groups are a good approximation of such neighborhoods—particularly in areas with relatively low population density. In more densely populated areas, however, neighborhood may be better estimated using larger geographies, like census tracts or clusters of census tracts (as is done in the Project on Human Development in Chicago Neighborhoods [PHDN]). Additionally, census boundaries are arbitrary and may have little correspondence with the socially defined spaces that would be recognized and understood as "neighborhoods" by the residents themselves. Therefore, administratively defined neighborhoods are often unlikely to be the most salient demarcations for individual health and well-being that we seek to understand when researching "neighborhood effects" on health (O'Campo 2003).

The decennial census attempts to be a total enumeration of the United States population, a largely impossible task. Population subgroups that are likely to be undercounted by the U.S. Census include children, renters (particularly in rural areas), racial and ethnic minorities (Rosenthal 2000), homeless persons, non-English-speaking people, individuals who distrust the government, and those who are mobile or were in transition during the census period. The differential census undercount of potentially vulnerable populations has important implications for social epidemiological research and is an important limitation in using these data.

Benefits of Using Census Data to Estimate Deprivation

Despite its limitations, using census data to approximate neighborhood effects, including those associated with neighborhood deprivation, will continue to be a common exposure assessment tool. Nationwide, census data are collected through a regular and systematic process and recorded with considerable accuracy. Substantial efforts are made by the U.S. government to obtain a legitimate census and assess population or geographic regions where inaccuracies are suspected (Rosenthal 2000). Census data are free and easily accessible to researchers, which makes them a logical data source for exposure or covariate variables.

Because census data are collected every decade, they are an important source of longitudinal data on the U.S. population. Until fairly recently, changing tract or block group numbers made linking data from multiple censuses difficult. For instance, a tract identified in the year 2000 census may not have existed previously, or a block group identified in previous years may have been incorporated into another tract and no longer exists in the year 2000 census, owing to population decline. Various companies have recently developed a variety of tools to address these problems and enable linking census data over decades to facilitate longitudinal analyses.

Summary

Using census data to approximate neighborhood effects continues to be an important method for social epidemiology. No other data source parallels the depth of geographic and temporal coverage provided by the U.S. Census. Having data available at multiple units of aggregation allows research to consider many levels of influence on individual and population health. Multiple approaches to reducing and analyzing census data have been used with considerable success. Although not without limitations, census data are likely to remain an important data source for sociodemographically characterizing places and estimating neighborhood effects.

References

Armhein, C. (1995). Searching for the elusive aggregation effect: Evidence from statistical simulations. *Environment & Planning, 27,* 105.

Barnett, S., Roderick, P., Martin, D., Diamond, I., & Wrigley, H. (2002). Interrelations between three proxies of health care need at the small area level: An urban/rural comparison. *Journal of Epidemiology and Community Health, 56,* 754–761.

Barry, J., & Breen, N. (2005). The importance of place of residence in predicting late-stage diagnosis of breast or cervical cancer. *Health and Place, 11,* 15–29.

Bell, D., Carlson, J., & Richard, A. (1998). The social ecology of drug use: A factor analysis of an urban environment. *Substance Use and Misuse, 33,* 2207–2217.

Berkman, L., & Macintyre, S. (1997). The measurement of social class in health studies: Old measures and new formulations. In M. Kogevinas, N. Pearce, M. Susser, & P. Bofetta (Eds.), *Social inequalities in cancer* (pp. 51–64). Lyon, FR: International Agency for Research on Cancer.

Berkman, L. F. (1995). The role of social relations in health promotion. *Psychosomatic Medicine, 57,* 245–254.

Blakely, T., Lochner, K., & Kawachi I. (2002). Metropolitan area income inequality and self-rated health—A multi-level study. *Social Science & Medicine, 54,* 65–77.

Borrell, L., Roux, A., Rose, K., Catellier, D., & Clark, B. (2004). Neighborhood characteristics and mortality in the artherosclerosis risk in communities study. *International Journal of Epidemiology, 33,* 398–407.

Buka, S. L., Brennan, R. T., Rich-Edwards, J. W., Raudenbush, S. W., & Earls, F. (2003). Neighborhood support and the birth weight of urban infants. *American Journal of Epidemiology, 157,* 1–8.

Burke, J., O'Campo, P., Peak, G., Gielen, A., McDonnell, K., & Trochim, W. (2005). An introduction to concept mapping as a participatory public health research methodology. *Qualitative Health Research, 15*(10), 1392–1410.

Carstairs, V., & Morris, R. (1989). Deprivation, mortality and resource allocation. *Community Medicine, 11,* 364–372.

Carstairs, V., & Morris, R. (1991). *Deprivation and health in Scotland.* Aberdeen, UK: Aberdeen University Press.

Caughy, M., O'Campo, P., & Patterson, J. (2001). A brief observational measure for urban neighborhoods. *Health and Place, 7,* 225–236.

Cohen, D., Spear, S., Scribner, R., Kissinger, P., Mason, K., & Wildgen, J. (2000). "Broken windows" and the risk of gonorrhea. *American Journal of Public Health, 90,* 230–236.

Cohen, D. A., Farley, T. A., & Mason, K. (2003). Why is poverty unhealthy? Social and physical mediators. *Social Science and Medicine, 57,* 1631–1641.

Cooper, R. (2001). Social inequality, ethnicity and cardiovascular disease. *International Journal of Epidemiology, 30,* S48–S52.

Cummins, S., Macintyre, S., Davidson, S., & Ellaway, A. (2005). Measuring neighbourhood social and material context: Generation and interpretation of ecological data from routine and non-routine sources. *Health and Place, 11,* 249–260.

Cunradi, C., Caetano, R., Clark, C., & Schafer, J. (2000). Neighborhood poverty as a predictor of intimate partner violence among white, black and Hispanic couples in the United States: A multilevel analysis. *Annals of Epidemiology, 10,* 297–308.

Department of Environment (1994). *Index of Local Conditions: An analysis based on 1991 Census Data.* London: Author.

Diez-Roux, A. V. (2001). Investigating neighborhood and area effects on health. *American Journal of Public Health, 91,* 1783–1789.

Dolk, H., Pattendon, S., & Johnson, A. (2001). Cerebral palsy, low birthweight and socioeconomic deprivation: Inequalities in a major cause of childhood disability. *Paediatric and Perinatal Epidemiology, 15,* 359–363.

Ewing, R., Schmid, T., Killingsworth, R., Zlot, A., & Raudenbush, S. (2003). Relationship between urban sprawl and physical activity, obesity, and morbidity. *American Journal of Health Promotion, 18,* 47–57.

Finch, B., Kolody, B., & Vega, W. (1999). Contextual effects of perinatal substance exposure among black and white women in California. *Sociological Perspectives, 42,* 141–156.

Forrest, R., & Gordon, D. (1993). *People and places: A 1991 census atlas of England.* Bristol, UK: SAUS.

Fremont, A. M., & Bird, C. E. (2000). Social and psychological factors, physiological processes and physical health. In C. E. Bird, P. Conrad, & A. M. Fremont (Eds.), *The Handbook of Medical Sociology* (pp. 334–352). Upper Saddle River, NJ: Prentice Hall.

Fullilove, M., Heon, V., Jimenez, W., Parsons, C., Green, I., & Fullilove, R. (1998). Injury and anomie: Effects of violence on an inner-city community. *American Journal of Public Health, 88,* 924–927.

Galea, S., Ahern, J., Vlahov, D., et al. (2003). Income distribution and risk of fatal drug overdose in New York City neighborhoods. *Drug and Alcohol Dependence, 70,* 139–148.

Geronimus, A. (1992). The weathering hypothesis and the health of African-American women and infants: Evidence and speculations. *Ethnicity and Disease, 2,* 207–221.

Geronimus A., Bound J., Waidmann T., Hillemeier M., Burns P. (1996). Excess mortality among blacks and whites in the United States. *New England Journal of Medicine, 335,* 1552–1558.

Gjelsvik, A., Zierler, S., & Blume, J. (2004). Homicide risk across race and class: A small area analysis in Massachusetts and Rhode Island. *Journal of Urban Health, 81,* 702–718.

Grisso, J., Schwarz, D., Hirschinger, N., Sammel, M., Brensinger, C., Santanna, J., et al. (1999). Violent injuries among women in an urban area. *New England Journal of Medicine, 341,* 1899–1905.

Hall, S., Ricketts, T., & Kaufman, J. (forthcoming). Measuring urban and rural areas in epidemiologic studies. *Journal of Urban Health.*

Hart, G., Larson, E., & Lishner, D. (2005). Rural definitions for health policy and research. *American Journal of Public Health, 95,* 1149–1155.

Heywood (1998). *Introduction to geographical information systems.* New York: Addison Wesley Longman.

James, R., & Mustard, C. (2004). Geographic location of commercial plasma donation clinics in the United States, 1980–1995. *American Journal of Public Health, 94,* 1224–1229.

Jarman, B. (1983). Identification of underprivileged areas. *British Medical Journal, 283,* 1705–1709.

Jarman, B. (1984). Underprivileged areas: Validation and distribution of scores. *British Medical Journal, 289,* 1587–1592.

Klassen, A., Curriero, F., Hong, J., Williams, C., Kulldorff, M., Meissner, H. I., et al. (2004). The role of area-level influences on prostate cancer grade and stage at diagnosis. *Preventive Medicine, 39,* 441–448.

Kramer, M. (1987). Determinants of low birth weight: Methodological assessment and meta-analysis. *Bulletin of the World Health Organization, 65,* 663–737.

Krieger, N., Chen, J., Waterman, P., Soobader, M-J., Subramanian, S., & Carson, R. (2003). Choosing area based socioeconomic measures to monitor social inequalities in low birth weight and childhood lead poisoning: The Public Health Disparities Geocoding Project (U.S.). *Journal of Epidemiology and Community Health, 57,* 186–199.

Krieger, N., Williams, D., & Moss, N. (1997). Measuring social class in U.S. public health research: Concepts, methodologies and guidelines. *Annual Review of Public Health, 18,* 341–378.

Kogan, M. (1995). Social causes of low birth weight. *Journal of the Royal Society of Medicine, 88,* 611–615.

Laraia, B. A., Messer, L., Kaufman, J. S., Caughy, M. O., O'Campo, P. O., Dole, N., & Savitz, D. A. (forthcoming). Direct observation of neighborhood attributes in an urban area of the U.S. south. *International Journal of Health Geographics* 2006.

Liberatos, P., Link, B. G., & Kelsey, J. L. (1988). The measurement of social class in epidemiology. *Epidemiologic Reviews, 10,* 87–121.

Link, B., & Phelan, J. (1996). Understanding sociodemographic differences in health: The role of fundamental social causes. *American Journal of Public Health, 86,* 471–473.

Macintyre S., Ellaway A., & Cummins S. (2002). Place effects on health: How can we conceputalise, operationalise and measure them? *Social Science & Medicine, 55,* 125–139.

Mares, A., Desai, R., & Rosenheck, R. (2005). Association between community and client characteristics and subjective measures of the quality of housing. *Psychiatric Service, 56,* 315–319.

Martens, P., Frohlich, N., Carriere, K., Derksen, S., & Brownell, M. (2002). Embedding child health within a framework of regional health: Population health status and sociodemographic indicators. *Canadian Journal of Public Health, 93,* S15–S20.

McEwen, B. S. (2000). Allostasis and allostatic load: Implications for neuropsychopharmacology. *Neuropsychopharmacology, 22,* 108–124.

Mellor, J., & Milyo, J. (2003). Is exposure to income inequality a public health concern? Lagged effects of income inequality on individual and population health. *Health Services Research, 38*, 137–151.

Messer, L. C., Kaufman, J. S., Dole, N., Savitz, D. A., & Laraia, B. A. (2006). Neighborhood crime, deprivation, and preterm birth. *Annals of Epidemiology, November 10 e-publication.*

Morenoff, J. D. (2003). Neighborhood mechanisms and the spatial dynamics of birthweight. *American Journal of Sociology, 108*, 976–1017.

O'Campo, P. (2003). Invited commentary: Advancing theory and methods for multilevel models of residential neighborhoods and health. *American Journal of Epidemiology, 157*, 9–13.

O'Campo, P., Rao, R., Gielen, A., Royalty, W., & Wilson, M. (2000). Injury-producing events among children in low-income communities: The role of community characteristics. *Journal of Urban Health, 77*, 34–49.

O'Campo, P., Xue, S., Wang, M-C., & Caughy, M. (1997). Neighborhood risk factors for low birth weight in Baltimore: A multilevel analysis. *American Journal of Public Health, 87*, 1113–1118.

Oliver L. (2001). Shifting boundaries, shifting results: The modifiable areal unit problem.

Parker, J., Schoendorf, K., & Kiely, J. (1994). Associations between measures of socioeconomic status and low birth weight, small for gestational age, and premature delivery in the United States. *Annals of Epidemiology, 4*, 271–278.

Patel, K., Eschbach, K., Rudkin, L., Peek, M., & Markides, K. (2003). Neighborhood context and self-rated health in older Mexican Americans. *Annals of Epidemiology, 13*, 620–628.

Pearl, M., Braveman, P., & Abrams, B. (2001). The relationship of neighborhood socioeconomic characteristics to birthweight among five ethnic groups in California. *American Journal of Public Health, 91*, 1808–1814.

Rauh, V., Andrews, H., & Garfinkel, R. (2001). The contribution of maternal age to racial disparities in birthweight: A multilevel perspective. *American Journal of Public Health. 2001, 91*, 1815–1824.

Robbins, J., & Webb, D. (2004). Neighborhood poverty mortality rates, and excess deaths among African Americans: Philadelphia 1999–2001. *Journal of Health Care for the Poor and Underserved, 15*, 530–537.

Robert, S., & Li, L. (2001). Age variation in the relationship between community socioeconomic status and adult health. *Research on Aging, 23*, 233–258.

Roberts, E. M. (1997). Neighborhood social environments and the distribution of low birthweight in Chicago. *American Journal of Public Health, 87*, 597–603.

Rosenthal, M. D. (2000). Striving for perfection: A brief history of advances and undercounts in the U.S. Census. *Government Information Quarterly, 17*, 193–208.

Ross, C. E., & Mirowsky, J. (2001). Neighborhood disadvantage, disorder and health. *Journal of Health and Social Behavior, 42*, 258–276.

Ruggles, S., Sobek, M., Alexander, T., et al. (2004). *Integrated public use microdata series* (Version 3.0). Minneapolis: Minnesota Population Center.

Salmond, C., Crampton, P., & Sutton, F. (1998). NZDep91: A New Zealand index of deprivation. *Australia New Zealand Journal of Public Health, 22*, 835–837.

Sampson R. (2003). The neighborhood context of well-being. *Perspectives in Biology and Medicine, 46*, S53–S64.

Sampson, R. J., & Raudenbush, S. W. (1999). Systematic social observation of public spaces: A new look at disorder in urban neighborhoods. *American Journal of Sociology, 105,* 603–651.

Sampson, R. J., Morenoff, J. D., & Gannon-Rowley, T. (2002). Assessing "neighborhood effects": social processes and new directions in research. *Annual Review of Sociology, 28,* 443–478.

Singh, G., & Siahpush, M. (2002). Increasing inequalities in all-cause and cardiovascular mortality among U.S. adults aged 25–64 years by area socioeconomic status, 1969–1998. *International Journal of Epidemiology, 31,* 600–613.

Singh, G., Miller, B., Hankey, B., Feuer, F., & Pickle, L. (2002). Changing area socioeconomic patterns in U.S. cancer mortality, 1950–1998: Part 1—All cancers among men. *Journal of the National Cancer Institute, 94,* 904–915.

Singh, G. K. (2003). Area deprivation and widening inequalities in U.S. mortality, 1969–1998. *American Journal of Public Health, 93,* 1137–1143.

Shenassa, E., Stubbendick, A., & Brown, M. (2004). Social disparities in housing and related pediatric injury: A multilevel study. *American Journal of Public Health, 94,* 633–639.

Stafford, M., & Marmot, M. (2003). Neighbourhood deprivation and health: Does it affect us all equally? *International Journal of Epidemiology, 32,* 357–366.

Stafford, M., Cummins, S., Macintyre, S., Ellaway, A., & Marmot, M. (2005). Gender differences in the associations between health and neighbourhood environment. *Social Science and Medicine, 60,* 1681–1692.

Statistica (2003). Principal components and factor analysis. In *StatSoft Electronic Textbook.* Retrieved March 16, 2005 from http://www.statsoft.com/textbook/stfacan.html.

Subramanian, S., Duncan, C., & Jones, K. (2001). Multilevel perspectives on modeling census data. *Environment and Planning, 33,* 399–417.

Tabachnick, B. G., & Fidell, L. S. (1996). *Using Multivariate Statistics* (chap. 13, pp. 635–708). Northridge: California State University, Harper Collins College.

Taylor, S., Repetti, R. L., & Seeman, T. (1997). Health psychology: What is an unhealthy environment and how does it get under the skin? *Annual Review of Psychology, 48,* 411–447.

Townsend, P., Phillimore, P., & Beattie, A. (1988). *Health and deprivation: Inequality and the North.* London: Croom Helm.

United States Census Bureau (1994). Geographical areas reference manual. Washington, DC: Department of Commerce.

United States Census Bureau (2000a). Appendix A. Census 2000 geographic terms and concepts. U.S. Census Bureau. Accessed on March 16, 2005, from http://www.census.gov/geo/www/tiger/glossry2.pdf

United States Census Bureau (2000b). Census 2000 final response rates: Public Information Office. Accessed June 3, 2005, from http://www.census.gov/dmd/www/response/2000response.html

Wang, F., & Luo, W. (2005). Assessing spatial and nonspatial factors for healthcare access: Towards an integrated approach to defining health professional shortage areas. *Health and Place, 11,* 131–146.

Welte, J., Wierczorek, W., Barnes, G., Tidwell, M., & Hoffman, J. (2004). The relationship of ecological and geographic factors to gambling. *Journal of Gambling Studies, 20,* 405–423.

Wilcox, M., Smith, S., Johnson, I., Maynard, P., & Chilvers, C. (1995). The effect of social deprivation on birthweight, excluding physiological and pathological effects. *British Journal of Obstetrics and Gynaecology, 102,* 918–924.

Wright, C., & Parker, L. (2004). Forty years on: The effect of deprivation on growth in two Newcastle birth cohorts. *International Journal of Epidemiology, 33,* 147–152.

Yen, I., & Syme, S. (1999). The social environment and health: A discussion of the epidemiologic literature. *Annual Review of Public Health, 20,* 287–308.

Yost, K., Perkins, C., Cohen, R., Morris, C., & Wright, W. (2001). Socioeconomic status and breast cancer incidence in California for different race/ethnic groups. *Cancer Causes and Control, 12,* 703–711.

Zierler, S., Krieger, N., Tang, Y., Coady, W., Siegfried, E., DeMaria, A., et al. (2000). Economic deprivation and AIDS incidence in Massachusetts. *American Journal of Public Health, 90,* 1064–1073.

PART THREE

DESIGN AND ANALYSIS

PART THREE

DESIGN AND ANALYSIS

CHAPTER TEN

COMMUNITY-BASED PARTICIPATORY RESEARCH: RATIONALE AND RELEVANCE FOR SOCIAL EPIDEMIOLOGY

Paula M. Lantz, Barbara A. Israel,
Amy J. Schulz, and Angela Reyes

Community-based participatory research (or CBPR) is an approach to research that consciously blurs the line between researchers and the "researched" (Gaventa 1981) or makes research "subjects" more than mere "objects" of research (Green and Mercer 2001). Community-based participatory research is a collaborative approach to research that engages partners from a community—geographic or otherwise defined—in all phases of the research process, with a shared goal of producing knowledge that will be translated into action or positive social change for the community (Green et al. 1997; Israel et al. 1998). In the realm of public health, CBPR efforts often focus on improving community health status or reducing social disparities in health or both (Israel et al. 1998). As such, CBPR is critically

The authors wish to acknowledge the contributions of the members of the Detroit Community-Academic Urban Research Center (URC), which was established in 1995 as part of the Urban Research Initiative of the CDC. The Detroit URC is a collaboration between the University of Michigan Schools of Public Health, Nursing, and Social Work; the Detroit Department of Health and Wellness Promotion; the Henry Ford Health System; and a number of community-based organizations including Communities in Schools, Community Health and Social Services, Detroit Hispanic Development Corporation, Detroiters Working for Environmental Justice, Friends of Parkside, Latino Family Services, Southwest Counseling and Development Services, and Warren/Conner Development Coalition. The authors also express gratitude to Sue Anderson for her assistance in the preparation of this chapter.

important to social epidemiology and its goal of identifying, understanding, and modifying the social determinants of health in populations.

Community-based participatory research has a long history as a research approach that aims to improve the well-being of people and their communities; it is not a new concept or approach (Freire 1970, 1973; Wallerstein and Duran 2003). Nonetheless, CBPR is receiving renewed attention in public health research and practice (O'Fallon and Dearry 2002). For example, the Institute of Medicine recently named CBPR as one of eight new competency areas essential for breadth in public health training (Viswanathan et al. 2004). Community-based participatory research is often discussed in the context of intervention or evaluation research (involving both experimental and quasi-experimental designs), where community members are fully engaged in the identification of a problem and the design and evaluation of potential interventions. As in the following description, however, CBPR has also been used to address basic research questions. As such, social epidemiologists engaged in observational research regarding health disparities and the social determinants of health can draw from the principles and processes of CBPR in their work as well.

In this chapter, we provide an overview of CBPR and its relevance to social epidemiology as a critical subfield of public health. We begin by defining CBPR and presenting an overview of what has been written about CBPR "principles" (or characteristics, grounded in theory and practice, about the way in which this approach to research ought to proceed). We then discuss the relevance of CBPR to social epidemiology, including what to consider when deciding whether or not to use a CBPR approach in a particular research endeavor. Next, we present some general guidance regarding the process of CBPR, including a discussion of some common challenges and facilitating factors that have been learned by those engaged in this type of work. Finally, we conclude by offering our perspective on some key issues and debates regarding CBPR in public health research.

Definition and Principles of CBPR

There are many partnership approaches to research in different disciplines variously referred to as "action research" (Reason and Bradbury 2001; Stringer 1996), "participatory research" (deKoning and Martin 1996; Green et al. 1995; Hall 1992; Park 1993; Tandon 1996), "participatory action research" (Whyte 1991), and "participatory community research" (Jason et al. 2004). Although these approaches have their differences, they all emphasize conducting research that actively involves members of the group or community being studied in the research process. Within the field of public health, the term "community-based participatory research" has been used increasingly to represent such collaborative approaches to research. Whereas there is no one definition, in our work we have defined CBPR as a partnership approach to research that equitably involves diverse partners (for example, academic researchers, health professionals, community members) in all steps of the research process, with all partners contributing their expertise, and in which influence, decision making, and ownership is shared (Israel et al. 1998, 2003). The overall goal of CBPR is to both increase knowledge and understanding of a given phenomenon (that is, address basic research questions) *and* to apply the knowledge gained to guide the development of interventions, policy, and social change aimed at improving the health of community members (Israel et al. 1998, 2003, 2005a). The term "participatory" is critical to this approach. It emphasizes the participatory processes involved and differentiates CBPR from other forms of community research, where the community is seen as a setting for conducting research but not an active partner in the process.

There is no one set of principles that will be applicable for all CBPR partnerships. Rather, the process of determining core values and principles that will guide collaborative efforts is essential in the development of individual partnerships. Recognizing this, we present the following synthesis of nine CBPR principles that have been discussed in the literature as useful for partnerships seeking to balance power and influence, research and practice. These principles reflect considerable experience in conducting participatory forms of research and are offered to help inform other partnerships as they develop sets of principles that are applicable to their unique contexts. The nine principles are summarized in Table 10.1 and explicated here (see Israel et al. 1998, 2003, and 2005a for more detailed examinations and discussions).

1. *Community-based participatory research recognizes community as a unit of identity.* The concept of units of identity refers to membership in, for example, a family, group, social network, or geographic neighborhood, and recognizes the importance of sense of identity with these units, which is created and recreated through social interactions (Hatch et al. 1993; Steuart 1993). A community, as a unit of identity, is defined by a sense of identification with and emotional connection to other members, through common values, norms, and symbol systems and shared interests and needs and commitment to meeting them (Steuart 1993). Communities of identity may have a common geographic boundary (for example, neighborhood) or may be dispersed geographically (for example, ethnic group). Any given city or town or geographic area may not be a community of identity; rather they may be an aggregate of individuals who do not share a common identity, or they may be made up of several overlapping communities of identity. Within the context of CBPR,

TABLE 10.1.   PRINCIPLES OF COMMUNITY-BASED PARTICIPATORY RESEARCH.

Principle 1:	CBPR recognizes community as a unit of identity.
Principle 2:	CBPR builds on strengths and resources within the community.
Principle 3:	CBPR facilitates a collaborative, equitable partnership in all phases of research, involving an empowering and power-sharing process that attends to social inequalities.
Principle 4:	CBPR promotes co-learning and capacity building among all partners.
Principle 5:	CBPR integrates and achieves a balance between knowledge generation and intervention for the mutual benefit of all partners.
Principle 6:	CBPR focuses on the local relevance of public health problems and ecological perspectives that attend to the multiple determinants of health.
Principle 7:	CBPR involves systems development through a cyclical and iterative process.
Principle 8:	CBPR disseminates results to all partners and involves them in the wider dissemination process.
Principle 9:	CBPR involves a long-term process and commitment to sustainability.

Source: Adapted from Israel et al. 1998, 2003, 2005a.

partnerships seek to identify and work within communities of identity, expanding beyond them as needed, to examine and address community identified public health issues.

   2. *CBPR builds on strengths and resources within the community.* An integral part of a CBPR effort is recognizing and building upon community strengths, assets, and resources (for example, individual skills, social networks, community-based organizations) to investigate research questions and address identified concerns (Israel et al. 1998, 2003; McKnight 1994; Steuart 1993).

   3. *CBPR facilitates a collaborative, equitable partnership in all phases of research, involving an empowering and power-sharing process that attends to social inequalities.* Drawing upon the expertise, interests, and time availability of the partners involved, CBPR efforts strive for all partners to participate in and share control and decision-making over the different steps in the research process—for example, problem definition, data collection, analysis and interpretation, dissemination, and application of findings to address community issues (deKoning and Martin 1996; Green et al. 1995; Israel et al. 1998, 2003; Park et al. 1993; Stringer 1996).

4. *CBPR promotes co-learning and capacity-building among all partners.* Acknowledging that all partners bring diverse skills, expertise, perspectives, and experiences to the partnership, CBPR is a co-learning process that promotes the reciprocal exchange of knowledge, skills, and competencies among the partners involved (deKoning and Martin 1996; Freire 1973; Israel et al. 1998, 2003; Stringer 1996; Suarez-Balcazar et al. 2004).

5. *CBPR integrates and achieves a balance between knowledge generation and intervention for the mutual benefit of all partners.* The goal of CBPR is to both contribute to science and integrate and balance the knowledge gained with the development of interventions and policies aimed at improving health in the communities involved (Green et al. 1995; Israel et al. 1998, 2003; Park et al. 1993). Within CBPR efforts, although they may not all include a direct intervention component, there is an emphasis on and commitment to translating research findings into actions that benefit the community (deKoning and Martin 1996: Green et al. 1995; Israel et al. 2003; Schulz et al. 1998).

6. *CBPR focuses on the local relevance of public health problems and ecological perspectives that attend to the multiple determinants of health.* Community-based participatory research emphasizes public health concerns of local relevance to the communities involved and uses an ecological approach that attends to individuals, their immediate context (for example, family, social network), and the broader contexts in which these are embedded (for example, community, society) (Bronfenbrenner 1990; Israel et al. 1998, 2003). Therefore, integral to CBPR efforts is the consideration of multiple determinants of health, such as biological, social, cultural, economic, and physical environmental factors (Israel et al. 1998, 2003; Suarez-Balcazar et al. 2004).

7. *CBPR involves systems development through a cyclical and iterative process.* Community-based participatory research involves all partners in a cyclical, iterative process aimed at systems development (for example, a partnership) in all steps of the research process (Altman 1995; Israel et al. 1998, 2003; Stringer 1996).

8. *CBPR disseminates results to all partners and involves them in the wider dissemination process.* A critical component of CBPR is the dissemination and collective interpretation of research findings to all partners and communities involved, in ways that are respectful, meaningful and applicable (Israel et al. 1998, 2003; Schulz et al. 1998). All partners also participate in the wider dissemination of results, for example, as co-presenters at conferences and co-authors of publications (Israel et al. 2003).

9. *CBPR involves a long-term process and commitment to sustainability.* To establish and maintain the trust needed and to address the multiple determinants of health, CBPR involves a long-term process and commitment to sustainability (Hatch et al. 1993; Israel et al. 2003; Mittelmark et al. 1993) that frequently requires extending beyond a single research project or funding period (Israel et al. 2003).

CBPR and Social Epidemiology

As described in the previous section, CBPR is not a specific method or research design. Rather, CBPR is an *approach* to or a *process* by which research using different types of designs and methods can proceed. As an approach to identifying research questions, attempting to answer them, and using the results for positive change, CBPR is of great relevance to social epidemiology in several significant ways. Community-based participatory research is applicable to a plethora of research questions, study designs and data collection efforts (both quantitative and qualitative), not only community intervention research (see Viswanathan et al. 2004 for a review of thirty health-related "noninterventional studies" that used a CBPR approach). In addition, CBPR is an approach to research that is more acceptable by communities of color and other marginalized groups who rarely see benefits from the research conducted in their communities and—for good reasons—have serious mistrust of researchers and the institutions they represent (Chavez et al. 2003). Thus, social epidemiologists engaged in a wide variety of research endeavors can do so with CBPR approaches.

We see four key types of social epidemiological research in which a CBPR approach could be implemented. First, CBPR can be useful in *descriptive research that attempts to identify or elucidate social determinants of health*. A wide variety of researchers engage in work that seeks to identify and explain social factors that promote and inhibit health. We are not suggesting that all of them need to use a CBPR approach in their research. For instance, is a CBPR approach called for if a social epidemiologist is going to analyze data from the National Health Interview Survey, a statewide tumor registry, or some other secondary data source? Having members of the population from which the data were gathered participate in identifying salient research questions, assessing data collection methods, and assisting in interpreting and disseminating the results could, in fact, improve the research effort. A CBPR approach is not often taken in secondary data analyses, however, especially if the data come from a large, dispersed geographic area.

Nonetheless, if the research approach involves collecting new data or analyzing existing data from community members with the purpose of better understanding the relationship between various social and community factors and health status, using a CBPR approach has the potential to significantly inform and improve the project. If primary data collection is going to occur, members of the community in question can offer valuable insight and expertise regarding the issues or problems that are of priority in the community and salient individual and community factors that might be investigated to better understand the priority problems. Community expertise can also provide useful direction regarding data collection strategies, operationalization of variables, and measurement approaches. For example, Zenk et al. (2005) describe specific contributions made by a CBPR partnership to the development of a neighborhood observational checklist, including the operationalization and interpretation of observed features of the local context. This included initial discussions about how best to observe vacant city lots in residential areas and record the amount of "dumped materials" in these spaces. Community members pointed out that residents often maintain such lots, keeping them free of dumped materials, mowing the grass, and planting flowers. In some cases, chairs and recreational equipment indicated residents' use of the space for social and recreational purposes. As a result of these discussions, more variables were added to the observational tool, reflecting a wider range of how vacant land is used than what has been captured by instruments used in previous studies.

Second, CBPR can also be a useful and productive approach in *research attempting to understand or elucidate disparities in health status or health-related risk factors.* Social epidemiologists often engage in research that seeks to understand and explain disparities in health and disease states or factors related to health. In this type of work, social epidemiologists often focus on populations that are disadvantaged or marginalized by socioeconomic position, race, ethnicity, or other social factors. The use of a CBPR approach ostensibly gives voice and power to these marginalized groups that are quite likely to have unique knowledge and valuable insights to contribute to the understanding of the causes and consequences of the disparities under investigation (Mullings et al. 2001; Stoeker and Beckwith 1992). Even if the research is purely descriptive (for example, it is attempting to identify patterns and differentials in some phenomenon by race, ethnicity, or social class), a participatory approach can help to reframe or refocus the research questions in ways that improve the research. Researchers, whose perspectives might be constrained by disciplinary lenses or other academic biases, can be challenged by community partners to think "outside the box" in new and creative ways. Also, in accordance with the principle of co-learning and capacity building, a CBPR approach to disparities research can serve to increase the knowledge or awareness of the existing causes or consequences of health disparities (or both) in a way that allows marginalized populations a voice in defining and creating knowledge about their own communities. This, in turn, serves the bigger goal of empowerment, whereby communities are empowered to define or elucidate their own problems and solutions (Freire 1970; Wallerstein and Duran 2003). Numerous studies have been conducted regarding social factors and processes related to health with a CBPR approach. See, for example, research carried out as part of the Eastside Village Health Worker Partnership in Detroit (Becker et al. 2002; Israel et al. 2002; Parker et al. 2001; Schulz et al. 2001; van Olphen et al. 2003b).

Third, social epidemiologists have also used a CBPR approach when conducting *research to identify or define needs, problems, and assets in specific communities*. It does not make intuitive sense to have people from *outside* of a community come into an area and define its issues, needs, or even its assets, regardless of how skilled and well-intentioned they may be. Those who live and work in the community are likely to have key insights about the dynamics in a specific community that may be difficult for outsiders to identify or understand, at least initially. The strength of CBPR is that it fosters collaboration between those from within a community—with their knowledge, history, and commitment—and researchers who have strengths and assets themselves, including the time, resources, and expertise to engage in a systematic assessment of a community's issues and priorities.

Wing (2002) and Farquhar and Wing (2003) described a case study in which a CBPR approach was used in community-driven environmental justice research in rural eastern North Carolina. The research was conducted in response to community members' concerns that corporate hog farming was producing air, water, and noise pollution that disproportionately affected low-income African American communities. An organized concerned-citizens group partnered with county health department staff and academic researchers to conduct a quantitative analysis of the distribution of industrialized hog operations in the state. The results showed that "hog operations were far more common in low-income communities and communities of color, that this concentration was more extreme for hog operations owned or operated by large corporations than for independent operations, and that the pattern was only partly explained by differences in population density" (Farquhar and Wing 2003, p. 225). The study also found that hog operations were more likely to be located in places where a significant portion of the population got their drinking water from household wells (Wing 2002). A subsequent community survey (also using a CBPR approach) documented that residents living near hog operations had a significantly higher rate of headaches, sore throats, burning eyes, respiratory symptoms, and diarrhea; and they also reported differences in quality of life because of noxious odors (Wing 2002).

Fourth, CBPR is an important approach in efforts *to design, implement, and evaluate interventions and policies* aimed at reducing the negative impact of particular social determinants of health or at reducing social inequalities in health (Springett 2003). Much of the published literature regarding CBPR involves examples of intervention research in which a participatory approach was used to identify a community need or problem, design an intervention—programmatic or policy response—evaluate the intervention, and make positive community change based on the research results. Just as community members are likely to be in the best position to define their own assets and needs, they are also likely to be the best judges of what types of interventions have the most potential in their communities. Community experts have the historical knowledge of programs or services that were tried in the past and what likely led to past successes and challenges. Community involvement in intervention development and pilot testing provides essential information not only regarding the content of the intervention but also its cultural appropriateness and the manner in which it will be implemented. For example, community members might tell you that community nutrition classes have the potential to be well-received but not if they are held at a specific municipal office as suggested, because of its location, negative attitudes towards the office based on widespread personal experiences, or other legitimate reasons.

A growing number of examples of how CBPR has been used to design and evaluate an intervention can be found in the public health literature. This includes social epidemiological studies employing experimental research designs (Oakes 2004). Examples of intervention research with a CBPR approach include the following projects: HIV Testing and Counseling for Latina Women in Los Angeles (Flaskerud and Nyamathi 2000; Flaskerud et al. 1997); Seattle Partners' adult vaccine intervention (Krieger et al. 2000); the Sierra Stanford Partnership in Northern California (Angell et al. 2003); and the Center for Urban Epidemiological Studies' policy research to promote reintegration of drug users leaving jail in New York City (van Olphen et al. 2003a). As another example, Lantz et al. (2003) described an evaluation in which staff and other representatives from Native American tribes and tribal consortia running federally-funded women's cancer-screening programs participated in all phases of a program evaluation, including the identification of evaluation priorities, data collection, and the interpretation and dissemination of results. Although tribal representatives were not involved with the design of the national intervention, they were full partners in a participatory evaluation of their local programs. Lantz et al. (2001, p. 693) wrote, "Tribal representatives and program staff have stated that they would not have participated in this [evaluation] had a participatory process not been used. . . . The participatory research process led to ownership of the results within participating tribal programs, which in turn has enabled them to document successes, educate new staff, learn from other programs, and reach out to mentor new programs."

Deciding Whether to Use a CBPR Approach

As described previously, there are many types of research in which social epidemiologists are engaged that could follow principles of CBPR. In addition, it is important to underscore that there are many different models regarding participation and how the participatory process within CBPR studies is implemented in practice (Green et al., 1995) For example, Stoeker (2003) suggests that a researcher can play the role of *initiator, consultant,* or *collaborator* in a project, depending on the situation and preferences of the community. Thus, there is no simple set of criteria that one can use to decide whether or not a specific type of CBPR approach is essential, merely advisable, or not necessary for a particular research endeavor. Nonetheless, we can offer a few points to consider in deciding whether to use a CBPR approach.

First, research that involves needs assessment or the identification of resources in a specific community can greatly benefit from approaches that engage community residents in the research process. Given that academically based researchers (including social epidemiologists) are not often from the community in which they are conducting research, they may not have an in-depth understanding of the local culture and community relations and dynamics—understandings that are central to social epidemiology, with its focus on how social processes and community conditions can influence health. Anthropologists, sociologists, epidemiologists, health educators, and other public health researchers have long recognized the value of key informants and insider knowledge in developing an understanding of community dynamics, including those that impact health (James 1994; Singer 1993, 1994; Steuart 1993). Actively engaging community residents in efforts to understand key social phenomenon related to health extends opportunities for dialogue and the exchange of insights and information regarding community concerns, social relationships, culture, and other contextual factors that influence the health of residents.

Second (and similarly), research focused on the development of interventions to address health concerns within local communities can also benefit from the active engagement of community members, whose perspectives regarding the local culture, community dynamics, and structural conditions that underlie health concerns are extremely valuable in considering how to bring about change. These insights are not limited to an understanding of within-community dynamics but can equally inform an understanding of local areas within broader social contexts (for example, understanding political relationships between urban communities and surrounding suburban neighborhoods). In addition, research seeking to evaluate the process or impact of intervention efforts can often benefit substantially by engaging community observers or participants in the prioritization of evaluation questions, the design of the evaluation, and in analysis and interpretation or implications drawn from the results.

At times, social epidemiologists might find that they will not be permitted access to or entrée into a community without giving community members a voice in or shared power regarding the project. For example, many Native American tribes are now requiring that a full participatory approach be used in any research regarding their people, land, or other resources, such that tribal people have a voice in and control over the research questions being investigated, the methods being used, the interpretation of results, and the dissemination of findings (Fisher and Ball 2003). Green and Mercer (2001) describe the "push from communities" demanding that research "show greater sensitivity to communities' perceptions, needs, and unique circumstances," and how CBPR is a critical part of how researchers are responding to this demand. In addition, a growing number of funders are developing funding mechanisms requiring that a CBPR approach be used to foster true community involvement and a convergence between research and community participation (Minkler et al. 2003). As such, it is becoming more common for researchers seeking funds for community-based public health projects to provide evidence in their proposal of a committed partnership and of the adoption of a participatory approach.

Finally, it is important to remember that social epidemiologists rarely conduct research simply for the sake of research. Rather, research is a means to a bigger end that often includes the production of knowledge from which action can be taken to improve health and reduce health status disparities. Thus, social epidemiologists should be able to articulate the bigger goals for a research project under consideration. If these goals include fostering positive changes in community health and well-being or expanding community capacity to produce knowledge and action, then it is essential to consider a CBPR approach (Gaventa 1993; Stoeker 2003).

The Process of CBPR

Community-based participatory research and its analogs (participatory action research, participatory evaluation research) have been described as part of a cyclical process that includes problem framing, planning, action, observation, and reflection, toward the goal more effective practice (Eng et al. 2005; Israel et al. 1998; King 1998; King and Lonnquist 1992; also, Nunneley Jr. et al., *Validating Standards for Action Research,* a paper presented March 1997 at the American Educational Research Association, Annual Meeting, Chicago.). The cyclical nature of the process allows knowledge and understanding to emerge over time and emphasizes that this process continually builds on, critiques, and extends prior knowledge and action. There are several steps or stages that can be identified within this ongoing process, regardless of the specific focus of the research and intervention efforts. These include the process of forming a partnership and maintaining it over time, assessing the community and its dynamics, identifying local health concerns, taking action to address identified concerns, and documenting or evaluating the effectiveness of the partnership itself and its actions to address health issues (Becker et al. 2005; Israel et al. 2001, 2005a).

The first step in the process—creating and maintaining a partnership—involves a number of issues, including the identification of the "community" (for example, geographic or a community of identity, and its boundaries) and the determination of who will represent that community. Attention is warranted to whether community representatives are formal or informal leaders and whether they are self-identified or identified through other means (for example, interviews with community residents). It is also important to determine the extent to which subgroups within the community are represented, with particular attention to race, class, gender, language, and other factors that may reflect dimensions of power and influence within the community and between community representatives, academic partners, and other members of the partnership. All of these factors influence the partnership dynamics as well as the effectiveness of the partnership in addressing research questions.

Creating and maintaining a partnership also involves attention to the process through which members will interact with each other (Becker et al. 2005; Israel et al. 2001). The process of creating a shared vision of the work that the partnership will undertake is essential to effective collaboration (Johnson and Johnson 2003). Attention to mechanisms that enable all partners to be involved in this process without overburdening them, and to the development and maintenance of trust and open communication, are central to the functioning of effective partnerships (Israel et al. 2005b; Johnson and Johnson 2003; Lasker and Weiss 2003; Lasker et al. 2001; Schulz et al. 2003b; Sofaer 2000). Researchers seeking to effectively engage community residents in analyzing, addressing, and evaluating efforts to address health challenges within their communities must be self-reflective about issues of race, gender, class, power, and privilege. Furthermore, they must develop both the skills and the readiness to address tensions and differences of perspective that may arise (Chavez et al. 2003; Minkler 2004; Nyden and Wiewel 1992).

The ability of partnerships to effectively resolve conflicts and address issues of power and equity are linked to trust and require the demonstration of trustworthiness on the part of partners—particularly, although not limited to, those from outside the community. Methods for addressing these and other issues of partnership formation and maintenance have been discussed in some detail elsewhere (Becker et al. 2005; Johnson and Johnson 2003; Wallerstein et al. 2005). The cyclical nature of the CBPR process described earlier in this section highlights the reality that these and other partnership issues are not limited to the initial stages of partnership formation. Rather, researchers engaged in CBPR must be prepared to attend to such issues throughout the life of CBPR efforts.

A second stage of CBPR is that of assessing the community itself, including for example, its history; relationships between groups within the community and between the community and neighboring communities; and the values, language, and communication and helping patterns of its residents (Eng et al. 2005; Kretzman and McKnight 1993; Steuart 1993). Within CBPR that have action or change as a priority, this stage of the process emphasizes attributes or dynamics within the community that may facilitate change (for example, identification of formal and informal leaders, community organizations, or other resources within the community). During this phase of the process, partners may draw upon multiple data collection methods, including for example participant observation, in-depth interviews, and review of historical documents, newspapers, and other media (Eng et al. 2005). Like the stage of forming and maintaining the partnership, partners may initiate this process at the beginning of a CBPR effort but continue to increase understanding of the life and dynamics of the community over time (Israel et al. 2005a).

Partners engaged in participatory research must also work together to define the research questions that will be addressed by the partnership. In this third stage, partners identify priority topics of concern as well as the specific research questions to be addressed. This process can be informed by existing data (for example, community morbidity or mortality records), priorities and concerns expressed by community key informants, systematic surveys of community residents, and other data collection methods alone or in combination (Christopher et al. 2005; Kieffer et al., 2005; Krieger et al. 2005; McQuiston et al. 2005; Zenk et al. 2005). Key here is the active involvement of partners from various perspectives and social locations. This helps to ensure that the process reflects the collective vision of the partners; is consistent with community norms, values, and interaction patterns; and benefits from the insights of community residents.

A fourth stage in the participatory research process involves the mutual commitment to take action to address the concerns that are identified through the preceding stages. Such actions can take many forms, including the design of specific individual or group interventions; efforts to promote community change; dissemination of study results within appropriate local, state, regional, or national venues; and efforts to change local, regional, or national policies that impact health. For example, the Community Action Against Asthma project, a CBPR effort in Detroit aimed at gaining an increased understanding of environmental triggers of childhood asthma, designed and implemented a family and household intervention that sought to reduce triggers in the home and alleviate asthma symptoms in children. At the same time, the project undertook basic research designed to assess the impact of air quality on asthma. On the basis of the finding that airborne particulate matter had a significant effect on children's asthma, the project engaged in community organizing to influence land-use decisions in the neighborhoods most negatively affected by air pollution. These efforts integrated the information gathered through community assessment as well as basic epidemiological research and were undertaken collaboratively by all members of the partnership as they worked together to develop and implement evidence-based interventions to improve health (Keeler et al. 2002; Parker et al. 2003).

The fifth stage involves the ongoing evaluation of both the partnership process (for example, the extent to which the partnership is following CBPR principles) and the extent to which CBPR efforts are successful in attaining research, intervention, and policy goals. Such evaluation is an important means by which members of the partnership—and external parties as well—may assess their impact or effectiveness. It is generally possible to determine whether and how well a partnership is achieving its process goals and intermediate outcomes long before it is possible to determine the partnership's impact on health outcomes, and such information can be used by the partnership to enhance its efforts and thereby the accomplishment of its long term goals (Israel et al. 2005b; Rossi et al. 1999; Schulz et al. 2003b; Weiss et al. 2002).

Common Pitfalls, Challenges, and Facilitating Factors in CBPR

As an approach to research, CBPR has much to offer the field of social epidemiology. It is also the case, however, that there are a number of challenges that researchers and community members alike may encounter in undertaking a CBPR approach. As more public health researchers and practitioners are engaging in this type of work and sharing their experiences, there is a growing literature on how to avoid common pitfalls and challenges. In this section, we summarize major themes from this literature and suggest that researchers considering or newly embarking upon a CBPR project engage in dialogue with their partners regarding how they might attempt to avoid or overcome them. Ideally these discussions should occur at the proposal-writing stage.

A common pitfall that can lead to tensions or misunderstandings among partners (and with potential funders and proposal reviewers) is conflating or mistaking an *advisory* process for a *participatory* process. Although there is no gold standard for what constitutes "participation" in CBPR, and most consider there to be a continuum regarding levels of community participation (Cornwall and Jewkes 1995), identifying community members to serve on a committee or board that meets several times a year to react to research plans and provide feedback and advice is not CBPR, as described here. Obtaining advice in this manner is not collaboration and does not reflect working in partnership with a community. The essential ingredient of participatory research involves the sharing of power and control over decisions and resources in *all* phases of the research process (Cornwall and Jewkes 1995; Israel et al. 1998, 2003).

Furthermore, although gathering data from community members in a way that gives them voice in defining problems and potential solutions is important, it does not constitute CBPR in and of itself. Conducting town hall meetings, focus groups, or individual interviews with community members to gather data on perceptions of problems and priorities are important and viable components of a collaborative research process. Gathering information in such ways, however, does not *alone* provide opportunities for active, ongoing engagement and influence in decisions related to the research. In the same vein, offering what might be an exciting new program or service to a community as part of an intervention research project also is not CBPR. Again, simply because one is working in a community and interacting with community members in various ways does not mean that one is engaged in participatory or collaborative research.

For those who are committed to a participatory process in which community members have equal power and voice in all phases of the research, there are obviously a number of challenges to this work. *Resource issues* are an omnipresent challenge in CBPR; and *time* is a very important resource. Making a commitment to a CBPR approach is also making a commitment to a very time-consuming process, for all involved (Israel et al. 1998). For researchers, engaging in a participatory process often means that the project will have an extended timeline and that a great deal of time will be devoted to meetings with community partners so that key decisions can be made in a participatory rather than unilateral fashion. If the researchers do not live or work in the community involved, the time required for travel to and from the community also can become significant. For community partners, research is yet another commitment and demand on time that is above and beyond their other obligations. For those participants who are representing a community-based organization or agency in a partnership, working on a CBPR project often means that they have added research responsibilities to a job that is already quite demanding. In addition, research institutions (including academia) and funders expect the research—and the resulting reports and publications—to proceed in a timely fashion. Community organizations expect their employees to be involved with the CBPR project but also to accomplish all their other work as well (Lantz et al. 2001). As such, institutional expectations related to time can also be quite challenging.

Money is also an important resource, and the distribution of it among the individuals and organizations involved in a CBPR endeavor is often a challenge. It is all too often the case that the time and effort of the researchers involved with a CBPR project are supported by the project budget, whereas the time and effort of community partners (whose primary goal is rarely research) is being donated or supported in a purely symbolic way. There are understandable reasons why the researchers and their institutions often receive more of the monetary resources than community partners and representatives, including how academic research is funded and valued. Furthermore, the traditional ways in which faculty, research staff, and graduate students are evaluated actually provide *disincentives* to engage in CBPR, which requires that researchers give up some control and add the need for more time and resources to the process. Nonetheless, resources need to be distributed in a way that supports the work and efforts of *all* partners and that participants believe is equitable.

Another challenge in conducting CBPR is *defining the community* and determining *who represents the community* (Israel et al. 1998, 2003; Minkler 2004) In working with a given community, there are a number of issues that need to be considered: Who represents the community? Who decides who community partners will be? To what extent are community partners involved as individuals or as representatives of community-based organizations? How "grassroots" are community members? And to what extent do community partners reflect and represent the community more broadly (Israel et al. 1998, 2003)?

One of the major strengths and benefits of using a CBPR approach is also one of the biggest challenges—*working with the diversity of partners involved*. This diversity includes cultural backgrounds with respect to ethnicity or race, social class, gender, sexual orientation, community or academic role, and academic discipline as well as differences in perspectives, priorities, values, beliefs, assumptions, and language (Israel et al. 1998, 2003). Given these multiple backgrounds and perspectives, participants may have different agendas, goals, expectations, experiences with and level of commitment to CBPR, conflicting loyalties, limited trust, lack of a common language, lack of multicultural understanding and humility (Tervalon and Murray-Garcia 1998), and little recognition of the need to create a culturally safe environment for all participants (Crampton et al. 2003; Ramsden 1997). Although these differences can lead to conflicts that need to be addressed, they provide a wide array of viewpoints, skills, and experiences that can be drawn upon to foster the successful integration and synergy of ideas and actions within the context of a CBPR project. Researchers must attend to the historical and ever-present role that privilege and racism play in trying to establish and maintain richly diverse CBPR partnerships (Chavez et al. 2003; Minkler 2004).

A final challenge is *creating a balance between research and change goals* that is mutually acceptable to all the partners involved (Israel et al. 1998; Minkler 2004). As described earlier, CBPR efforts can address basic research questions, intervention research questions, or both types of questions. Challenges arise when there is a difference among partners in the emphasis and value placed on some types of research and data as compared with others. For example, some researchers may prefer that more data be collected than some community partners, and researchers and community partners may differ in their interest in examining basic research questions versus the development and evaluation of interventions. This is not a situation of deciding whether to conduct research versus action; rather it is a matter of creating a balance and staying committed to the overarching goal that the research will benefit the community involved. For example, in the Healthy Environments Partnership, the partners agreed that the focus would be on the investigation of a basic research question: the contributions of social and physical environments to cardiovascular disease risk among Detroit residents. Whereas the focus of this effort was on basic etiological research, it was undertaken within the context of long-term relationships and mutual commitment to ensuring that the research findings would be disseminated and translated into subsequent interventions and policy change (Schulz et al., unpublished manuscript. *Social and physical environments and disparities in risk for cardiovascular disease: The Healthy Environments Partnership conceptual model.*)

Although engaging in CBPR is hard work with some serious challenges, a number of facilitating factors have been identified, as reported in the growing journal and book literature on participatory and collaborative research (see Israel et al. 1998, 2003; Minkler and Wallerstein 2003). There are also published evaluations of participatory coalitions and partnerships, where the focus is on the process by which a partnership was convened and how it engaged in its work (Eisinger and Senturia 2001; Freudenberg 2001; Lantz et al. 2001; Parker et al. 2003; Schulz et al 2003b). From this burgeoning literature, we discuss in this section some of the identified facilitating factors for CBPR.

A critically important facilitating factor for CBPR is *trust* (Israel et al. 1998). Community members often do not trust the motives or intentions of researchers. There is a legacy of mistrust of research in many communities of color in the United States, fueled by the historical reality of the Tuskegee Syphilis Study and many other research projects that have raised serious ethical concerns (Freimuth et al. 2001; Gamble 1997; Schulz et al. 2003a). This mistrust is also fueled by the fact that social research regarding community issues and problems is rarely fed back to the community or used as a springboard for community change. The result is that many community members believe that research "uses" the community to benefit researchers and their institutions but does nothing for the community itself and can actually cause harm (Israel et al. 1998). Thus, an important facilitating factor for CBPR is establishing and maintaining trust among community partners and researchers by assuring that the research will be beneficial to the community and that this is not "research as usual." Community partners have to believe that the research is indeed going to address concerns that are salient to the community and that it is going to benefit the community in some tangible and important way. Building trust with communities takes time and is dependent on both the words and the actions of the researchers (Lantz et al. 2001). Many of the other facilitating factors described in this section are important to the CBPR process precisely because they help to promote and facilitate relationships that are based on trust, mutual respect, and a shared commitment to positive social change.

This includes a facilitating factor that is well-recognized in the literature: the need to pay significant attention to the *process* by which the group or partnership is engaging in CBPR (Becker et al. 2005; Israel et al. 2001; Lantz et al. 2001; Schulz et al. 2003b). It is important that process not be taken for granted, because it is fundamental to CBPR that all participants are comfortable and satisfied with the process by which the group is making decisions and engaging in its work. Processes for how decisions will be made and how work will be accomplished need to be decided upon and implemented, with an infrastructure put in place to support them. It is recommended that partnerships develop and follow mutually agreed-upon CBPR principles, operating norms, dissemination guidelines, and so forth, all of which pay attention to process issues (see Israel et al. 1998, 2003; Metzler et al. 2003). These processes and procedures do not have to be as formal as by-laws or rules. What is important is that they are the result of open discussion and consensus-building among the partners, that they are documented, and that there is a commitment to revisit them periodically to either ensure that they are being followed or to discuss whether they need to be revised or both.

A third facilitating factor is commitment to *equitable resource distribution*. A true participatory approach fairly compensates community partners and organizations for their time, contributions, and expenses. Equitable distribution does not mean equal distribution; it is up to a particular partnership to decide what constitutes a fair or equitable distribution of resources. Many types of resources (especially money) are distributed through a budgetary process. In a CBPR effort, community partners should participate in budget planning and approval or both. In addition, proposal reviewers and funders look carefully at the budgets, especially when reviewing a project that purports to be CBPR. A budget in which every minute of time, every mile driven, every telephone call made, and every office supply used by an academic or research partner is covered but only trivial and largely symbolic amounts of money are going to academic partners raises serious red flags. In addition to money, there are a number of other resources that can be distributed among the partners to ensure equity, such as training, technical assistance, the ownership of data, and opportunities for participation in national conferences and publications. Although any one CBPR project may not be able to achieve complete equity, over time and multiple projects, it is critical that all partners perceive that resources are distributed equitably.

A number of additional facilitating factors have been identified in the CBPR literature, including those reviewed in detail by Israel et al. (1998): (1) building upon a prior history of work or collaboration with a community and positive relationships that already exist; (2) identifying key community experts and representatives with whom to partner; (3) identifying and articulating common goals and objectives for the work of the collaboration; (4) having democratic leadership and decision-making processes; and (5) creating infrastructure and having the involvement of support staff, which frequently are the "glue" that holds a partnership together. In a recent review of the literature, Viswanathan et al. (2004) discussed several strategies that have been used to "remove barriers to community participation in research," including the use of educational experiences such as workshops or community forums in which both community members and researchers participate to share understanding and expertise, the creation of a written plan detailing the types of expertise required from *all* partners at each phase of the project (including the publication, dissemination, and action phases), and the hiring of local people for project coordination and other staff positions. It is beyond the scope of this chapter to review all of the facilitating factors and strategies in detail. Rather, we emphasize that there is a large published literature to which social epidemiologists can turn for guidance and constructive advice for all phases of the CBPR process.

Discussion

In this chapter, we have provided a general overview of CBPR and its relevance for social epidemiology. We have discussed the principles of CBPR, major steps in the process, common challenges, and facilitating factors. We view CBPR as a viable and important approach to research for those social epidemiologists who aim to foster positive health change and to reduce health disparities, especially in communities or populations that are marginalized by social class, race, ethnicity, geography, or other social factors. A CBPR approach—which focuses on the production of research that is of interest and use to a community and that emphasizes community participation and ownership in all phases—can facilitate and enhance the critical translation of research into interventions and other types of policy action (Themba and Minkler 2003). In this section, we address two critical issues that are sometimes raised regarding CBPR: (1) whether using a CBPR approach compromises the integrity of the research process and (2) whether CBPR "works."

CBPR and Science

A number of interrelated concerns regarding CBPR and scientific integrity have been raised. The involvement of community members in CBPR as a key and dominant stakeholder is viewed by some as a threat to the objectivity of the research endeavor (Cornwall and Jewkes 1995). A related concern is that CBPR approaches may "water down" or compromise the research process in an effort to make research more accessible, resulting in research that it is not as rigorous or sophisticated as it could be. This includes concerns about the ability to detect intervention effectiveness, especially if the research design does not include a control group (Krieger et al. 2005). Another concern is that a participatory research process—which blurs the lines between the research process and research "subjects"—produces results that are specific to the process used and thus are not generalizable beyond the community involved.

It is clearly the case that decisions made within the context of CBPR require respectful, honest, and careful discussion of the implications of various research designs, framing of research questions, and the implementation of the research for the integrity of the results. Such conversations require the development of trust; the demonstration of trustworthiness; and the time, energy, and commitment to engage different opinions and perspectives; and it is important that partners do not shortchange this process. We also need to recognize that there are multiple perspectives on "What is science?" and on what constitutes valid research designs and methodologies in social science research (Green and Mercer 2001; Sullivan et al. 2003). Questions raised about the scientific integrity of CBPR afford an opportunity for dialogue, in which the successful conclusion of some of these conversations may be an "agreement to disagree." It is also important, however, to probe the assumptions that may underlie some of the aforementioned concerns. The assumption that research conducted by academically trained researchers will be more "objective" or less problematic than research incorporating the insights and knowledge of community residents is one that bears consideration. Indeed, there are many examples of academic research that were erroneously motivated by stereotypes or other types of misinformation about groups or communities. Thus, questions raised about the scientific integrity of CBPR afford an opportunity for dialogue about research writ large and the criteria and conditions under which valid and generalizable knowledge is produced.

As an *approach* to conducting research, CBPR has the potential to be as good or as bad as the research design, data collection methods, analysis, and interpretation of results allow. We do recognize that inviting and listening to community voices regarding priorities and preferences and that sharing power and control in the research process can significantly influence the choices made at every phase. Such concerns should not be taken lightly. Nonetheless, as noted previously, the concerns raised about CBPR are relevant to *all* research, whether participatory or not. For instance, program evaluators readily acknowledge that stakeholder politics can influence the evaluation questions, the study design, and interpretation and dissemination of results regardless of whether or not a participatory approach is being used (Quinn Patton 1997). It is also the case that CBPR in the realm of public health has employed the full range of research designs (for example, cross sectional, longitudinal, experimental) and data collections methods (qualitative and quantitative) available to researchers. In the area of CBPR intervention research, the designs used have ranged from primarily qualitative analysis without a control group to randomized controlled trials (Viswanathan et al. 2004). It is true that researchers often have to make choices that compromise the ideal research design or data collection approach. Again, this is a challenge that is not unique to CBPR, but a common part of dealing with resource constraints, political situations, and stakeholder realities when conducting research in human populations.

It is likely that a CBPR approach to research can actually enhance or improve the research endeavor in multiple ways, including the selection of research questions that are more salient for the community, improved variable operationalization and data collection strategies, improved interventions with greater potential for success, and enhanced dissemination of results in ways that are constructive and meaningful for community change. This is not to argue that some research approaches are "better" than others. Rather, we are recognizing that there are multiple perspectives on judging scientific quality (Israel et al. 1998; Reason and Bradbury 2001) and that all research strategies have strengths and limitations that need to be considered.

But Does it Work?

This, however, leads us to a second concern raised by some as an important rhetorical question: Does CBPR work? In other words, what is the evidence that a participatory approach to public health research is effective and worthwhile? Because CBPR is an approach to research rather than an intervention in and of itself, this is a challenging question. A better question might be: Does CBPR produce research results that are more likely to meet the long-term goals of creating interventions that address important community issues, identifying the mechanisms by which health disparities are created and perpetuated, and enhancing community capacity to identify and address salient issues on a long-term basis? Although this is also a difficult question to answer, a growing empirical literature suggests that this is indeed the case.

In a recent evidence-based review of the CBPR literature related to health sponsored by the Agency for Healthcare Research and Quality (Viswanathan et al. 2004), the review team found evidence of enhanced research quality in eleven of the twelve completed intervention studies reviewed. This included documented evidence of enhanced participant recruitment in eight studies, improved research methods in four studies, improved variable measurement in three studies, and improved intervention outcomes in two studies. This literature review also concluded that "very little evidence of diminished research quality resulting from CBPR was reported" (Viswanathan et al. 2004, p. 41). An additional conclusion was that forty-seven of the sixty CBPR studies analyzed for the review reported evidence of enhanced community capacity as an outcome of the CBPR project, with nine studies also documenting increased capacity among researchers. These findings suggest that there is indeed "value added" from using a participatory approach in health-related research. Thus, the accumulating evidence regarding CBPR underscores our fundamental point that it is an approach that is well worth implementing in a number of social epidemiological research contexts.

Conclusion: "Push Beyond the Research"

Community-based participatory research—as a collaborative approach to research that has as its ultimate goals the improvement of community health and the enhanced capacity of community members to define and address their own health needs—is something with which all social epidemiologists should be familiar. To be clear, we are *not* arguing that one either "believes" in CBPR and follows its principles in all research endeavors or one does not. A social epidemiologist could decide to use a CBPR approach in some research projects but that it is not necessary, desired, or feasible in other work. As described earlier in this chapter, there are inherent challenges in doing CBPR, many of which present significant barriers to committing to this research approach. Nonetheless, there are myriad benefits to and strengths in using a CBPR approach in research that has as its goals the improvement of community health and an increased ability to use research as a mechanism for positive social change. Thus, it is incumbent upon social epidemiologists—working to further understand the social determinants of community health, the causes of social inequalities in health over the life course, and effective ways to reduce disparities and improve health in disadvantaged, marginalized populations—to use research processes that involve and incorporate the knowledge, experience, and strengths of the communities most affected. As Zachary Rowe, a community activist and member of the Detroit Community-Academic Urban Research Center, has stated (Schulz et al. 2003a, p. 293): "It's not enough to come into a community and do research. The community is not about research—that's a university or academic perspective. The community is about solving problems or challenges that it's facing . . . The research can aid in that process. So, as much as possible, we have to push beyond the research."

References

Altman, D. G. (1995). Sustaining interventions in community systems: On the relationship between researchers and communities. *Health Psychology, 14*(6), 526–536.

Angell K. L., Kreshka, M. A., McCoy, R., et al. (2003). Psychosocial intervention for rural women with breast cancer. *Journal of General Internal Medicine, 18*(7), 499–507.

Becker, A. B., Israel, B. A., & Allen, A. (2005). Strategies and techniques for effective group process in community-based participatory research partnerships. In B. A. Israel, E. Eng, A. J. Schulz, & E. Parker (Eds.), *Methods in community-based participatory research for health.* San Francisco: Jossey-Bass.

Becker, A. B., Israel, B. A., Schulz, A. J., et al. (2002). Predictors of perceived control among African American women in Detroit: Exploring empowerment as a multilevel construct. *Health Education and Behavior, 29*(6), 699–715.

Bronfenbrenner, U. (1990). *The ecology of human development: Experiments by nature and design.* Cambridge, MA: Harvard University Press.

Chavez, V., Duran, B. M., Baker, Q. E., Avila, M. M., & Wallerstein, N. (2003). The dance of race and privilege in community based participatory research. In M. Minkler & N. Wallerstein (Eds.), *Community-based participatory research for health* (pp. 81–97). San Francisco: Jossey-Bass.

Christopher, S., Burhansstipanov, L., & Knows His Gun-McCormick, A. (2005). Using a community-based participatory research approach to develop an interviewer training manual with members of the Apsáalooke Nation. In B. A. Israel, E. Eng, A. J. Schulz, & E. Parker (Eds.), *Methods in community-based participatory research for health.* San Francisco: Jossey-Bass.

Cornwall, A., & Jewkes, R. (1995). What is participatory research? *Social Science and Medicine, 41,* 1667–1676.

Crampton, P., Dowell, A., Parkin, C., & Thompson, C. (2003). Combating effects of racism through a cultural immersion medical education program. *Academic Medicine, 78*(6), 595–598.

deKoning, K., & Martin, M. (Eds.) (1996). *Participatory research in health: Issues and experiences.* London: Zed Books Ltd.

Eisinger, A., & Senturia, K. (2001). Doing community-driven research: A description of Seattle Partners for Healthy Communities. *Journal of Urban Health, 78*(3), 519–534.

Eng, E., Moore, K., Rhodes, S.D., Griffith, D., Allison, L., Shirah, K., et al. (2005). Insiders and outsiders assess who is "the community": Participant observation, key informant interview, focus group interview, and community forum. In B. A. Israel, E. Eng, A. J. Schulz, & E. Parker (Eds.), *Methods in community-based participatory research for health.* San Francisco: Jossey-Bass.

Farquhar, S., & Wing, S. (2003). Methodological and ethical considerations in community-driven environmental justice research: Two case studies from rural North Carolina. In M. Minkler & N. Wallerstein (Eds.), *Community-based participatory research for health* (pp. 221–241). San Francisco: Jossey-Bass.

Fisher, P. A., & Ball, T. J. (2003). Tribal participatory research: Mechanisms of a collaborative model. *American Journal of Community Psychology, 32*(3–4), 207–216.

Flaskerud, J. H., Nyamathi, A. M., & Uman, G. C. (1997). Longitudinal effects of an HIV testing and counseling programme for low-income Latina women. *Ethnicity and Health, 21*(1–2), 89–103.

Flaskerud, J. H., & Nyamathi, A. M. (2000). Collaborative inquiry with low-income Latina women. *Journal of Healthcare for the Poor and Underserved, 11*(3), 326–342.

Freimuth, V. S., Quinn, S. C., Thomas, S. B., Cole, G., Zook, E., and Duncan, T. (2001). African Americans' views on research and the Tuskegee Syphilis Study. *Social Science and Medicine, 52*(5), 797–808.

Freire, P. (1970). *Pedagogy of the oppressed*. New York: Seabury Press.

Freire, P. (1973). *Education for critical consciousness* (2nd ed.). New York: Continuum.

Freudenberg, H. (2001). Case history for the Center for Urban Epidemiologic Studies in New York City. *Journal of Urban Health, 78*(3), 508–518.

Gamble, V. N. (1997). The Tuskegee Syphilis Study and women's health. *Journal of the American Medical Women's Association, 52*(4), 195–196.

Gaventa, J. (1981). Participatory action research in North America. *Convergence, 14*, 30–42.

Gaventa, J. (1993). The powerful, the powerless, and the experts: Knowledge struggles in an information age. In P. Park, M. Brydon-Miller, B. L. Hall, & T. Jackson (Eds.), *Voices of change: Participatory research in the United States and Canada* (pp. 21–40). Westport, CT: Bergin and Garvey.

Green, L. W., & Mercer, S. L. (2001). Can public health researchers and agencies reconcile the push from funding bodies and the pull from communities? *American Journal of Public Health, 91*(12), 1926–1929.

Green, L. W., George, M. A., Daniel, M., et al. (1997). Background on participatory research. In: D. Murphy, M. Scammell, & R. Sclove (Eds.), *Doing community-based research: A reader* (pp. 53–66). Amherst, MA: Loka Institute.

Green, L. W., George, M. A., Daniel, M., Frankish, C. J., Herbert, C. J., Bowie, W. R., et al. (1995). *Study of participatory research in health promotion*. Vancouver: University of British Columbia, Royal Society of Canada.

Habermas, J. (1974). *Theory and practice*. (J. Biertel, Trans.). London: Heinemann.

Hall, B. (1992). From margins to center? The development and purpose of participatory research. *The American Sociologist, 23*(4), 15–28.

Hatch, J., Moss, N., Saran, A., Presley-Cantrell, L., & Mallory, C. (1993). Community research: Partnership in black communities. *American Journal of Preventive Medicine, 9* (Suppl. 6), 27–31.

Israel, B. A., Eng, E., Schulz, A. J., & Parker, E. A. (2005a). Introduction. In B. A. Israel, E. Eng, A. J. Schulz, & E. Parker (Eds.), *Methods in community-based participatory research for health*. San Francisco: Jossey-Bass.

Israel, B. A., Farquhar, S. A., Schulz, A. J., et al. (2002). The relationship between social support, stress, and health among women on Detroit's East Side. *Health Education and Behavior, 29*(3), 342–360.

Israel, B. A., Lantz, P. M., McGranaghan, R., Kerr, D., & Guzman, J. R. (2005b). Documentation and evaluation of community-based participatory research partnerships: The use of in-depth interviews and closed-ended questionnaires. In B. A. Israel, E. Eng, A. J. Schulz, & E. Parker (Eds.), *Methods in community-based participatory research for health*. San Francisco: Jossey-Bass.

Israel, B. A., Lichtenstein, R., Lantz, P. M., McGranaghan, R., Allen, A., Guzman, J. R., et al. (2001). The Detroit Community-Academic Urban Research Center: Development, implementation and evaluation. *Journal of Public Health Management and Practice, 7*(5), 1–19.

Israel, B. A., Schulz, A. J., Parker, E. A., & Becker, A. B. (1998). Review of community-based research: Assessing partnership approaches to improve public health. *Annual Review of Public Health, 19*, 173–202.

Israel, B. A., Schulz, A. J., Parker, E. A., Becker, A. B., Allen, A. J., & Guzman, J. R. (2003). Critical issues in developing and following community-based participatory research principles. In M. Minkler & N. Wallerstein (Eds.), *Community-based participatory research for health* (pp. 56–73). San Francisco: Jossey-Bass.

James, S. A. (1994). *Addressing the public health needs of a diverse America, Annual Minority Health Conference.* Ann Arbor: University of Michigan.

Jason, L. A., Keys, C. B., Suarez-Balcazar, Y., Taylor, R. R., & Davis, M. I. (Eds.) (2004). *Participatory community research: Theories and methods in action.* Washington, DC: American Psychological Association.

Johnson, D. W., & Johnson, F. P. (2003). *Joining together: Group theory and group skills* (8th ed.). Boston, MA: Allyn and Bacon.

Keeler, G. J., Dvonch, T., Yip, F. Y., Parker, E. A., et al. (2002). Assessment of personal and community-level exposures to particulate matter among children with asthma in Detroit, Michigan, as part of Community Action Against Asthma (CAAA). *Environmental Health Perspectives, 110* (Suppl. 2), 173–81.

Kieffer, E. C., Salabarría-Peña, Y., Odoms-Young, A., Willis, S., Baber, K., & Guzman, J. R. (2005). The application of focus group methodologies to community-based participatory research. In B. A. Israel, E. Eng, A. J. Schulz, & E. Parker (Eds.), *Methods in community-based participatory research for health.* San Francisco: Jossey-Bass.

King, J. A. (1998). Making sense of participatory evaluation practice. *New Directions for Evaluation, 80*, 57–67.

King, J. A., & Lonnquist, M. (1992). *A review of writing on action research: 1944–present.* Minneapolis, MN: Center for Applied Research and Educational Improvement.

Kretzmann, J. P., & McKnight, J. L. (1993). *Building communities from the inside out: A path toward finding and mobilizing a community's assets.* Chicago: ACTA Publications.

Krieger, J. W., Castorina, J. S., Wall, M. L., et al. (2000). Increasing influenza and pneumo-coccal immunization rates: A randomized controlled study of a senior center-based intervention. *American Journal of Preventive Medicine, 18*(2), 123–31.

Krieger, J. W., Allen, C., Roberts, J., Ross, L. C., & Takaro, T. K. (2005). What's with the wheezing: Methods used by the Seattle-King County Healthy Homes Project to assess exposure to indoor asthma triggers. In B. A. Israel, E. Eng, A. J. Schulz, & E. Parker (Eds.), *Methods in community-based participatory research for health.* San Francisco: Jossey-Bass.

Lantz, P. M., Orians, C. E., Liebow, E., Joe, J. R., Burhansstipanov, L., Erb, J., et al. (2003). Implementing women's cancer screening programs in American Indian and Alaska Native Populations. *Health Care for Women International, 24*, 674–696.

Lantz, P. M, Viruell-Fuentes, E., Israel, B. A., Softley, D., & Guzman, J. R. (2001). Can communities and academia work together on public health research? Evaluation results from a community-based participatory research partnership in Detroit. *Journal of Urban Health, 78*(3), 495–507.

Lasker, R. D., & Weiss, E. S. (2003). Broadening participation in community problem solving: A multidisciplinary model to support collaborative practice and research. *Journal of Urban Health, 80*(1), 14–60.

Lasker, R. D., Weiss, E. S., & Miller, R. (2001). Partnership synergy: A practical framework for studying and strengthening the collaborative advantage. *The Milbank Quarterly, 79*(2), 179–205.

McKnight, J. L. (1994). Politicizing health care. In P. Conrad & R. Kern (Eds.), *The sociology of health and illness: Critical perspectives* (4th ed., pp. 437–441). New York: St. Martin's Press.

McQuiston, C., Parrado, E. A., Olmos, J. C., & Bustillo, A. M. (2005). Community-based participatory research and ethnography: The perfect union. In B.A. Israel, E. Eng, A. J. Schulz, & E. Parker (Eds.), *Methods in community-based participatory research for health.* San Francisco: Jossey-Bass.

Metzler, M. M., Higgins, D. L., Beeker, C. G., Freudenberg, N., Lantz, P. M., Senturia, K. D., et al. (2003). Addressing urban health in Detroit, New York City, and Seattle through community-based participatory research partnerships. *American Journal of Public Health, 93*(5), 803–811.

Minkler, M. (2004). Ethical challenges for the "outside" researcher in community-based participatory research. *Health Education and Behavior, 31*(6), 684–697.

Minkler, M., Blackwell, A. G., Thompson, M., & Tamir, H. (2003). Community-based participatory research: Implications for public health funding. *American Journal of Public Health, 93*(8),1210–1213.

Minkler, M., & Wallerstein, N. (2003). *Community-based participatory research for health.* San Francisco: Jossey-Bass.

Mittelmark, M. B., Hunt, M. K., Heath, G. W., & Schmid, T. L. (1993). Realistic outcomes: Lessons from community-based research and demonstration programs for the prevention of cardiovascular diseases. *Journal of Public Health Policy, 14*(4), 437–462.

Mullings, L., Wali, A., McLean, D., Mitchell, J., Prince, S., Thomas, D., et al. (2001). Qualitative methodologies and community participation in examining reproductive experiences: The Harlem Birth Right Project. *Maternal & Child Health Journal, 5*(2), 85–93.

Nyden, P. W., & Wiewel, W. (1992). Collaborative research: Harnessing the tensions between researcher and practitioner. *American Sociologist, 24*(4), 43–55.

Oakes, J. M. (2004). The (mis)estimation of neighborhood effects: Causal inference for a practicable social epidemiology. *Social Science & Medicine, 58,* 1929–1952.

O'Fallon, L. R., & Dearry, A. (2002). Community-based participatory research as a tool to advance environmental health sciences. *Environmental Health Perspectives, 110* (Suppl. 2), 155–159.

Park, P. (1993). What is participatory research? A theoretical and methodological perspective. In P. Park, M. Brydon-Miller, B. Hall & T. Jackson (Eds.), *Voices of change: Participatory research in the United States and Canada* (pp. 1–19). Westport, CT: Bergin and Garvey.

Parker, E. A., Israel, B. A., Williams, M., et al. (2003). Community action against asthma: Examining the partnership process of a community-based participatory research project. *Journal of General Internal Medicine, 18*(7), 558–567.

Parker, E. A., Lichtenstein, R. L, Schulz, A. J., et al. (2001). Disentangling measures of individual perceptions of community social dynamics: Results of a community survey. *Health Education and Behavior, 28*(4), 462–486.

Quinn Patton, M. (1997). *Utilization-focused evaluation: The new century text.* Thousand Oaks, CA: Sage Publications.

Ramsden, I. (1997). Cultural safety: Implementing the concept. The social force of nursing and midwifery. In P. T. Whaiti, M. McCarthy, & A. Durie (Eds.), *Mai I Rangiatea: Maori Wellbeing and Development* (pp. 113–125). Auckland: Auckland University Press, Bridget Williams Books.

Reason, P., & Bradbury, H. (Eds.) (2001). *Handbook of action research: Participative inquiry and practice.* London: Sage.

Rossi, P. H., Freeman, H. E., & Lipsey, M. W. (1999). *Evaluation: A systematic approach* (6th ed.). Thousand Oaks, CA: Sage.

Schulz, A. J., Caldwell, C. H., & Foster, S. (2003a). "What are they going to do with the information?" Latino/Latina and African American perspectives on the Human Genome Project. *Health Education and Behavior, 30*(2), 151–169.

Schulz, A. J., Israel, B. A., & Lantz, P. M. (2003b). Instrument for evaluating dimensions of group dynamics within community-based participatory research partnerships. *Evaluation and Program Planning, 26*(3), 249–262

Schulz, A. J., Israel, B. A., Selig, S. M., Bayer, I. S., & Griffin, C. B. (1998). Development and implementation of principles for community-based research in public health. In R. H. MacNair (Ed.), *Research strategies for community practice* (pp. 83–110). New York: Haworth Press.

Schulz, A. J., Parker, E., Israel, B. A., et al. (2001). Social context, stressors, and disparities in women's health. *Journal of the American Medical Women's Association, 56*(4), 143–149.

Singer, M. (1993). Knowledge for use: Anthropology and community-centered substance abuse research. *Social Science and Medicine, 37*(1), 15–25.

Singer, M. (1994). Community-centered praxis: Toward an alternative non-dominative applied anthropology. *Human Organization, 53*(4), 336–344.

Sofaer, S. (2000). *Working together, moving ahead: A manual to support effective community health coalitions.* New York: Baruch College School of Public Affairs.

Springett, J. (2003). Issues in participatory evaluation. In M. Minkler & N. Wallerstein (Eds.), *Community-based participatory research for health* (pp. 263–288). San Francisco: Jossey-Bass.

Steuart, G. W. (1993). Social and cultural perspectives: Community intervention and mental health. *Health Education Quarterly, 20*(Suppl. 1), 99–111.

Stoeker, R. (2003). Are academics irrelevant? Approaches and roles for scholars in community based participatory research. In M. Minkler & N. Wallerstein (Eds.), *Community-based participatory research for health* (pp. 98–112). San Francisco: Jossey-Bass.

Stoeker, R., & Beckwith, D. (1992). Advancing Toledo's neighborhood movement through participatory action research: Integrating activist and academic approaches. *Clinical Sociology Review, 10,* 198–213.

Stringer, E. T. (1996). *Action research: A handbook for practitioners.* Thousand Oaks, CA: Sage.

Suarez-Balcazar, Y., Davis, M. I., Ferrari, J., Nyden, P., Olson, B., Alvarez, J., et al. (2004). University-community partnerships: A framework and an exemplar. In L. A. Jason, & C. B. Keys (Eds.), *Research: Theories and methods in action* (pp. 105–120). Washington, DC: American Psychological Association.

Sullivan, M., Chao, S., Allen, C. A., Koné, A., Pierre-Louis, M., & Krieger, J. W. (2003). Community-researcher partnerships: Perspectives from the field. In M. Minkler & N. Wallerstein (Eds.), *Community-based participatory research for health* (pp. 113–130). San Francisco: Jossey-Bass.

Tandon, R. (1996). The historical roots and contemporary tendencies in participatory research: Implications for health care. In P. Reason & H. Bradbury (Eds.), *Participatory research in health: Issues and experiences* (2nd ed., pp. 19–26). London: Zed Books.

Tervalon, M., & Murray-Garcia, J. (1998). Cultural humility vs. cultural competence: A critical distinction in defining physician training outcomes in medical education. *Journal of Health Care for the Poor and Underserved, 9*(2), 117–125.

Themba, M. N., & Minkler, M. (2003). Influencing policy through community based participatory research. In M. Minkler & N. Wallerstein (Eds.), *Community-based participatory research for health* (pp. 349–370). San Francisco: Jossey-Bass.

van Olphen, J., Freudenberg, N., Galea, S., Palermo, A. G., & Ritas, C. (2003a). Advocating policies to promote community reintegration of drug users leaving jail: A case study of first steps in a policy change campaign guided by community based participatory research. In M. Minkler & N. Wallerstein (Eds.), *Community-based participatory research for health* (pp. 371–389). San Francisco: Jossey-Bass.

van Olphen, J., Schulz, A. J., Israel, B. A., et al. (2003b). Religious involvement, social support, and health among African-American women on the east side of Detroit. *Journal of General Internal Medicine, 18*(7), 549–57.

Viswanathan, M., Ammerman, A., Eng, E., Gartlehner, G., Lohr, K. N., et al. (July, 2004). *Community-based participatory research: Assessing the evidence.* Evidence Report/Technology Assessment No. 99 (Prepared by RTI and University of North Carolina Evidence-based Practice Center under Contract No. 290–02–0016). AHRQ Publication 04-E022–2. Rockville, MD: Agency for Healthcare Research and Quality.

Wallerstein, N., & Duran, B. (2003). The conceptual, historical, and practice roots of community-based participatory research and related participatory traditions. In M. Minkler & N.Wallerstein (Eds.) (2003) *Community-based participatory research for health.* San Francisco: Jossey-Bass.

Wallerstein, N., Duran, B. M., Minkler, M., & Foley, K. (2005). Developing and maintaining partnerships with communities. In B. A. Israel, E. Eng, A. J. Schulz, & E. Parker (Eds.), *Methods in community-based participatory research for health.* San Francisco: Jossey-Bass.

Weiss, E. S., Anderson, R. M., & Lasker, R. D. (2002). Making the most of collaboration: Exploring the relationship between partnership synergy and partnership functioning. *Health Education and Behavior, 29*(6), 683–698.

Whyte, W. F. (1991). *Participatory action research.* Newbury Park, CA: Sage.

Wing, S. (2002). Social responsibility and research ethics in community-driven studies of industrialized hog production. *Environmental Health Perspectives, 108,* 225–231.

Zenk, S., Schulz, A. J., House, J. S., Benjamin, A., & Kannan, S. (2005). Application of community-based participatory research in the design of an observational tool: The neighborhood observational checklist. In B. A. Israel, E. Eng, A. J. Schulz, & E. Parker (Eds.), *Methods in community-based participatory research for health.* San Francisco: Jossey-Bass.

CHAPTER ELEVEN

NETWORK METHODS IN SOCIAL EPIDEMIOLOGY

Peter V. Marsden

Networks of interpersonal relationships can be important mediators between conditions in the social environment and health-related outcomes. Risks of contracting a disease that spreads through personal contact are influenced not only by individual behaviors but also by the behaviors of close contacts and by social proximity to already-infected persons. Social relationships that structure flows of information and social support may also affect the course and outcomes of disease. Networks are central to several social processes affecting health-related behaviors, including the shaping and enforcement of norms, the production or amelioration of stress, and the regulation of access to information, resources, and opportunities (Berkman and Kawachi 2000, p. 7).

This chapter introduces methods for measuring and analyzing social networks, drawing on the social network approach per se as well as studies in social epidemiology that have used network techniques. It first highlights some exemplar studies that demonstrate the potential importance of networks in epidemiological research. After reviewing some basic network concepts, it describes common research designs that incorporate network data, data collection methods, instruments, common indices based on network data, and methods used

Author's Note: Writing was supported in part by grant R-01 AG24448–01 from the National Institute on Aging, National Institutes of Health. For helpful comments, I am grateful to Nicholas A. Christakis, Paul D. Cleary, and Hector P. Rodriguez.

to obtain such structural measures. It then introduces methods for studying rare populations and developing interventions that draw on network ideas. Finally, it highlights important ethical issues that arise in network-based health research.

Background

The Alameda County study (Berkman and Syme 1979) was among the earliest to call attention to the importance of networks for social epidemiology. Berkman and Syme found a substantial association between all-cause mortality and a Social Network Index including four types of social affiliations, reporting age-adjusted relative risks of 2.8 and 2.3 among women and men, respectively. With a prospective design, the Tecumseh Community Health Study (House et al. 1982) corroborated many of Berkman and Syme's findings; associations were considerably stronger among men than among women. These studies pointed to networks as structural sources of social support and helped to stimulate a vital, ongoing body of research on social support and health (for example, Cohen and Syme 1985; Cohen et al. 2000).

Recent studies link social networks to a wide variety of health behaviors and outcomes. For example, Cohen et al. (1997) report greater susceptibility to common colds among persons with relatively few types of social relationships compared with those having greater network diversity. Unger and Chen (1999) link the presence of smokers in an adolescent's social network to earlier initiation of smoking, whereas Ennett and Baumann (1993) find smoking to be more common among adolescents isolated from peer group structures. Ennett et al. (1999) show that runaway and homeless youth citing no social relationships are more apt to engage in risky behaviors than those claiming social ties. Valente et al. (1997) report higher contraceptive use among women who perceive that their network contacts use and approve of contraception.

The onset of the HIV epidemic highlighted sexual contact networks as settings for disease transmission together with other social relationships that place people at high risk, such as needle-sharing among injection drug users. Klovdahl (1985) mapped a network of sexual contacts among homosexual men, called attention to the potential of a network approach to add insight into a disease outbreak, and suggested that understanding social network structures might aid in the design of effective interventions. Extensive information on both risk networks (sexual and needle exchange) and social networks has since been assembled in several large-scale network studies. Notable among these are the National Health and Social Life Survey (NSHLS; Laumann et al. 1994); the National Longitudinal Study of Adolescent Health (Add Health; Bearman et al. 2004); a Colorado Springs study of prostitutes, injecting drug users, and their personal associates (Klovdahl et al. 1994); and a New York City study of interrelated drug injectors (Friedman et al. 1997). Such studies examine both the behavioral networks directly involved in disease transmission and the social networks that influence opportunities, norms, and practices surrounding risky behavior.

Berkman and Glass (2000) posit five principal mediating pathways through which social relationships may influence health. Prominent among these is social support, which has emotional, instrumental, appraisal (assistance in decision-making), and informational aspects (House and Kahn 1985). Different forms of support flow through different ties (Wellman and Wortley 1990). Not all social ties are necessarily supportive; indeed, some may be burdensome. Some models maintain that the availability of social support has a generally salutary influence on health. Other "buffering" models assert that support has a conditional effect, moderating the severity of response to a stressor. Beyond social support, networks may also offer access to tangible resources such as financial assistance or transportation. They can also convey social influence by defining norms about such health-related behaviors as smoking or diet or via social controls promoting (for example) adherence to medication regimens. The increased social engagement associated with network ties can contribute to attachment and a better-defined social identity (Thoits 1983). Finally, networks may be direct channels of exposure to infectious disease agents.

Basic Network Concepts

Networks are often depicted as a set of points (representing persons)[1] linked by a set of lines (representing relationships), as in the illustrative 11-element network shown in Figure 11.1. Data on individual characteristics of persons in the network usually accompany the relational data; for example, the square points in Figure 11.1 might be men and the circular ones women, whereas the shaded points could represent persons having a support resource or disease condition. The subnetwork consisting of a point, those points directly linked to it, and the relationships among them is known as an egocentric network. The egocentric network for point I, for example, includes I, G, J, and K.

Relationships may be reciprocal, as illustrated by two-headed arrows, or unilateral. Often only the presence or absence of relationships is measured, but ties can vary in strength; Figure 11.1 uses variations in line weights to depict such

[1]Network studies can and do measure relationships between social entities other than persons, notably organizations. The most common application, however, is to interpersonal networks.

FIGURE 11.1. AN 11-ELEMENT NETWORK.

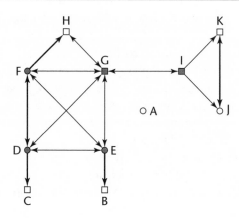

differences. In multi-relational networks, two or more types of relationships may be present between each pair of points. Points in a network may be directly or indirectly connected to one another. In Figure 11.1, point D is indirectly connected to point H via points F and G as intermediaries. Points G and I lie along many such indirect "paths" joining other points and are relatively central within this network. Point A, in contrast, is an isolate.

The "density" of a network is the proportion of pairs of points connected by lines; network density in Figure 11.1 is just over 0.2. Studies often seek to identify network subgroups conceived as densely connected subnetworks. Points D, E, F, and G in Figure 11.1 constitute a "clique," having all possible direct relationships with one another; because points H and I are either directly or indirectly connected to D, E, F, and G, they are part of a six-element "component." The remaining points (A, B, C, J, and K) are not in this component because no relationships lead from them to points in the component. The G–I relationship is a "bridge" between the D–E–F–G clique and the J–K dyad.

Certain structural properties of networks play a central role in mathematical models of disease spread that relax the assumption of random or "full" mixing (Morris 1993; Newman 2002). One of these is the degree distribution given by the number of connections of each network element with others. Positively skewed degree distributions—found in centralized networks—are common. Other important properties involve segregation of social ties. Among these are *homophily*, a tendency to form relationships with socially similar others, and *transitivity*, a tendency toward closure that results in clustering within a network. To the extent that there is selective mixing, diffusion may be more rapid within subgroups but slower in a network as a whole.

Network Data and Network Measures

The vast majority of network studies in social epidemiology rely on data from surveys and questionnaires. The objective is to characterize the context in which diseases propagate or in which health-related behaviors develop. Network measures thought to influence health outcomes provide data for mathematical models of disease spread or appear as explanatory variables in statistical models for the incidence or prevalence of conditions or behaviors.

Some studies measure social affiliations or network properties with relatively standard survey questions. Others use instruments specifically designed to elicit detailed data about networks. Studies of "egocentric" or "personal" networks concentrate on the social relationships surrounding a given person. "Whole network" studies instead attempt to measure relationships among all elements of a closed population. Less common are intermediate "partial" network studies, such as the "random walk" design (McGrady et al. 1995), which samples chains of connected elements in large, open populations. Data on subjects and their relationships collected via these designs are subsequently combined into indices that measure features of networks.

Survey Measures of Social Affiliations

Social integration is sometimes measured directly by asking survey respondents to report about specific social relationships or make summary "global" characterizations of their sets of social ties. Three of the four components of Berkman and Syme's (1979) Social Network Index, for example, were standard survey items measuring marital status and membership in churches and other voluntary groups. House and Kahn (1985, p. 90) view measures of the presence or absence, quantity, and frequency of major relationships as essential items for studies of social support.

Also common are relatively simple dyadic measures. Lowenthal and Haven (1968, p. 22) show that an item measuring presence of a confidante—"Is there anyone in particular you confide in or talk to about yourself or your problems?"—is associated with morale. Dean and Tausig (1986, p. 124) use a variant on this item: "During the past six months, have you had anyone that you could trust and talk to?" Multiple-item indices of social relationships combine responses to several such questions; for example, Cohen et al. (1997) measure social network diversity with reports of involvement in twelve types of relationships.

Global measures of networks ask respondents for summary judgments about their sets of friends, relatives, neighbors, coworkers, or other role relations. For example, Berkman and Syme (1979, p. 188) measure contacts with friends and relatives with overall reports of the number, intensity, and frequency of such ties:

> How many close friends do you have?
>
> How many relatives do you have that you feel close to?
>
> How often do you see these people each month?

Global measures make considerable cognitive demands on survey respondents; the item on "close friends," for instance, requires that a respondent define both "friend" and "close," enumerate, and aggregate. Perhaps as a result, Sudman (1985) shows that there is considerable response variance in global estimates of network size compared with more time-consuming network measurements based on recognition or free recall.

Summary measures of social affiliation are relatively efficient in that they require little interview time and often display robust associations with phenomena of interest. It can be difficult to distinguish different mechanisms or pathways affecting health behaviors with such measures, however, because they usually assess only overall levels of affiliation. Brissette et al. (2000) recommend supplementing affiliation measures by assessing intervening variables such as self-concept or self esteem that are thought to be influenced by different network processes. Other approaches that elicit more detailed data about social networks are discussed in the following sections.

Egocentric Network Data and Measures

An egocentric network instrument measures the network in the locality of a given subject. Such instruments can be used within standard sample survey designs, usually relying on the sampled respondent (ego) to report all requisite data. The most widely-used protocol consists of two types of survey questions: "name generators" that elicit specific persons ("alters") within the respondent's network, and "name interpreters" that provide content about alters and their relationships to the respondent. Dyadic or network-level indices constructed with such data are then used to predict measures of (for example) health behaviors, knowledge, or beliefs.

Egocentric instruments pose questions about individual alters and relationships rather than asking respondents to make summary judgments about their networks. This improves data quality but lengthens administration time; extensive egocentric instruments can require twenty minutes or more of interview time, so social networks must be a focal feature of studies that include them.

Name Generator Items. Most egocentric instruments establish network boundaries by eliciting names of alters with whom a respondent has a criterion social relationship, such as friendship, usually via free recall. Questions used for this purpose are known as name generators.[2] The criterion relationship may be behavioral, affective, or role-related, varying with the substantive focus of a study. Reference periods (for example, the past six months) are often specified; some instruments use multiple name generators (Campbell and Lee 1991). Most egocentric network studies include only alters with whom the ego has a direct relationship.

The Ennett et al. (1999, p. 66) study of runaway and homeless youth used a frequency-of-contact name generator, asking respondents to name alters "you see a lot or spend most of your time with now." The NHSLS elicited recent sexual partnerships with the item "How many people, including men and women, have you had sexual activity with, even if only one time?" and a one-year reference period (Laumann et al. 2004, p. 28). A study of perceived risks for HIV/AIDS and preventive strategies among rural Malawians (Smith and Watkins 2005) elicited alters with whom respondents had "chatted" about AIDS. Bond et al. (1999) measured egocentric networks for unmarried urban migrants in Thailand with two name generators: one elicited persons with whom a respondent likes to spend free time; the other, boyfriends or girlfriends, sex partners, and lovers. The Social Support Questionnaire (Sarason et al. 1983) uses twenty-seven name generators, asking for persons from whom the subject receives various forms of social support, such as consolation or help in a crisis situation.

The number of alters elicited by a name generator depends on the criterion relationship specified: more intimate relational contents tend to produce fewer alters (Campbell and Lee 1991). Because answering repetitive follow-up name-interpreter questions about alters can burden respondents, the number of alters followed up is often limited (to, for example, three or five). Limiting the number of alters truncates variation in network size, however, so it is desirable to record the full number of alters elicited by the name generator even when such limitations are imposed. Probes or aided recall devices are sometimes used with name generator items; for example, the NHSLS used a life history calendar while eliciting lifetime sexual partners (Laumann et al. 2004).

Name Interpreter Items. Data on the form and content of an egocentric network are obtained with name interpreter questions that request descriptions of those

[2]A related elicitation strategy (Kahn and Antonucci 1980) presents respondents with a "target sociogram" with three concentric circles, asking that they place alters "who are important in your life right now" in central or peripheral locations on the basis of closeness.

alters and relationships elicited by a name generator. These include proxy reports about characteristics or behaviors of alters, descriptions of relationships with alters, and reports on ties between pairs of alters.

Name interpreters reflect a study's substantive emphasis. Relatively generic items include sociodemographic descriptions of alters in terms of age, education, race, and sex. Such questions can also ask about the respondent-alter tie, often including role relations (for example, kinship, friendship, coworker, or neighbor status), intensity and closeness, duration, and frequency of contact. Additional data on egocentric network structure can be obtained with questions about relationships between pairs of alters, often relying on a matrix format. The General Social Survey egocentric network instrument, for example, asked if each pair of alters was "especially close" and if the alters were "total strangers" (Marsden 1987).

Studies can also include name interpreters tailored to their objectives. The NHSLS, for instance, asked about sexual practices with "primary" and "secondary" sexual partners as well as the partner's number of recent sexual partners and the concurrency of other partnerships with the respondent-partner sexual relationship (Laumann et al. 2004). Ennett et al. (1999) measured alters' alcohol and drug use, alter pressures on respondents to engage in risky behaviors, and provision of four types of social support.

Egocentric network studies usually obtain all data about alters from respondents, so research into the quality of name interpreter data is important. Studies that contact some alters to obtain independent reports on their characteristics and their relationships to respondents are therefore valuable; Marsden (1990, pp. 450–453; 2005, pp. 17–18) reviews findings from some such studies. Respondent knowledge of certain data on alters may be limited. For example, although the Kenyan village women studied by White and Watkins (2000) made high-quality proxy reports on observable alter characteristics, responses about alters' contraceptive behaviors (an often-secret datum in the village setting) were less concordant with alter self-reports. Responses about alters were often anchored on respondents' own behavior. Shelley et al. (1995) found that HIV+ informants deliberately restricted dissemination of information about their HIV status. Such examples indicate that investigators should consider what respondents are likely to know about alters when formulating name interpreters.

Measures Based on Egocentric Data. Name interpreter data support construction of a wide variety of egocentric network indicators. Some are dyadic measures. For example, Youm and Laumann (2002) use four name interpreters (free time spent together, jealous conflict, and so forth) to measure potential social control within sexual partnerships. Morris et al. (1995) focus on the regularity of sexual relationships between Thai men and commercial sex partners, showing that condom use declines with regularity.

Other indices are based on the full set of alters elicited by a name generator. Two very common network-level measures are network size (number of alters) and local network density (the extent to which pairs of alters in an egocentric network are interconnected). Dense, closed networks are thought to have high control potential (Youm and Laumann 2002) and to contribute to secure identity formation. Haines and Hurlbert (1992) suggest that dense egocentric networks reduce stress exposure because they tend to include stronger ties. More open, sparse egocentric networks, in contrast, widen network range and broaden access to diverse sources of informational support.

Respondent-specific summary statistics on the distribution of alter or dyadic characteristics measure network composition and heterogeneity: the extent to which an egocentric network is composed of kin; its heterogeneity in terms of age, race and ethnicity, or sex; or the average intensity of respondent-alter relationships (Marsden 1987). Smith and Watkins (2005) use the average level of worry about contracting AIDS among discussion partners to predict a focal respondent's concern. Ennett et al. (1999) measure norms and sanctions surrounding risky behavior with data on the presence of risky behaviors and the perceived pressures to engage in them among alters. Caraël et al. (2004) use name interpreter data on the timing of recent sexual partnerships to calculate a respondent-level index of concurrency. Social support scales often aggregate descriptions or evaluations across alters; Hirsch's (1980) Social Network List, for example, measures overall support as the mean satisfaction rating across alters with whom a respondent interacts.

"Mixing matrices" giving relative frequencies of intergroup contact can be constructed with egocentric data by cross-classifying respondent and alter measurements. Laumann and Youm (1999), for example, classify heterosexual partnerships in the NHSLS by race or ethnicity and level of sexual activity, finding levels of contact between "core" and "peripheral" activity groups to be higher among African-Americans than among whites and linking differences in mixing patterns to racial differences in the prevalence of sexually transmitted diseases.

Other Egocentric Network Instruments. Social network specialists have developed some egocentric network instruments that do not rely on name generators and interpreters; these have not yet been widely used in social epidemiology. The "position generator" (Lin et al. 2001) elicits relationships to specific social locations such as occupations or ethnic groups rather than to specific alters, yielding measures of network composition and range. The "resource generator" (Van Der Gaag and Snijders 2005) measures individual social capital by ascertaining whether a respondent's personal relationships provide access to specified resources (for example, knowledge about financial matters, medical or legal advice, aid with shopping or household jobs). These instruments yield more limited data about egocentric networks than do more extensive name generator-interpreter instruments but can be administered more efficiently.

Whole Network Studies

In a "whole network" study, data are collected on relationships linking all elements in a closed population such as a school or community. Whole network studies depart from standard survey designs, deliberately clustering participants in geographic or social space. They measure egocentric networks for each population element but also allow modeling of group-level social structure. They can ascertain the relative centrality or prominence of population elements, map patterns of indirect connectedness, and identify subgroups of interrelated elements.

Boundary Specification. The crucial first step in a whole network study is to specify criteria for inclusion in the network to be studied. Boundaries are often based on some criterion of membership in a formally or informally defined group. The Add Health study included all students in each of a sample of high schools (Bearman et al. 2004). Ennett and Baumann (1993) studied ninth-grade students in five schools. Valente et al. (1997) studied discussion networks within nine voluntary groups (known as *tontines*) in Cameroon.

Other studies rely on referrals or relational criteria, either exclusively or in combination with other information, to determine membership in a network. Bond et al. (1999) used snowball sampling methods to delineate networks in department store and entertainment settings. The Colorado Springs study of persons at high risk for heterosexual transmission of AIDS (Klovdahl et al. 1994) began with subjects identified at a health department clinic and a drug treatment program. It continued using staff outreach efforts and later recruited partners of women engaged in prostitution and injecting drug users. A study of injecting drug users in a Brooklyn neighborhood (Neaigus et al. 1995) used chain referrals from initial participants to supplement a sample initially identified by observation and informant interviews. Neaigus et al. do not claim to have identified a closed network of drug users; they note some limitations of referral methods, including both subject reluctance to reveal names of contacts and genuine lack of knowledge about names.

Data Collection Methods. Whole network studies often collect data with survey and questionnaire methods, though other means are occasionally used. An important difference from egocentric studies is that subjects need not be asked to provide name interpreter data on alters or relationships among alters, because alters are sought out as subjects as part of the design. This lowers respondent burden substantially.

When inclusion in the network under study can be determined in advance with a membership list or other enumeration, whole network data on respondent-alter relationships can be assembled with recognition rather than recall methods. A roster listing persons in the network is compiled and presented to respondents, who then specify those on the list with whom they have a given relationship. This improves data quality substantially; studies reviewed by Brewer (2000) suggest that respondents overlook substantial fractions of their contacts when performing recall tasks.

Bond et al. (1999) use roster methods when gathering data in dormitory settings, whereas Bearman et al. (2004, p. 205) encouraged Add Health respondents to refer to a student directory when designating friends in their schools. Other studies of school networks, however, rely on recall (Ennett and Baumann 1993; Urberg et al. 1997). Brewer (2000) recommends that studies using recall include nonspecific probes and multiple name generators to prompt memory for relationships.

Whole network studies often limit the number of alters that respondents may cite. For example, Ennett and Baumann (1993) asked for three best friends, and Valente et al. (1997) limited nominations to five discussion partners. Such limitations are sometimes necessary as a practical matter to control respondent burden. They are best avoided, however, because truncation introduces error into both egocentric and group-level network measures (Holland and Leinhardt 1973).

Measures Based on Whole Network Data. Data from a whole network study can be used to measure dyadic, egocentric, and network-level properties. Urberg et al. (1997) focus on tobacco and alcohol use by the first-elicited friend as an indicator of best-friend influence. Egocentric network measures can be constructed by combining network data and self-reports of respondent characteristics. Indeed, whole-network data allow construction of more refined egocentric measurements; for example, Bearman and Moody (2004), using Add Health data, measure egocentric network openness as the fraction of persons reached by two-step indirect ties that are not also direct contacts.

Whole network data are distinctive, however, because they support construction of measures that describe group-level structure that depend on indirect as well as direct links between network elements. Some methods used in social epidemiology focus on identifying clusters of persons who are relatively densely related to one another. Others are concerned with measuring the relative centrality of persons within a network.

Network subgroups may be defined with many criteria; see Scott (2000, chap. 6) or Wasserman and Faust (1994, chap. 7). The most stringent definition of a "clique" requires that each member of such a subgroup be linked to each other member. A somewhat weaker standard is that each member of a subgroup be related to at least two other members and that at least one-half of the individual's relationships be with other subgroup members. Ennett and Baumann (1993) and Urberg et al. (1997) use such a subgroup definition in their studies of schools. Even less restrictive standards define membership in a "2-core" or a "connected component." Klovdahl et al. (1994) show that a large fraction of participants in the Colorado Springs study were in such a component, linked to one another by either direct or indirect channels.

A crucial question for social epidemiology is how clique, core, or component membership is associated with other data. In the Colorado Springs study, few HIV+ persons were found in the large connected component; hence the social context did not promote transmission (Rothenberg et al. 1998). By contrast, in the New York City study of injecting drug users, persons in the large interconnected subgroup were more apt to be infected with HIV and to engage in risky behavior; there the authors conclude that this may be a "core group" that can maintain and broaden transmission (Friedman et al. 1997).

The relative centrality of nodes within a network can be measured in numerous ways with whole network data (Scott 2000, chap. 5; Wasserman and Faust 1994, chap. 5). Two widely used definitions are egocentric network size ("degree" centrality) and the extent to which a given network element lies along indirect chains or paths linking other elements ("betweenness" centrality). Central network elements are often found to be more prominent or influential than are peripheral ones. Klovdahl (1985) argued that central individuals could play especially crucial roles in disease epidemics. Potterat et al. (2004) used whole network methods to map networks in the Colorado Springs study, finding that the few HIV-infected persons in the large interconnected component were in peripheral locations and arguing that this contact pattern helped to account for the low incidence of disease in that study.

Additional Applications of Network Methods

Network-related ideas have many applications beyond providing contextual measures for use in statistical and mathematical models. Two are highlighted here: studying rare populations and network interventions.

Rare and Hard-to-Count Populations

It is difficult to estimate the size and composition of many populations of interest to social epidemiologists, such as AIDS victims or intravenous drug users. Many such groups are numerically small and composed of persons with stigmatizing conditions or behaviors that they may wish to conceal. Social network data on patterns of contact between randomly sampled persons and those in the rare population offer some insight into such questions. Laumann et al. (1993) used reports about whether survey respondents know people with AIDS to estimate the sex, race or ethnic, age, and regional distributions of U.S. AIDS cases in the early 1990s, concluding that surveillance systems may have understated prevalence among whites and Midwestern residents. Killworth et al. (1998) use sample survey data on contacts with many subpopulations of known size (for example, diabetics, adoptive parents) as well as one of unknown size (HIV+ persons) to develop "scale up" estimates of the size of an unknown population. Their method produced a higher seroprevalence estimate than did then-current Centers for Disease Control figures; Killworth et al. note the dependence of their approach on accurate respondent knowledge of alter characteristics.

Related methods can be used to locate subjects in special or unlisted populations. Multiplicity sampling (Sudman and Kalton 1986) asks randomly sampled survey respondents whether they have a particular relationship (for example, relative, coworker) to anyone having the characteristic defining the population of interest. Persons elicited are subsequently approached as study subjects. If the relationships that link initial respondents and potential subjects are well-defined, the relative chances of contacting any particular subject can be specified, resulting in a probability sample from the special population. In contrast, "respondent-driven sampling" (RDS; Heckathorn 1997) does not require random sampling at the first stage. Respondent-driven sampling is a chain-referral sampling method that provides incentives to early respondents for both referring and recruiting later ones. Heckathorn demonstrates that when continued over several stages, RDS leads to a sample that is independent of the initial "seed" informants. The approach is suitable for sampling from an interconnected population; it would not be effective for drawing a national sample.

Interventions

Many suggest that a network approach holds the potential to increase the effectiveness of interventions. Rothenberg and Narramore (1996) observe that a network approach is implicit in control efforts involving mandatory reporting and contact tracing. They suggest that such programs could be improved by overt use of network concepts and data. Klovdahl (1985) argues that knowledge of network channels could direct intervention efforts toward those individuals and relationships best situated to reduce disease spread. Recommendations based on a study of "core" and "bridge" populations in the Thai AIDS epidemic (Morris et al. 1996) exemplify such a strategy. It suggests three groups toward which safe-sex campaigns might be profitably oriented: young men, who have high contact with both commercial sex workers (CSWs, a core group) and uninfected non-commercial partners; truckers who often have concurrent sexual relationships with CSWs, wives, and other non-commercial partners; and young women not engaged in commercial sex, who may be at high risk because of the practices of their sexual partners.

Others argue that social networks may be an effective vehicle for delivering interventions. Neaigus et al. (1994) contend that intervening on networks may have multiplier effects in the form of social pressure and support for behavior change. They suggest intervening on intact networks of at-risk individuals and encouraging those at risk to form ties with others not at risk. Latkin (1995) describes a network-level intervention that sought to reduce drug-injection risk behaviors; among other things, he suggests that network interventions may aid in both gaining access to and recruiting participants and also promote retention. Latkin et al. (1996) show that subjects receiving an intervention accompanied by self-designated network members exhibited greater reductions in needle-sharing at eighteen-month follow-up than did those treated individually.

Valente et al. (2003) demonstrated the potential utility of using network approaches to intervention in an experimental study of a school-based, peer-led tobacco prevention program. The intervention made a greater difference when group leaders were selected based on network centrality rather than designated by teachers and also when students were assigned to groups based on network data rather than at random or by teachers.

Ethical and Human Subjects Issues in Network Studies

Network studies in social epidemiology often seek highly sensitive medical or behavioral information about subjects and their associates. This highlights important questions about obtaining informed consent, the criteria defining participation in a study, and steps needed to guard the confidentiality of data. Woodhouse et al. (1995) discuss such issues with reference to the Colorado Springs study (Klovdahl et al. 1994).

Special vigilance about protecting confidentiality is warranted, because both behavioral and network data could be of interest to parties not involved in the research, such as employers, insurance companies, or law enforcement agencies. Some studies can obtain Federal Certificates of Confidentiality to protect subjects against subpoenas or prosecution as a result of participation in research (Klovdahl 2005). For all studies, extensive steps to guard the possibility of disclosure are necessary. Klovdahl (2005, pp. 125–126) recommends segmentation of data instruments, minimizing the number of project personnel having access to identifying or linking information, and using highly secure computers not connected to any network, among other precautions. The NHSLS implemented many of these measures (Laumann et al. 1994, pp. 71–73), destroying all identifying information about its respondents upon verifying interviews and limiting the geographic detail in public release files to guard against deductive disclosure. Destroying identifiers, however, precludes longitudinal studies.

Network studies almost always assemble information about "third parties"—associates or alters linked to subjects. Currently there is debate about whether third parties are to be regarded as research subjects from whom informed consent must be obtained (Klovdahl 2005; Morris 2004, p. 3). Under some conditions (Klovdahl 2005, pp. 128–132), institutional review boards can grant waivers of consent for third parties. In any event, investigators are obligated to protect such "secondary subjects" against harm through disclosure of research data and to make the case that risks to such subjects are minimal and outweighed by potential benefits. Some (Woodhouse et al. 1995) have suggested that researchers may have more affirmative obligations to secondary subjects in the event that it is found that the behavior of primary subjects places them at risk.

Conclusion

This overview of network methods has stressed approaches that have attracted interest from social epidemiologists. Sources such as Scott (2000) and Wasserman and Faust (1994) present general and more extensive guides to contemporary social network analysis; recent developments are covered in Carrington et al. (2005). Marsden (1990, 2005) reviews issues of study design and measurement at greater length. Valente (1995) focuses on network models for diffusion. Cohen et al. (2000) reviews recent developments in social support research, with special attention to measurement and intervention. Morris (2004) contains reports on several of the major network epidemiological studies, which offer detail on their implementation as well as their design and measurement strategies.

There are many challenges for future network studies in this field. Many associations between network measures and health phenomena have been documented, but some of these may reflect endogeneity of the network phenomena—if, for instance, healthier persons are able to maintain more extensive network connections—rather than social influence. Longitudinal network studies can help to address such issues, but they are complex to conduct because both principal respondents and network alters must be tracked over time. Many questions about the pathways or mechanisms that underlie observed associations remain open even when the directionality of influence is clear. Inquiry into how designation of network boundaries, nonresponse, and missing or erroneous data affect network analyses is much needed.

Such challenges are well worth pursuing. Research to date offers a persuasive case that social network environments play an important role in producing health-related outcomes. Indeed, some contend that their importance could be much greater than recognized to date, once the "collateral health consequences" or network-mediated "externalities" associated with health events or health policy interventions are better understood (Christakis 2004).

References

Bearman, P. S., & Moody, J. (2004). Suicide and friendships among American adolescents. *American Journal of Public Health, 94,* 89–95.

Bearman, P. S., Moody, J., Stovel, K., & Thalji, L. (2004). Social and sexual networks: The National Longitudinal Study of Adolescent Health. In M. Morris (Ed.), *Network epidemiology: A handbook for survey design and data collection* (pp. 201–220). New York: Oxford University Press.

Berkman, L. F., & Glass, T. (2000). Social integration, social networks, social support, and health. In L. F. Berkman & I. Kawachi (Eds.), *Social Epidemiology* (pp. 137–173). New York: Oxford University Press.

Berkman, L. F., & Kawachi, I. (2000). A historical framework for social epidemiology. In L. F. Berkman & I. Kawachi (Eds.), *Social Epidemiology* (pp. 3–12). New York: Oxford University Press.

Berkman, L. F., & Syme, S. L. (1979). Social networks, host resistance and mortality: A nine-year follow-up study of Alameda County residents. *American Journal of Epidemiology, 109,* 186–204.

Bond, K. C., Valente, T. W., & Kendall, C. (1999). Social network influences on reproductive health behaviors in urban northern Thailand. *Social Science & Medicine, 49,* 1599–1614.

Brewer, D. D. (2000). Forgetting in the recall-based elicitation of personal networks. *Social Networks, 22,* 379–403.

Brissette, I., Cohen, S., & Seeman, T. E. (2000). Measuring social integration and social networks. In S. Cohen, L. G. Underwood, & B. H. Gottlieb (Eds.), *Social support measurement and intervention: A guide for health and social scientists* (pp. 53–85). New York: Oxford University Press.

Campbell, K. S., & Lee, B. A. (1991). Name generators in surveys of personal networks. *Social Networks, 13,* 203–221.

Caraël, M., Glynn, J. R., Lagarde, E., & Morison, L. (2004). Sexual networks and HIV in four African populations: The use of standardized behavioral survey with biological markers. In M. Morris (Ed.), *Network epidemiology: A handbook for survey design and data collection* (pp. 58–84). New York: Oxford University Press.

Carrington, P. J., Scott, J., & Wasserman, S. (2005). *Models and methods in social network analysis.* New York: Cambridge University Press.

Christakis, N. A. (2004). Social networks and collateral health effects. *British Medical Journal, 329*, 184–185.

Cohen, S., Doyle, W. G., Skoner, D. P., Rabin, B. S., & Gwaltney, J. M. (1997). Social ties and susceptibility to the common cold. *Journal of the American Medical Association, 277*, 1940–1944.

Cohen, S., & Syme, S. L. (Eds.) (1985). *Social support and health.* New York: Academic Press.

Cohen, S., Underwood, L. G., & Gottlieb, B. H. (Eds.) (2000). *Social support measurement and intervention: A guide for health and social scientists.* New York: Oxford University Press.

Dean, A., & Tausig, M. (1986). Measuring intimate support: The family and confidant relationships. In N. Lin, A. Dean, & W. Ensel (Eds.), *Social support, life events, and depression* (pp. 117–128). Orlando, FL: Academic Press.

Ennett, S. T., Bailey, S. L., & Federman, E. B. (1999). Social network characteristics associated with risky behaviors among runaway and homeless youth. *Journal of Health and Social Behavior, 40,* 63–78.

Ennett, S. T., & Baumann, K. E. (1993). Peer group structure and adolescent cigarette smoking: A social network analysis. *Journal of Health and Social Behavior, 34*, 226–326.

Friedman, S. R., Neaigus, A., Jose, B., Curtis, R., Goldstein, M., Idefonso, G., et al. (1997). Sociometric risk networks and risk for HIV infection. *American Journal of Public Health, 87,* 1289–1296.

Haines, V. A., & Hurlbert, J. (1992). Network range and health. *Journal of Health and Social Behavior, 33*, 254–266.

Heckathorn, D. D. (1997). Respondent-driven sampling: A new approach to the study of hidden populations. *Social Problems, 44,* 174–199.

Hirsch, B. J. (1980). Natural support systems and coping with major life changes. *American Journal of Community Psychology, 8*, 159–172.

Holland, P. W., & Leinhardt, S. (1973). The structural implications of measurement error in sociometry. *Journal of Mathematical Sociology, 3*, 85–111.

House, J., Robbins, C., & Hetzner, H. (1982). The association of social relationships and activities with mortality: Prospective evidence from the Tecumseh Community Health Study. *American Journal of Epidemiology, 116*, 123–140.

House, J. S., & Kahn, R. L. (1985). Measures and concepts of social support. In S. Cohen & S. L. Syme (Eds.), *Social support and health* (pp. 83–108). New York: Academic Press.

Kahn, R. L., & Antonucci, T. C. (1980). Convoys over the life course: Attachment, roles, and social support. *Life-Span Development and Behavior, 3*, 253–286.

Killworth, P. D., Johnsen, E. C., McCarty, C., Shelley, G. A., & Bernard, H. R. (1998). A social network approach to estimating seroprevalence in the United States. *Social Networks, 20*, 23–50.

Klovdahl, A. S. (1985). Social networks and the spread of infectious diseases: The AIDS example. *Social Science & Medicine, 21*, 1203–1216.

Klovdahl, A. S. (2005). Social network research and human subjects protection: Towards more effective infectious disease control. *Social Networks, 27,* 119–137.

Klovdahl, A. S., Potterat, J. J., Woodhouse, D. E., Muth, J. B., Muth, S. Q., & Darrow, W. W. (1994). Social networks and infectious disease: The Colorado Springs Study. *Social Science & Medicine, 38*, 79–88.

Latkin, C. (1995). A personal network approach to AIDS prevention: An experimental peer group intervention for street-injecting drug users: The SAFE Study. In R. H. Needle, S. L. Coyle, S. G. Genser, & R. T. Trotter, (Eds.), *Social networks, drug abuse and HIV transmission* (pp. 181–195). Rockville, MD: National Institute on Drug Abuse.

Latkin, C. A., Mandell, W., Vlahov, D., Oziemkowska, M., & Celentano, D. D. (1996). The long-term outcome of a personal network-oriented HIV prevention intervention for injection drug users: The SAFE Study. *American Journal of Community Psychiatry, 24,* 341–364.

Laumann, E. O., Gagnon, J. H., Michael, R. T., & Michaels, S. (1994). *The social organization of sexuality: Sexual practices in the United States.* Chicago: University of Chicago Press.

Laumann, E. O., Gagnon, J. H., Michaels, S., Michael, R. T., & Schumm, L. P. (1993). Monitoring AIDS and other rare population events: A network approach. *Journal of Health and Social Behavior, 34,* 7–22.

Laumann, E. O., Mahay, J., Paik, A., & Youm, Y. (2004). Network data collection and its relevance for the analysis of STDs: The NHSLS and CHSLS. In M. Morris, (Ed.), *Network epidemiology: A handbook for survey design and data collection* (pp. 27–41). New York: Oxford University Press.

Laumann, E. O., & Youm, Y. (1999). Racial/ethnic group differences in the prevalence of sexually transmitted diseases in the United States: A network explanation. *Sexually Transmitted Diseases, 26,* 250–261.

Lin, N., Fu, Y., & Hsung, R. (2001). The position generator: Measurement techniques for investigations of social capital. In N. Lin, K. Cook, & R. S. Burt (Eds.), *Social capital: Theory and research* (pp. 57–71). New York: Aldine de Gruyter.

Lowenthal, M. F., & Haven, C. (1968). Interaction and adaptation: Intimacy as a critical variable. *American Sociological Review, 33,* 20–30.

Marsden, P. V. (1987). Core discussion networks of Americans. *American Sociological Review, 52,* 122–131.

Marsden, P. V. (1990). Network data and measurement. *Annual Review of Sociology, 16,* 435–463.

Marsden, P. V. (2005). Recent developments in network measurement. In P. J. Carrington, J. Scott, & S. Wasserman, (Eds.), *Models and methods in social network analysis* (pp. 8–30). New York: Cambridge University Press.

McGrady, G. A., Marrow, C., Myers, G., Daniels, M., Vera, M., Mueller, C., et al. (1995). A note on implementation of a random-walk design to study adolescent social networks. *Social Networks, 17,* 251–255.

Morris, M. (1993). Epidemiology and social networks: Modeling structured diffusion. *Sociological Methods and Research, 22,* 99–126.

Morris, M. (Ed.) (2004). *Network epidemiology: A handbook for survey design and data collection.* New York: Oxford University Press.

Morris, M., Podhisita, C., Wawer, M. J., & Handcock, M. S. (1996). Bridge populations in the spread of HIV/AIDS in Thailand. *AIDS, 10,* 1265–1271.

Morris, M., Pramualratana, A., Podhisita, C., & Wawer, M. J. (1995). The relational determinants of condom use with commercial sex partners in Thailand. *AIDS, 9,* 507–515.

Neaigus, A., Friedman, S. R., Curtis, R., Des Jarlais, D. C., Furst, R. T., Jose, B., et al. (1994). The relevance of drug injectors' social and risk networks for understanding and preventing HIV infection. *Social Science and Medicine, 38,* 67–78.

Neaigus, A., Friedman, S. R., Goldstein, M., Goldstein, M., Ildefonso, G., Curtis, R., et al. (1995). Using dyadic data for a network analysis of HIV infection and risk behaviors among injecting drug users. In R. H. Needle, S. L. Coyle, S. G. Genser, & R. T. Trotter

(Eds.), *Social networks, drug abuse and HIV transmission* (pp. 20–37). Rockville, MD: National Institute on Drug Abuse.

Newman, M. E. J. (2002). Spread of epidemic disease on networks. *Physical Review E, 66,* 016128.

Potterat, J. J., Woodhouse, D. E., Muth, S. Q., Rothenberg, R. B., Darrow, W. W., Klovdahl, A. S., et al. (2004). Network dynamism: History and lessons of the Colorado Springs study. In M. Morris (Ed.), *Network epidemiology: A handbook for survey design and data collection* (pp. 87–114). New York: Oxford University Press.

Rothenberg, R., & Narramore, J. (1996). The relevance of social network concepts to sexually transmitted disease control. *Sexually Transmitted Diseases, 23,* 24–29.

Rothenberg, R., Potterat, J. J., Woodhouse, D. E., Muth, S. Q., Darrow, W., & Klovdahl, A. S. (1998). Social network dynamics and HIV transmission. *AIDS, 12,* 1529–1536.

Sarason, I. G., Levine, H. M., Basham, R. B., & Sarason, B. R. (1983). Assessing social support: The social support questionnaire. *Journal of Personality and Social Psychology, 44,* 127–139.

Scott, J. (2000). *Social network analysis: A handbook.* Thousand Oaks, CA: Sage.

Shelley, G. A., Bernard, H. R., Killworth, P., Johnsen, E., & McCarty, C. (1995). Who knows your HIV status? What HIV+ patients and their network members know about each other. *Social Networks, 17,* 189–217.

Smith, K. P., & Watkins, S. C. (2005). Perceptions of risk and strategies for prevention: Responses to HIV/AIDS in rural Malawi. *Social Science & Medicine, 60,* 649–660.

Sudman, S. (1985). Experiments in the measurement of the size of social networks. *Social Networks, 7,* 127–151.

Sudman, S., & Kalton, G. (1986). New developments in the sampling of special populations. *Annual Review of Sociology, 12,* 401–429.

Thoits, P. A. (1983). Multiple identities and psychological well-being: A reformulation and test of the social isolation hypothesis. *American Sociological Review, 48,* 174–187.

Unger, J. B., & Chen, X. (1999). The role of social networks and media receptivity in predicting age of smoking initiation: A proportional hazards model of risk and protective factors. *Addictive Behaviors, 24,* 371–381.

Urberg, K. A., Değirmencioğlu, S. M., & Pilgrim, C (1997). Close friend and group influence on adolescent cigarette smoking and alcohol use. *Developmental Psychology, 33,* 834–844.

Valente, T. W. (1995). *Network models of the diffusion of innovations.* Creskill, NJ: Hampton Press.

Valente, T. W., Hoffman, B. R., Ritt-Olson, A., Lichtman, K., & Johnson, C. A. (2003). Effects of a social-network method for group assignment strategies on peer-led tobacco prevention programs in schools. *American Journal of Public Health, 93,* 1837–1843.

Valente, T. W., Watkins, S. C., Jato, M. N., van der Straten, A., & Tsitsol, L. M. (1997). Social network associations with contraceptive use among Cameroonian women in voluntary associations. *Social Science and Medicine, 45,* 677–687.

Van Der Gaag, M., & Snijders, T.A.B. (2005). The resource generator: Social capital quantification with concrete items. *Social Networks, 27,* 1–29.

Wasserman, S., & Faust, K. (1994). *Social networks: Methods and applications.* New York: Cambridge University Press.

Wellman, B., & Wortley, S. (1990). Different strokes from different folks: Community ties and social support. *American Journal of Sociology, 96,* 558–588.

White, K., & Watkins, S. C. (2000). Accuracy, stability, and reciprocity in informal conversational networks in Kenya. *Social Networks, 22,* 337–355.

Woodhouse, D. E., Potterat, J. J., Rothenberg, R. B., Darrow, W. W., Klovdahl, A. S., & Muth, S. Q. (1995). Ethical and legal issues in social network research: The real and the ideal. In R. H. Needle, S. L. Coyle, S. G. Genser, & R. T. Trotter (Eds.), *Social networks, drug abuse and HIV transmission* (pp. 131–143). Rockville, MD: National Institute on Drug Abuse.

Youm, Y., & Laumann, E. O. (2002). Social network effects on the transmission of sexually transmitted diseases. *Sexually Transmitted Diseases, 29,* 689–697.

CHAPTER TWELVE

IDENTIFYING SOCIAL INTERACTIONS: A REVIEW

Lawrence E. Blume and Steven N. Durlauf[1]

. . . political economy . . . does credit to thought because it finds the laws underlying a mass of contingent occurrences. It is an interesting spectacle to observe here how all the interconnections have repercussions on others, how the particular spheres fall into groups, influence others and are helped or hindered by these. This interaction, which seems at first sight incredible since everything seems to depend on the arbitrary will of the individual . . . bears a resemblance to the planetary system, which presents only irregular movements to the eye, yet whose laws can nevertheless be recognized.

G.W.F. HEGEL, ELEMENTS OF THE PHILOSOPHY OF RIGHT[2]

Whereas economics has long focused on how individual decisions are interconnected via markets, growing interest has developed for the last decade or so in understanding how social factors beyond the marketplace affect individual decisions and outcomes. Economic analysis now incorporates a range of

[1]Corresponding author. Blume: Department of Economics, Cornell University, Uris Hall, Ithaca, NY; Durlauf: Department of Economics, 1180 Observatory Drive, Madison WI, 53706-1393. The John D. and Catherine T. MacArthur Foundation, National Science Foundation and University of Wisconsin Graduate School have provided financial support. We thank J. Michael Oakes for immensely helpful comments on a previous draft and Buz Brock for many comments on this work. Ethan Cohen-Cole, Giacomo Rondina, and Histaoshi Tanaka have provided splendid research assistance.
[2]Allen Wood translation, Cambridge University Press, 1991, pg. 228.

dimensions in which individuals interact directly with one another rather than indirectly via the effects of individuals on market prices. As noted by Manski (2000), the emergence of the social interactions literature parallels the rise of game theory, in which the key primitive assumptions are based on modeling how the behaviors of others affect an individual relative to general equilibrium theory, which focuses on the analysis of conditions under which markets can coordinate many individual decisions via a price system. Such direct interdependences in behaviors and outcomes are known in the economics literature as social interactions.

Economic research on social interactions has proceeded along theoretical as well as empirical lines.[3] In terms of abstract theory, the social interactions research has followed two main directions. A first direction is the description of how interdependent decisions produce different aggregate configurations. Early examples of this work include Blume (1993, 1995), Brock (1993), and Durlauf (1993); more recent research includes Brock and Durlauf (2001a, 2001b, 2005 [forthcoming], 2006 [forthcoming]), Bisin et al. (2004), and Horst and Scheinkman (2004). This sort of research investigates the appropriate specification of individual decision-making in the presence of social influences and the consequent implications of these influences for the behavior of population aggregates. One important message from this work is that the incorporation of social interactions into economic models is fully compatible with standard economic reasoning, in which individuals make purposeful decisions subject to constraints. A second direction evaluates the role of social interactions in determining how groups form. Research of this type includes Bénabou (1996), Durlauf (1996), and Hoff and Sen (2005). Perhaps unsurprisingly, the canonical example of endogenous group formation is residential neighborhoods; in fact, in economics, social interaction effects and neighborhood effects are used interchangeably.[4] These general structures have been used to develop theoretical descriptions of phenomena ranging from spatial unemployment patterns (Oomes 2003) to welfare dependence (Lindbeck et al. 1999) to economic development and the transition from underdeveloped to modern economies (Kelly 1997). These "applied theory" studies have typically been motivated by various empirical claims that seem hard to understand using other types of economic models. The sources of social interactions in various types of theoretical models are themselves varied. Some models assume that there are

---

[3]Surveys of different aspects of the economic approach to social interactions include Becker and Murphy (2000), Brock and Durlauf (2001b), Durlauf (2004), and Manski (2000). See also Sampson et al. (2004) for a sociological perspective.

[4]Following Akerlof (1997), individuals may be conceptualized as located in a general social space in which groups of commonly interacting individuals constitute a neighborhood.

primitive psychological reasons why individuals wish to conform to the behavior of others, whereas others focus on the information transmission that occurs when one person observes what others choose to do.

In parallel to this theoretical work, many empirical studies of social interactions now exist. Among the conventional economic phenomena that have been studied are public assistance use (Aizer and Currie 2004; Bertrand et al. 2000), labor market behavior (Conley and Topa 2002; Topa 2001; Weinberg et al. 2004), agricultural contract specification (Young and Burke 2001), and urban economics (Ioannides and Zabel 2003a, 2003b; Irwin and Brockstaed 2002). In addition, interest in social interactions has led economists to study phenomena that are traditionally in the domain of other social sciences, such as crime (Glaeser et al. 1996; Sirakaya 2004), choice of medical techniques by physicians (Burke et al. 2004), and smoking (Krauth 2003, 2004; Soetevent and Kooreman 2004).

A third component of the new social interactions research program has been the systematic investigation of econometric issues. This econometric work primarily focuses on the determination of conditions under which various types of social interactions may be econometrically identified.[5] Identification arguments in this context amount to asking under what conditions on data and model can the role of social interactions effects be distinguished from other influences on behavior. Thus, identification analysis represents a key link between theory and empirics.

The econometric research program on the identifiability of social interactions was initiated in Manski (1993), a seminal paper that still warrants careful study; recent contributions include Brock and Durlauf 2001a, 2001b, 2005 [forthcoming], 2006 [forthcoming]; Glaeser et al. 1996; Graham 2005; Graham and Hahn 2004; Moffitt 2001; and Soetevent and Kooreman 2004. Although the general econometrics of social interactions has not developed to the same extent as the theoretical and empirical literatures, there now exists a fairly wide range of results on identification.

In this chapter, we review some of the identification results that have been developed in the econometrics literature on social interactions. We will focus on two statistical frameworks in which social interactions have been embedded: linear models and binary choice models. The discussion avoids formal proofs in order to highlight major conceptual issues. The results we describe are not specific to economic contexts and so presumably may be useful for social epidemiologists as well.

Section Two describes the two statistical social interactions models that we will analyze. Section Three describes the identification problems that arise when

[5]There is also some work on estimation and computation issues, cf. Bisin et al. (2002).

model errors are independent and identically distributed. This is a useful baseline for understanding how identification problems arise that are intrinsic to the structure of the behavioral process. Section Four discusses how self-selection of individuals into groups affects identification. Section Five analyzes identification in the presence of unobserved group effects. Section Six relates the econometrics literature on social interactions to some aspects of the social epidemiology literature. Hierarchical models and models that incorporate social capital are studied. Section Seven provides summary and conclusions.

Basic Models

To understand the main identification problems that arise in empirical studies of social interactions, we start with some notation and baseline models. These models, although not exhaustive, cover much of the economic social interactions literature and illustrate the main identification problems faced by a researcher attempting to adduce evidence that social interactions matter.

Individuals are denoted by i and groups are denoted by g. Each individual is a member of a single group; the composition of these groups is known to the researcher. In other words, prior to the statistical exercise, a researcher has determined the relevant environment in which social interactions are present. This is a standard assumption in social interactions analyses. For example, a researcher investigating the role of residential neighborhoods typically makes an ex ante decision on how neighborhoods are measured (for example, via census tracts). The analysis of social interactions when there is uncertainty about the correct specification of the relevant social groups has not been pursued, to our knowledge, although work such as Conley and Topa (2002) has attempted to compare the predictive power of different conceptions of neighborhoods defined in a general social space. In principle, one can incorporate model uncertainty about the correct social group for individuals into the econometric analysis of social interactions (see Brock et al. 2003, for one way to proceed), but the implications for identification have not been explored; this seems an important area for future research.

Each individual makes a choice ω_i. These choices are assumed to depend on a combination of individual-specific and group-specific factors. The individual-specific factors come in two types: X_i, deterministic (to the modeler) characteristics associated with individual i, and ε_i, random and unobservable (to the modeler) characteristics associated with i. In the econometric analog to the theoretical model of choice under social interactions, ε_i corresponds to the random error in a regression. We assume in both the theoretical and econometric discussion that these random terms are independent and identically distributed across individuals. This means that the within-group distribution of ε_i does not depend on the individual's characteristics or the identity of the group of which he is a member

$$F_{\varepsilon_i|X_i,Y_g} = F_\varepsilon. \tag{1}$$

The assumption of independent and identically distributed (i.i.d.) errors will be relaxed in some directions when we discuss econometrics.

Group-specific factors are partitioned into Y_g, predetermined with respect to decisions by individuals concerning ω) group-level characteristics, and $m_{i,g}^e$, the expected average choice in the group. In the economics social interactions literature, the role of Y_g in affecting individuals is known as a contextual effect, whereas the role of $m_{i,g}^e$ is known as an endogenous effect and plays a central role in the discussion to follow. Contextual effects thus describe how the characteristics of others affect an individual's decisions, whereas endogenous effects describe how the behaviors of others affect an individual's decision or choice. The importance of this distinction is that endogenous effects are usually understood to be reciprocal and thus create feedbacks between individual decisions. Although behavioral endogeneity is rarely considered in other social sciences, from the economics perspective, social interactions have not been modeled at a deeper level than the endogenous or contextual effect distinction. An important open research question is whether attention to particular generative mechanisms, such as social interactions as a mechanism for information transmission, could facilitate identification.

The use of expected average choice rather than the realized average choice is made for analytical convenience. The assumption makes most sense for larger groups where the behaviors of the rest of group are not directly observable. The assumption that individuals react to expected rather than actual behaviors is not critical for the bulk of the identification analysis we describe; we will indicate where the assumption matters. See Graham (2005) and Soetevent and Kooreman (2004) for analysis of social interactions in small groups where all behaviors are observed.

To make this abstract description concrete, we follow discussion in Durlauf (2006 [forthcoming]) and consider the example of modeling the determinants of schooling outcomes among children. One class of explanations may focus on how parental characteristics affect these outcomes, as more successful parents are able to provide more educational resources to their children, provide role models that enhance their children's aspirations, and so forth. These sorts of determinants are captured by the vector X_i. In contrast, other theories might focus on the role of contextual influences, such as how the sorts of occupations observed across adults within a residential neighborhood affect student aspirations or how the distribution of incomes across families within the community affects decisions on the level of expenditures on education. These sorts of factors are captured by the vector Y_g.

A final set of explanations may derive from direct interdependence between the educational outcomes of children; for example, high outcomes by one student may be induced by the desire of the student to perform as well as his peers. This type of explanation is captured by $m_{i,g}^e$.

How do these different factors combine to determine individual choices? We consider two formal frameworks. The first is a basic linear model with social interactions, originally studied in Manski (1993), in which outcomes are described by a linear model:

$$\omega_i = k + cX_i + dY_g + Jm_{i,g}^e + \varepsilon_i. \tag{2}$$

Note that k and J are scalars whereas c and d are vectors[6]. This model is typically not derived from a fully articulated decision problem for individual agents, but this can be done in principle. The model has the important virtue that it is easily interpreted as a regression and so may be directly taken to data, where the goal of the analysis is to estimate the parameters k, c, d, and J. Claims about social interactions are, from the econometric perspective, equivalent to statements about the values of d and J. The statement that social interactions matter is equivalent to the statement that at least some element of the union of the parameters in d and J is nonzero. The statement that contextual social interactions are present means that at least one element of d is nonzero. The statement that endogenous social interactions matter requires that J be nonzero.

A second useful model is the binary choice model with social interactions studied in detail by Brock and Durlauf (2001a, 2001b). Following Brock and Durlauf (2001a, 2001b), choices are coded so that they lie in the set $\{-1, 1\}$. For example, -1 can denote *had a child while a teenager,* whereas 1 denotes *did not have a child while a teenager,* if one is studying teenage fertility. This model is directly derived from an individual decision problem. Each choice is associated with a payoff level $V_i(\omega_i)$. The difference between the payoffs for the two choices is assumed to be additive in the different factors that have been defined, that is,

$$V_i(1) - V_i(-1) = k + cX_i + dY_g + Jm_{i,g}^e - \varepsilon_i. \tag{3}$$

Individual i chooses 1 if and only if $V_i(1) - V_i(-1) > 0$, which is to say that an individual acts rationally in the sense that she makes the choice that makes her best off. Because

$$\Pr(V_i(1) - V_i(-1) \geq 0) = \Pr(\varepsilon_i \leq k + cX_i + dY_g + Jm_{i,g}^e)$$
$$= F_\varepsilon(k + cX_i + dY_g + Jm_{i,g}^e), \tag{4}$$

[6]Throughout, coefficient vectors such as c are row vectors whereas variable vectors such as X_i are column vectors.

$\Pr(\omega_i = 1 \mid X_i, \Upsilon_g, g)$, the probability that i chooses 1, is defined by

$$\Pr(\omega_i = 1 \mid X_i, \Upsilon_g, g) = F_\varepsilon(k + cX_i + d\Upsilon_g + \mathcal{J}m_{i,g}^e). \tag{5}$$

Neither the linear model nor the binary choice model has any empirical content without restricting how individuals form expectations about the average behavior of others. Otherwise, any set of observed behaviors could be reconciled with any set of model parameters by appropriate choices of $m_{i,g}^e$. In economics, the standard approach to closing the social interactions model is the requirement that expectations be consistent with the structure of the choices in the model. This property, known as self-consistency, means that the subjective expectation of the average choice in one's group corresponds to the mathematical conditional expectation of the average choice, m_g, given the information set of each agent. We assume these information sets include the values of X_i for other agents within i's group, the value of Υ_g, as well as the equilibrium expected choice level that occurs for the individual's group. Agents are assumed to be unable to observe the choices of others or their random payoff terms ε_i. Alternative information assumptions will not affect the qualitative properties of the model. For the linear in means model, self-consistency means that

$$m_{i,g}^e = m_g = \frac{k + cX_g + d\Upsilon_g}{1 - \mathcal{J}} = \frac{k + d\Upsilon_g}{1 - \mathcal{J}} + \frac{cX_g}{1 - \mathcal{J}} \tag{6}$$

where X_g is the average of X_i within g. In simple terms, the mathematical expectation of average behavior in a group depends linearly on the average of the individual determinants of behavior, X_g, and the contextual effects that each member experiences in common, Υ_g.

For the binary choice model, self-consistency means that

$$m_{i,g}^e = m_g = 2 \int F_\varepsilon(k + cX + d\Upsilon_g + \mathcal{J}m_g) \, dF_{X|g} - 1 \tag{7}$$

where recall that $F_{X|g}$ is the empirical within-group distribution of X. The description of a process for individual choices combined with its associated self-consistency condition fully specifies a model.

From the perspective of economic theory, there is an important difference between the linear and binary choice models of social interactions: multiple equilibria can exist for the latter but not the former. A model exhibits multiple equilibria if its microeconomic structure is compatible with more than one aggregate outcome. For the models we have described, the only aggregate outcome of interest is the expected average choice level m_g. It is evident for the linear model that once one knows the individual and group characteristics within a group, there is only one expected average choice level that is consistent; equation (6) maps these characteristics into a single m_g. In contrast, equation (7) can produce more than one solution for m_g. In general, as shown in Brock and Durlauf (2006 [forthcoming]), for each value of Y_g and $F_{X,g}$ for a given group, there will exist a threshold H (which depends on these values) such that if $J > H$, then there are at least three solutions to equation (7) whereas if $J < H$ then the solution to equation (7) is unique.[7]

More precise results may be obtained if one specifies the functional forms for $F_{X,g}$ and F_ε; these different cases are analyzed in Brock and Durlauf (2001a, 2001b, 2005 [forthcoming], 2006 [forthcoming]). For example, suppose that

$$F_\varepsilon(z) = \frac{1}{1 + \exp(-z)} \tag{8}$$

so that the model errors are negative exponentially distributed, and that $k + cX_i + dY_g = h$, so that this component of the payoff differential between the two choices is constant across group members. For this special case,

$$\Pr(\omega_i = 1 \,|\, X_i, Y_g, g) = \frac{\exp(h + Jm_{i,g}^e)}{\exp(h + Jm_{i,g}^e) + \exp(-h - Jm_{i,g}^e)}. \tag{9}$$

Under self-consistency, the expected average choice level m_g within a group must obey

$$m_g = \tanh(h + Jm_g). \tag{10}$$

In equation (10), $\tanh(x) = \frac{\exp(x) - \exp(-x)}{\exp(x) + \exp(-x)}$. For this case, one can show formally that if $J < H$, then the equilibria is unique whereas if $J > H$ there are three equilibria, of which only the two extremal equilibria (in terms of the magnitude of m_g) are stable under dynamic analogs of the model. This special case is of interest since the assumption (8) corresponds to the logit regression model for binary choice.

Blume and Durlauf (2003) extend this work by considering a dynamic analog of the binary choice model with social interactions. This paper studies the stability of the self-consistent equilibria in the static model and finds that over time, a dynamic analog of this model will have the property that the population spends most of its time in the vicinity of the equilibrium that maximizes average utility (that is, the equilibrium whose mean choice has the same sign as h). One question that has not been examined is whether the far-from-steady state behavior of the model can provide additional information on social interactions that is not

---

[7]The knife edge case $J = H$ is conventionally ignored in theoretical studies, because it is presumably a probability 0 possibility.

present in a steady state. This is intuitively plausible because far-from-steady state behavior will obey a different probability process from steady state behavior, even though it derives from the same microeconomic foundations.

The assumption that each agent reacts to the mean behavior of the population is restrictive. Within the economic theory literature, there has been considerable attention to models in which interactions are local. In such models, agents are located in some sort of social space and interact only with those agents that, according to some metric, are near the agent. This type of work was pioneered in Föllmer (1974). Blume (1993, 1995) provides a rigorous analysis of models of this type, employing formal game theoretic arguments; Kirman (1997) is a valuable survey. As far as we know, empirical analogs of such models have not been formally investigated with respect to identification.

Identification and the Reflection Problem

In this section, we consider how the various determinants of individual behavior may be revealed empirically. We focus on a cross-section of data where individuals are sampled across a set of groups. The objective of a statistical exercise is to estimate the parameters k, c, d, and J; identification arguments will focus on whether more than one set of values for these parameters generate identical probability statements about ω_i. When discussing binary choice models, it is understood that identification means identification up to scale (that is to say that the parameters k, c, d, and J are identified means that any alternative set of parameters that produces the same probability statements about w_i must be a multiple of the initial parameter set). The reason for this is that if one were to multiply all the parameters in equation (3) by a nonzero constant, individual behavior would be unchanged, because the choice is based on the comparison of the utility levels for each of the choices, not their absolute values.

The available data to a researcher are assumed to be ω_i, X_i and Y_g, the individual choices and associated individual-specific contextual effects, as well as $F_{X|g}$ and $F_{\omega|g}$, the empirical distribution functions for the individual characteristics and individual outcomes within each group of which the individuals are members. We do not consider whether other data can facilitate identification. One obvious candidate is price data on group memberships (for example, housing or rental prices for different neighborhoods.) Work by Ekeland et al. (2002, 2004) and Nesheim (2002) suggest that such data may be very valuable from the perspective of hedonic pricing models.

The first problem that arises in the study of social interactions is the classic identification problem: under what conditions on the data, if any, can the different parameters in the linear model (2) or the binary choice model (5) (or both) be distinguished from an alternative set of parameters? Intuitively, the reason why identification may not hold is that the distinct roles of the endogenous effects and the contextual effects may be difficult to disentangle, because the two types of effects move together. This comovement occurs because, when beliefs are self-consistent, the contextual variables Y_g help to determine the endogenous variable m_g as indicated by the self-consistency conditions (6) and (7). Thus the identification problem for social interactions bears much resemblance to the elementary identification problem that occurs in linear regressions when the regressors are not linearly independent.

Does the fact that endogenous and contextual social interaction effects are, by the logic of social interaction models, correlated lead to a failure of identification? In the case of the linear regression model, the answer is yes. Specifically, without prior information about the relationship between the individual-specific characteristics X_i and the group-level characteristics Y_g, the linear model of social interactions is not identified. The possibility for non-identification was first recognized by Manski (1993). To see why identification may fail for this model, assume, following Manski's original argument, that $Y_g = X_g$. This means that every contextual effect is the average of a corresponding individual characteristic. In this case, equation (6) reduces to

$$m_g = \frac{k + (c + d)Y_g}{1 - J},\tag{11}$$

which means the regressor m_g in model (2) is linearly dependent on the other regressors (that is, the constant and Y_g). This linear dependence means that identification fails: the comovements of m_g and Y_g are such that one cannot disentangle their respective influences on individuals. Manski (1993) named this failure the *reflection problem;* metaphorically, if one observes that ω_i is correlated with the expected average behavior in a neighborhood, (11) indicates it may be possible that this correlation is due to the fact that m_g may simply reflect the role of Y_g in influencing individuals.

Are there versions of the linear model where the reflection problem does not hold? The answer is yes. To see why it is possible for some linear models with social interactions to be identified, suppose that we relax the assumption that $X_g = Y_g$. In this case, as indicated by equation (6), it is possible that m_g is not linearly dependent on the constant and Y_g. The reason for this is the presence of the term $\frac{cX_g}{1-J}$ in equation (6). This term can break the reflection problem. This will happen if the $\frac{cX_g}{1-J}$ term is such that it is not linearly dependent on a constant and Y_g; when this is so, m_g cannot be linearly dependent on the other regressors in equation (6). A necessary condition for this to happen is that there exists at least one regressor in X_i whose group-level average does not appear in Υ_g. For example, identification can be achieved if an individual's age affects educational outcomes, but we are willing to rule out in advance that the average age of his peers influences him, once we have controlled for other characteristics of the peers. Formal conditions for identification in the linear model with social interactions are given in Brock and Durlauf (2001a, 2001b).

Although the reflection problem arises naturally in the linear model, it does not necessarily generalize to alternative data structures, such as the binary choice model we have described. For the binary choice model, formal statements of conditions for identification appear in Brock and Durlauf (2001a, 2001b) for the case when the random terms ε_i are logistically distributed and in Brock and Durlauf (2006 [forthcoming]) for general distribution functions. The logic of the reflection problem as it emerges in the linear model indicates why identification will not fail for the binary choice model. Equation (7) indicates that for the binary choice model, m_g cannot be a linear function of the other regressors in equation (5). This is intrinsic to the model when there is sufficient variation in X_i and Υ_g, because probabilities are bounded between zero and one; m_g (which is a weighted average of the individual-specific choice probabilities) *cannot* be linearly dependent on X_i and Υ_g when these vectors have sufficiently wide supports. This finding does not depend on the fact that the error distribution is known; see Brock and Durlauf (2005 [forthcoming]) for a proof. Furthermore, identification will generally hold for other nonlinear models, such as nonlinear regressions and duration data models; Brock and Durlauf (2001b) discuss these cases.

Of course, identification will even fail for nonlinear models if the elements that comprise X_i and Υ_g are themselves linearly dependent; however, this source of non-identification does not seem natural in most contexts. One example where this would happen is a world where (1) $\Upsilon_g = X_g$, and (2) individuals are perfectly segregated by X_i (so that each person in a group has the same value of X_i). Perfect segregation means that $X_g = X_i$, which in turn implies that $\Upsilon_g = X_i$.

Therefore, the two key messages for identification of social interactions with i.i.d. errors are: (1) for linear models, identification requires that there exist individual specific characteristics; and (2) identification will hold under standard conditions for nonlinear models.

Social Interactions and Self-Selection

For contexts such as residential neighborhoods, it is natural to believe that assumption (1), which states that individuals are randomly assigned to groups, is not tenable. The natural reason for this is that in many contexts, group membership is itself a choice variable. One does not think of families as being randomly allocated across neighborhoods; rather, families choose neighborhoods subject to constraints such as rent levels and personal income. For environments in which self-selection is present, the consistency of various statistical methods for estimating social interactions may be affected. Specifically, the presence of self-selection can mean that the expected value of the random term ε_i, conditional on the individual's characteristics and group memberships, may no longer be zero. If one observes a poor family living in a rich neighborhood, one would reasonably infer that the level of parental investment in children is higher than other families. If this investment contains an unobservable component, then it will be part of the ε_i term. Following this logic, for a model of educational attainment, the conditional value of ε_i for a child who is part of a poor family in a rich neighborhood is positive.

If one ignores self-selection in estimation, then one may produce spurious evidence of social interactions. For example, if poorer neighborhoods tend to contain relatively less ambitious parents than affluent neighborhoods and if lack of ambition on the part of parents leads to lower educational performance by children, then the failure to account for this self-selection could lead to the false conclusion that poor neighborhoods causally affect education. Generally, if neighborhoods are (partially) stratified according to unobservable individual-level characteristics that affect outcomes, then the danger of finding spurious evidence of social interactions will be present.

There is a vast literature in economics on accounting for self-selection in statistical exercises and it is covered in virtually any graduate microeconometrics textbook; see Cameron and Trivedi (2005) for a recent example. One solution to self-selection is the use of instrumental variables. In this approach, the problem of self-selection is interpreted as the presence of correlation between the regression errors in a model and the model regressors; the previous example of parental ambition produces such a correlation. The study by Evans et al. (1992) is a well known example of the use of instrumental variables to account for self-selection; this study concluded that controlling for self-selection eliminated the statistical significance of neighborhood effects for the data that were analyzed. Of course, there is no reason why this must be the case; in a similar exercise, Rivkin (2001) finds that estimates of social interactions increase in magnitude when instrumental variables are used. One important point to note here is that the identification of valid instruments is often quite hard (see Heckman [1997] for discussion in the context of treatment effects analysis and Brock and Durlauf [2001c] for discussion using aggregate data to study economic growth). Intuitively, one often finds that asserted instruments, although predetermined with respect to a behavioral equation, nevertheless are likely to violate the requirement of uncorrelatedness with the equation error, once one considers a complete description of the behavioral decisions of the agents under study.

Within econometrics, the deepest analyses of self-selection are based on explicitly modeling the self-selection and including it as part of the statistical analysis. Unlike the instrumental variables approach, this has interesting implications for identification, at least for the linear model; Brock and Durlauf (2001b) first recognized this possibility. To understand their argument, rewrite the regression error in the linear model as

$$\omega_i = cX_i + dY_g + \mathcal{J}m_g + E(\varepsilon_i | X_i, Y_g, F_{X|g}) + \xi_i. \tag{12}$$

This expression exploits Heckman's (1979) idea that in the presence of self-selection, the regression residual ε_i no longer has a conditional mean of zero. Following the logic behind Heckman's classic selection correction, equation (12) can be consistently estimated if one adds a term proportional to $E(\varepsilon_i | X_i, Y_g, F_{X|g})$ to equation (12) before estimation; denote this estimate as $\kappa \overline{E(\varepsilon_i | X_i, Y_g, F_{X|g})}$. Heckman's great insight was that one can construct such a term. Hence, from this perspective, controlling for self-selection amounts to estimating

$$\omega_i = cX_i + dY_g + \mathcal{J}m_g + \rho\kappa\overline{E(\varepsilon_i | X_i, Y_g, F_{X|g})} + \xi_i. \tag{13}$$

Thus, accounting for self-selection necessitates considering identification for this regression, as opposed to equation (2).

The property of interest for the identification of social interactions is that the term $\kappa\overline{E(\varepsilon_i | X_i, Y_g, F_{X|g})}$ can help facilitate identification. To see this, consider two possibilities for the underlying conditional expectation $E(\varepsilon_i | X_i, Y_g, F_{X|g})$. One possibility is that

$$E(\varepsilon_i | X_i, Y_g, F_{X|g}) = \phi(m_g) \tag{14}$$

In this case, the presence of the regressor $\kappa\overline{E(\varepsilon_i | X_i, Y_g, F_{X|g})}$ in equation (13) means that the model is no longer linear in m_g. Assuming $\phi(\cdot)$ is invertible, then the self-consistent solution for m_g is

$$m_g = \psi(k + (c + d)Y_g) \tag{15}$$

where $\psi(\cdot)$ is the inverse of $1 - \phi(\cdot)$. Equation (15) illustrates that for this case, self-selection converts a linear model that is not identified into a nonlinear (in m_g) model in which m_g cannot be linearly dependent on a constant term and Y_g. The key point is that self-selection induces an intrinsic nonlinearity into the determinants of individual behavior and so converts the linear model into a nonlinear one.

Alternatively, suppose that

$$E(\varepsilon_i \mid X_i, \, Y_g, \, F_{X|g}) \; = \; \phi(X_i, \, Y_g) \qquad\qquad (16)$$

In this case, $\phi(X_i, \, Y_g)$ functions as an additional individual-specific regressor whose group level average does not appear in equation (13). Hence, following the argument about identification in linear models that was developed in the previous section, the presence of the regressor with a nonzero coefficient can allow for identification to occur. This approach to identification has been successfully used in Ioannides and Zabel (2003b) to identify social interaction effects in housing.[8]

The incorporation of self-selection into social epidemiology analyses seems, from the vantage point of econometrics, of first-order significance. Self-selection issues have proven to be of enormous importance in understanding a range of issues involving questions of policy evaluation. A major component of James Heckman's profound contributions to economics revolves around developing ways to draw inferences when self-selection is present. See Heckman (2001) for an extraordinary survey.

In accounting for self-selection, it is important to recognize that it can occur with respect to *unobservable* variables. In the context of job training programs, for example, program participation and completion are likely to be associated with the abilities and ambitions of an individual. This contrasts with the sort of analysis that is associated with causal inference in which selection is assumed to occur with respect to observables. The latter does not necessarily affect inferences; for example in the linear model, selection on observables does not affect analysis of the linear model (2) so long as $E(\varepsilon_i \mid X_i, \, Y_g, \, F_{X|g}) = 0$. Much of the statistical literature on causal effects focuses on self-selection on observables; as Heckman (1996) makes clear, such an approach is often inadequate as it is typical that "persons making decisions have more information about the outcomes than the statisticians studying them" (p. 461). This is clearly the case for group memberships.

It seems that there has been some confusion in the social epidemiology literature on the implications for self-selection in empirical analysis when selection occurs on unobservables. Subramanian (2004), in criticizing arguments of Oakes (2004), who argues that self-selection invalidates many claims in the social epidemiology literature, suggests that self-selection issues "are partially tractable and

---

[8]An important unanswered research question is how one can employ semiparametric estimates of $\overline{\kappa E(\varepsilon_i \mid X_i, \, Y_g, \, F_{X|g})}$ to help identify social interactions models; existing theoretical results on identification (Brock and Durlauf 2001b, 2006 [forthcoming]; Ioannides and Zabel (2003b) construct estimates based on parameter assumptions about the distribution of the error ε_i in equation (2) as well as the selection question that is combined with equation (2) to produce the estimated $\overline{\kappa E(\varepsilon_i \mid X_i, \, Y_g, \, F_{X|g})}$.

one potential strategy is through applying creative multilevel structures" (p. 1963). His example seems to suggest that movements across neighborhoods can provide information on the presence of social interactions. Such a claim is untenable unless one models the decision to change neighborhoods. The value of the self-selection correction $E(\varepsilon_i \mid X_i, Y_g, F_{X|g})$ will depend on the characteristics of a neighborhood and thus will differ for a given individual when that individual is observed in different neighborhoods. Perhaps this is reading too much into the discussion in Subramanian (2004). What is known from the econometrics literature, however, is that one cannot make arguments about what is or is not identified without formal analysis; terms such as "partially tractable" are only meaningful in the context of a fully articulated model.

We also disagree with Oakes (2004) to the extent that he advocates randomized experiments as clearly superior to other data sets in uncovering social interactions. His argument that such data sets can overcome self-selection problems is of course correct; however, as illustrated in the discussion of equations (12) through (16), self-selection can, when correctly modeled, facilitate identification. This should not be surprising. Self-selection describes another behavior by individuals beyond the behavioral choice ω_i—the choice of group membership. This second choice has implicit information about the social interactions the group produces. Whereas exploration of how this additional information may be exploited has only just begun, it seems potentially important.

Unobserved Group Effects

The second major deviation from the baseline social interactions model concerns the possibility that unobserved group effects exist. This case has received attention in the linear case in Brock and Durlauf (2001b), Graham and Hahn (2004), and Graham (2005) and in the binary choice case in Brock and Durlauf (2005 [forthcoming]). To be concrete, if one is interested in whether residential neighborhoods produce social interactions that affect offspring educational performance, a natural candidate for an unobservable is the average quality of schools, at least some component of which is unobservable to the econometrician.

Similar to the case of self-selection, the presence of the unobservable group effects can, if not accounted for, lead to spurious conclusions concerning the presence of social interactions. Why? Suppose that more affluent parents choose neighborhoods with higher school quality. If one then calculates the correlation between student outcomes and average neighborhood income, this correlation will be positive not because of any influence of the incomes of others on a given student, but because average parental income is itself correlated with school quality. Notice one would not necessarily regard these effects as unobserved types of social interactions. For example, variations in school quality may derive from variation in the quality of teachers, which is driven by community attributes such as the opportunities for spousal employment that have nothing to do with social influences on children.

Algebraically, the introduction of unobserved group effects is simple. Denoting the fixed effect as α_g, the original linear model is modified to

$$\omega_i = k + cX_i + dY_g + \mathcal{J}m_g + \alpha_g + \xi_i. \tag{17}$$

In parallel, the payoff comparison in the original binary choice model is modified to

$$V_i(1) - V_i(-1) = k + cX_i + dY_g + \mathcal{J}m^e_{i,g} + \alpha_g - \varepsilon_i \tag{18}$$

so that the conditional probability that 1 is chosen is modified from equation (3) to

$$\Pr(\omega_i = 1 \mid X_i, Y_g, \alpha_g) = F_\varepsilon(k + cX_i + dY_g + \mathcal{J}m^e_{i,g} + \alpha_g) \tag{19}$$

with the new self-consistency condition

$$m_g = 2 \int F_\varepsilon(k + cX + dY_g + \mathcal{J}m_g + \alpha_g)\, dF_{X\mid g} - 1. \tag{20}$$

Unobserved group effects are usually best regarded as fixed effects, because there is typically no plausible reason to believe the effects are orthogonal to observable group characteristics. In contrast, suppose that group memberships are generated endogenously and individuals observe α_g when groups are formed. If so, then there will presumably be some relation between α_g and those characteristics of individuals and the associated groups that are observed by the econometrician. Returning to our neighborhoods and education example, because families will presumably care about teacher quality when selecting neighborhoods, this will induce correlations between unobserved (to the econometrician) school quality and variables such as average income of parents. In our view, the problem of unobserved group characteristics is the most serious impediment to developing persuasive evidence of social interactions.

For linear models, identification in cross-sections is impossible when fixed effects are present. Any pattern of outcomes in the linear model without unobserved fixed effects can be replicated one for one by an identical model with no social interactions and unobserved group effects. One simply sets $\alpha_g = dY_g + \mathcal{J}m_g$. Identification of social interactions in linear models with unobserved group effects can occur for alternative data structures and models.

One way to achieve identification with unobserved fixed effects involves using panel data. In this approach, the assumption is that the unobservable group effects are time invariant, whereas other determinants of behavior are not. The basic idea in the panel approach is to consider a time indexed analog to equation (17), that is,

$$\omega_{i,t} = k + cX_{i,t} + dY_{g,t} + Jm_{g,t} + \alpha_g + \xi_{i,t} \tag{21}$$

and construct differences of the form

$$\begin{aligned}
\omega_{i,t} - \omega_{i,t-1} &= c(X_{i,t} - X_{i,t-1}) + d(Y_{g,t} - Y_{g,t-1}) \\
&\quad + J(m_{g,t} - m_{g,t-1}) + \xi_{i,t} - \xi_{i,t-1}
\end{aligned} \tag{22}$$

As equation (22) illustrates, taking first differences of $\omega_{i,t}$ can eliminate the unobserved fixed effect α_g. This approach is employed, for example, in Hoxby (2000a, 2000b). The validity of this approach, of course, depends on the validity of the assumption that α_g does not vary over time. For this reason, differencing generally cannot be used to account for self-selection in panels; the time-indexed version of the self-selection correction analyzed in Section Four will normally vary across time, as it is a function of $X_{i,t}$ and $Y_{g,t}$.

Alternatively, one can follow Graham (2005) and assume that α_g is a random effect rather than a fixed effect. Of course, to do this, one needs to be able to defend the random effect assumption; for Graham, the assumption is tenable because the data he studies involves random assignments of students to classrooms. This approach also necessitates restricting the analysis to the effort to identify some social interactions (that is, conducting the analysis without distinguishing between endogenous and contextual effects). The following is a variant of Graham's approach, which corresponds to the framework we have been using.[9] Considering the regression

$$\omega_i = k + dY_g + \alpha_g + \varepsilon_i, \tag{23}$$

we assume that Y_g is a scalar for convenience. If there are no social interactions present (that is, $d = 0$) then

$$\mathrm{var}(\omega_i) = \mathrm{var}(\varepsilon_i) + \mathrm{var}(\alpha_g). \tag{24}$$

Note that the random effect assumption means that $\mathrm{cov}(Y_g, \alpha_g) = 0$. In contrast, if social interactions are present, then

$$\mathrm{var}(\omega_i) = \mathrm{var}(\varepsilon_i) + \mathrm{var}(dY_g) + \mathrm{var}(\alpha_g). \tag{25}$$

---

[9]Graham (2005) considers the model $\omega_i = k + J\bar{\omega}_g + \alpha_g + \varepsilon_i$ and exploits data from an experiment in which students were assigned to classrooms of different sizes, leading to differences in the variance of $\bar{\omega}_g$, which is partially determined, of course, by the number of members of g. Computation of the value of J is more elaborate than the calculation of d that we illustrate, but the idea is the same.

Now suppose that groups come in two types: those such that Υ_g is drawn from a distribution with variance $\bar{h}$, and those such that Υ_g is drawn from a distribution with variance $\underline{h}$. By assumption $\bar{h} > \underline{h}$, one can construct an estimate of the social interactions parameter d.

$$\text{var}\left(\omega_i | \text{var} \Upsilon_g = \bar{h}\right) - \text{var}\left(\omega_i | \text{var} \Upsilon_g = \underline{h}\right)$$

$$= d^2(\bar{h} - \underline{h}) \Rightarrow d = \sqrt{\frac{\text{var}\left(\omega_i | \text{var} \Upsilon_g = \bar{h}\right) - \text{var}\left(\omega_i | \text{var} \Upsilon_g = \underline{h}\right)}{\bar{h} - \underline{h}}} \quad (26)$$

The idea of using variance differences to identify social interactions is also employed in Glaeser et al. (1996); this analysis focuses on what may be learned about social interactions from aggregated data.

In using tests of this type, it is important that a researcher be able to justify the assumption that the distribution of α_g does not vary across groups. It is not clear that this is so, even if group memberships are randomly assigned. For example, in Graham's analysis, in which students are observed in classrooms with different numbers of classmates, the assumption implicitly means that the variance of teacher quality does not depend on the number of students who are being taught.

In moving from linear models to binary choice models, some new results emerge. For binary choice models, one can develop evidence of social interactions for cross-section data even in the presence of group-level fixed effects. Panel methods can help with identification as well; these are discussed in Brock and Durlauf (2005 [forthcoming]). Brock and Durlauf (2005 [forthcoming]) show that, unlike the linear model case, it is also possible to learn something about social interactions from cross-section data.

The reason why cross-section data on binary choices may produce evidence in support of or against social interactions is that the binary choice model can produce multiple equilibria only if endogenous social interaction effects are present. If the available data require the existence of multiple equilibria, this in turn implies the existence of endogenous social interactions. To develop this argument, we assume that there is random assignment of individuals across groups

$$F_{X|g} = F_X. \quad (27)$$

Brock and Durlauf (2005 [forthcoming]) consider various relaxations of this assumption, but the bulk of the analysis in that paper is conducted under equation (27), as may be seen when one examines the formal proofs underlying the subsequent discussion.

The translation of multiple equilibria into data restrictions is somewhat complicated. A major intuition as to why multiple equilibria are associated with endogenous social interactions is that the multiple equilibria can produce what Brock and Durlauf refer to as *pattern reversals*. Assume that $d > 0$ so that increasing any element in Y_g increases, other things equal, the probability that an individual in g chooses 1. One can always measure the elements of Y_g this way, so long as one knows the direction of the effects of its elements. A pattern reversal occurs for groups g and g' if

$$Y_g < Y_{g'} \text{ and } m_g > m_{g'}. \tag{28}$$

Recall that m_g can be computed, because it is the conditional expectation of the same average of within-group choices $\overline{\omega}_g$, so pattern reversals represent restrictions on data. For the identification of social interactions, pattern reversals are important because they may derive from the presence of endogenous social interactions producing multiple equilibria. Why? Intuitively, multiple equilibria can produce a pattern reversal because group g can coordinate on a high m_g equilibrium whereas group g' does not, so that the effect of the higher value of Y on the average outcome in the group is negated.

The difficulty with using this heuristic argument is that without any restrictions on α_g, pattern reversals can occur without multiple equilibria being present. Brock and Durlauf (2005 [forthcoming]) thus attempt to identify weak restrictions associated with α_g such that pattern reversals imply the existence of multiple equilibria and hence endogenous social interactions. This type of argument does not identify the value of the endogenous social interactions parameter J; rather it shows that the value is nonzero and large enough to produce multiple equilibria. As such, it is a form of partial identification (see Manski 2003).

What sorts of assumptions allow for partial identification of J via pattern reversals? One potentially appealing assumption is a stochastic monotonicity restriction on the group level unobservables. Suppose that if $Y_g > Y_{g'}$ then the conditional distribution of unobservables in g', $F_{\alpha_{g'}|Y_{g'}}$ is first-order stochastically dominated by $F_{\alpha_g|Y_g}$. In this case, subject to various technical conditions described in Brock and Durlauf (2005 [forthcoming]), the pattern reversal defined by equation (28) will imply that endogenous social interactions exist.

Another route toward partial identification of social interactions is via unimodality versus multimodality comparisons. Suppose that Y_g is constant across groups, X_i is constant across all individuals within and across groups, and $\alpha_g = 0$. In this case, it is easy to see that m_g will take on a single value when there are no endogenous social interactions and will take on one of a finite set of values when there are multiple equilibria due to social interactions. Suppose that $dF_{\alpha_g|Y_g}$ is unimodal for all Y_g. In this case, m_g will be multimodal, with each equilibrium representing a possible value. This leads to the intuition that multiple equilibria may occur when one relaxes the assumption that Y_g and X_i are constant.

The translation of this intuition into data restrictions turns out to be fairly hard. One reason for this is straightforward: if α_g exhibits multimodality, then there is no link between multiple equilibria and unimodality of the other variables. Hence it is necessary to assume that $dF_{\alpha_g|Y_g}$ is unimodal for all Y_g; however, even in this case, it turns out that multimodality of m_g conditional on Y_g is neither a necessary nor a sufficient condition for the existence of multiple equilibria. The reason for this is that the relationship between m_g and Y_g is nonlinear as indicated by equation (20), and this nonlinearity can induce multimodality. Brock and Durlauf (2005 [forthcoming]) overcome this problem by considering $dF_{Y_g|m_g}$ rather than $dF_{m_g|Y_g}$. Specifically, they show that unimodality of $dF_{\alpha_g|Y_g}$ implies that there must exist a vector π such that $dF_{\pi Y_g|m_g}$ is unimodal if there are no endogenous social interactions. This is the correct way to think about pattern reversals and multimodality. When social interactions are present, a given m_g may be associated with more than one value of Y_g.

In our judgment, the identification of social interactions effects in the presence of unobserved group effects represents the major existing impediment to developing evidence of the role of social influences. The reason for this is that in the contexts in which social interactions are usually studied, there are typically many unobserved group characteristics that can be argued to plausibly affect individual outcomes. One example was given for the relationship between educational outcomes and neighborhoods. For another example, the ability to infer a relationship between social factors and crime rates requires careful attention to the possibility of differential police resources across neighborhoods. Further work on identification for the case of unobserved group effects is thus of great importance.

Some Implications for Social Epidemiology

In this section, we relate some of our analysis to the treatment of social interactions in the social epidemiology literature.

The Reflection Problem and Endogenous Social Interactions

As far as we know, with the exception of Oakes (2004) there has been no attention to the reflection problem in the social epidemiology literature. The reason for this seems to derive from differences between the economic and epidemiological concepts of individual outcomes. In the economics contexts, choices are purposeful and so it is natural to attempt to identify direct interdependences in decisions, whether they are due to a primitive psychological preference for conformity or information transmission that occurs via the behaviors of others. In contexts such as health outcomes (for example, coronary heart disease), such factors do not directly occur. That being said, it does seem that consideration of endogenous social interactions would augment epidemiological studies. In the context of health outcomes, endogenous social interactions can affect behaviors that in turn affect health. So, to the extent that exercise levels are influenced by social interactions, if exercise affects health, one has an endogenous influence.

Does the explicit evaluation of endogenous versus contextual effects matter? If one is interested in understanding causal mechanisms, the answer is clearly yes. There are, however, certain dimensions along which the answer is no. Suppose that one is interested in changing the value of an element in X_i for each of the members of a group. The effect of this in the linear model is fully characterized by the reduced form for individual behavior (that is, the combination of equation [2] with equation [6])

$$\omega_i = \frac{k}{1-\mathcal{J}} + cX_i + \frac{d}{1-\mathcal{J}}\Upsilon_g + \frac{\mathcal{J}c}{1-\mathcal{J}}X_g + \varepsilon_i \tag{29}$$

The regression is known in the econometrics literature as a reduced form as it relates ω_i to a set of predetermined variables. The coefficients in this regression are, as analyzed in Manski (1993), all identified under standard linear independence conditions on the regressors X_i and Υ_g, even if one cannot identify the distinct roles of contextual and endogenous effects. So, if all one wants to do is generate predictions of the effect of a change in some predetermined variable (that is, an element of X_i or Υ_g) on an individual[10], this regression is sufficient. For example, if one is interested in the effects on student outcomes from redistricting schools and if school district define the groups through which social interactions occur, then the effects of the policy change on students may be determined without distinguishing between the respective roles of contextual effects and endogenous effects; the effects can be determined via equation (29); the reduced form is thus sufficient for prediction of policy effects.

In contrast, the distinction between contextual effects and endogenous effects must be accounted for to understand the implications of changing elements of X_i or Υ_g. In the binary choice model, if one omits the endogenous effect in estimating equation (5), then the estimates of the remaining parameters will not be consistent and cannot be interpreted as a reduced form. If one considers the effects of redistricting on binary choices such as graduation, one potentially important effect may derive through the effect of the redistricting on the number of equilibria.

---

[10]By *predetermined variables*, we refer to variables that are determined at the time the choices ω_i are made.

Hierarchical Models

Unlike economics, social interactions are generally modeled in the social epidemiology literature with hierarchical models (that is, models in which contextual effects alter the coefficients that link individual characteristics to outcomes). The reason for this again seems to be a different conceptualization of the meaning of social interactions in economics in comparison with other social sciences. Hierarchical models seem, in our reading, to be motivated by a view of social groups as defining ecologies in which decisions are made and matter because different ecologies induce different mappings from the individual determinants of these behaviors and choices (see Raudenbush and Sampson 1999). Economics, in contrast, regards the elements that comprise endogenous and contextual social interactions as directly affecting the preferences, constraints, and beliefs of agents and so treats them as additional determinants to individual specific characteristics, X_i. The specific modeling choices in terms of either allowing for coefficients to linearly depend on group characteristics—as occurs in hierarchical models— or the direct embedding of group characteristics in decision rules as suggested by the role they are hypothesized to play—as occurs in economics—follow from these different conceptions of why group memberships matter.

For hierarchical models, there has been little attention to identification problems of the sort that have been analyzed in the social interactions literature, although these arguments are clearly germane. This subsection explores identification of hierarchical models. One formulation that seems consistent with the logic of hierarchical models is

$$\omega_i = k_i + c_i X_i + \mathcal{J}_i m_g + \varepsilon_i \tag{30}$$

where self-consistency of beliefs has been imposed, and

$$k_i = k + d\Upsilon_g, \, c_i = c + \Upsilon_g' \Pi_c, \, \mathcal{J}_i = \mathcal{J} + \pi_{\mathcal{J}} \Upsilon_g. \tag{31}$$

In equation (31), Π_c is a matrix. We omit any random terms in equation (31) for simplicity. This formulation assumes that the endogenous effect directly affects outcomes whereas the contextual effect works via the individual behavioral coefficients. This model can easily be translated into the original linear framework we have analyzed. The hierarchical model described by equations (30) and (31) is thus equivalent to the linear model

$$\omega_i = k + c X_i + d\Upsilon_g + \mathcal{J} m_{i,g}^e + \Upsilon_g' \Pi_c X_i + \pi_{\mathcal{J}} \Upsilon_g m_{i,g}^e + \varepsilon_i. \tag{32}$$

Hence, the difference between the linear model used in economics and the hierarchical structure is the addition of the terms $\Upsilon_g' \Pi_c X_i$ and $\Upsilon_g m_{i,g}^e$.

Can this model exhibit the reflection problem? The self-consistent solution to equation (32) is

$$m_g = \frac{k + cX_g + dY_g + Y_g' \prod_c X_g}{1 - \mathcal{J} - \pi_{\mathcal{J}} Y_g} \tag{33}$$

where, as before, X_g is the within group average of X_i. The reflection problem originally emerged when the Y_g vector equaled the within-group averages of X_i. If we impose this, then equation (33) becomes

$$m_g = \frac{k + cX_g + dY_g + Y_g' \prod_c Y_g}{1 - \mathcal{J} - \pi_{\mathcal{J}} Y_g}. \tag{34}$$

Equation (34) makes clear that the relationship between m_g and the other regressors is nonlinear; furthermore, the presence of $Y_g' \prod_c Y_g$ in the numerator and $-\pi_{\mathcal{J}} Y_g$ in the denominator ensures that linear dependence will not hold, except for hairline cases, so long as there is sufficient variation in X_i and Y_g. In other words, the hierarchical model will be identified under standard conditions on X_i and Y_g.

This hierarchical model with contextual and endogenous social interactions will not exhibit multiple equilibria even though the model contains nonlinearities. The nonlinear structure of the model, however, distinguishes it from the linear model in that the reflection problem can be overcome without prior information about the relationship between X_g and Y_g. And equally important, because hierarchical models are nonlinear, this means that the failure to account for the possibility of endogenous effects will lead to inconsistent estimates, so that the misspecified model cannot be used to evaluate the effects of changes in different variables or the effects on individual outcomes of altering group memberships (for example, by changing school district boundaries).

This is apparent from equation (34). The equilibrium effect of a change in Y_g on m_g is nonlinear when endogenous effects are present (that is, when the vector $\pi_{\mathcal{J}}$ is nonzero). This means that the effect of a change in contextual effects on the expected average behavior of the system will differ according to the initial value of Y_g. If the system defined by equations (30) and (31) is estimated under the assumption that $\pi_{\mathcal{J}} = 0$, then the resultant estimates will not provide a model in which counterfactuals may be accurately evaluated. Predictions based on the erroneous assumption of no endogenous effects can be highly misleading, although the extent to which this is true will depend on context.

Social Capital

A large number of social epidemiology papers study the role of social capital in determining various health-related outcomes. These studies often use aggregated data at levels ranging from residential neighborhoods to larger units; see Lochner et al. (2003) and Kawachi et al. (1997) for examples in which social capital is used to understand mortality. In this approach, average group outcomes are regressed against various group level controls and a measure of social capital. The general social capital literature has been subjected to criticism owing to the lack of conceptual precision in defining, let alone measuring, social capital (see Durlauf 2002a, 2002b; Portes 1998, 2000), but our purpose here is to evaluate identification.

To do this, we consider the case where social capital is endogenous. What this means is that each individual chooses a level of social capital SC_i in addition to the outcome of interest ω_i. Notice that even for outcomes such as mortality that are not themselves choice variables, behaviors that contribute to the outcome—such as exercise, diet, and willingness to take risks—are endogenous, so the identification analysis we have employed seems relevant. Furthermore, the notion that social capital is endogenous does not necessarily imply that the individual choices that produce social capital are conscious ones. One may adopt a level of personal honesty in dealing with others based on norms of honesty in a community without being consciously aware that one has done so.

Our discussion will focus only on the linear model, in order to use results in Durlauf (2002a). The introduction of social capital thus leads to a two equation linear model that generalizes equation (2)

$$\omega_i = k + cX_i + dY_g + \mathcal{J}_1 m_g + \mathcal{J}_2 s_g + \varepsilon_i \tag{35}$$

and

$$SC_i = \bar{k} + \bar{c}X_i + \bar{d}Y_g + \bar{\mathcal{J}}_1 m_g + \bar{\mathcal{J}}_2 s_g + \eta_i. \tag{36}$$

These two equations describe the joint determination of the outcome of interest and social capital. In these equations, SC_i denotes the level of social capital associated with individual i, and s_g denotes the expected average level of social capital in the group. The terms $\bar{k}, \bar{c}, \bar{d}, \bar{\mathcal{J}}_1$, and $\bar{\mathcal{J}}_2$ are all coefficients in the social capital equation; regressors in the two equations are assumed to be the same. As before, we employ expected rather than realized levels for aggregate outcome variables for simplicity.

Durlauf (2002a) provides conditions for identification of this model. The main findings are that this joint social interactions/social capital model suffers from an analogous reflection problem to the original social interactions model. Identification requires prior information to restrict the presence of particular terms in the equations. In particular, to identify the parameters of equation (35), it is necessary that there exist *two* elements of X_i whose group level analogs are not elements of Y_g.

In many contexts in which social capital is analyzed, individual level data are not available. If one only has group level data available, then the equations that may be studied are parallel to the individual model; that is,

$$\omega_g = k + d\Upsilon_g + \mathcal{J}_1 m_g + \mathcal{J}_2 s_g + \varepsilon_g \qquad (37)$$

where ω_g is the sample average within group g of ω_i and

$$SC_g = \bar{k} + \bar{d}\Upsilon_g + \bar{\mathcal{J}}_1 m_g + \bar{\mathcal{J}}_2 s_g + \eta_g. \qquad (38)$$

To identify the social capital effect (that is, the coefficient $\mathcal{J}_2$), with aggregate data, it is necessary to distinguish it from the contextual effects Υ_g as well as the endogenous effect m_g. Formal conditions for identification are given in Durlauf (2002a). One requirement for identification is that one must be able to identify two elements of Υ_g that appear in the social interaction equation (38) but do not appear in the outcome equation (37) (that is, the coefficients in equation (37) are a priori known to equal zero). Unless these two elements exist, SC cannot be linearly independent of both Υ_g and m_g.

Durlauf (2002a) argues that such prior information is generally implausible. One reason for this relates to the definitional ambiguities for social capital. Without a clear definition, it is hard to see how one can argue that an aggregate variable affects its aggregate level without directly affecting the aggregate outcome ω_g. If one is willing to assume that $\mathcal{J}_1 = 0$, then one still needs at least one element of Υ_g to affect social capital without affecting the aggregate outcome, which again requires justification. We are not aware of any empirical application where this defense is actually made.

This discussion illustrates some reasons why empirical claims on the role of social capital in influencing individuals and especially for groups are, in our judgment, often very weak. Empirical studies of social capital rely on implicit assumptions about which variables influence individuals and groups that, in our view, can be highly unappealing. This negative conclusion should not be interpreted as a dismissal of the social capital concept; weaknesses in current empirical practice in no way imply social capital is uninteresting or unimportant. Durlauf and Fafchamps (2004) discuss routes by which social capital inferences may be strengthened.

Conclusions

Although the econometrics literature on social interactions is still quite new, progress has been made in understanding important aspects of identification. Much remains to be done, in particular with respect to comprehensive studies of dynamic versus cross-section environments. Still, considerable progress has been made in understanding when social interactions can or cannot be identified in various data sets.

In conclusion, we note that terms such as "propensity score" and "causality" did not earlier appear anywhere in this essay. This omission is not inadvertent. From the perspective of the social interactions, the causality research program pioneered in the statistics literature has had little impact. The reason for this is that social interactions models in economics have been conceptualized as fully articulated descriptions on individual behavior, as opposed to efforts to identify the effects of changing certain factors, as occurs in the analysis of treatment effects. As such, social interactions econometrics reflects standard economic reasoning. From the social interactions perspective, one does not naturally think of a group as a treatment, but rather as a constrained choice by the individual. When one worries about selection on unobservables, one moves away from the sorts of assumptions, such as strong ignorability, that are important in the causality literature. Perhaps the most important message of this chapter is that there are perspectives on the inference of social interactions that are not well captured from the perspective of purely statistical literatures and may be addressed only by careful consideration of the behavioral foundations that underlie a statistical model specification.

References

Aizer, A., & Currie, J. (2004). Networks or neighborhood? Correlations in the use of publicly-funded maternity care in California. *Journal of Public Economics, 88*, 2573–2585.

Akerlof, G. (1997). Social distance and economic decisions. *Econometrica, 65*, 1005–1027.

Becker, G., & Murphy, K. (2000). *Social economics.* Cambridge, MA: Harvard University Press.

Bénabou, R. (1996). Equity and efficiency in human capital investment: The local connection. *Review of Economic Studies, 63*, 237–264.

Bertrand, M., Luttmer, E., & Mullainathan, S. (2000). Network effects and welfare cultures. *Quarterly Journal of Economics, 115*, 1019–1055.

Bisin, A., Horst, U., & Ozgur, O. (2004). *Rational expectations equilibria of economies with local interactions* (mimeo). New York University.

Bisin, A., Moro, A., & Topa, G. (2002). *The empirical content of models with multiple equilibria* (mimeo). New York University.

Blume, L. (1993). The statistical mechanics of strategic interaction. *Games and Economic Behavior, 5*, 387–424.

Blume, L. (1995). The statistical mechanics of best-response strategy revision. *Games and Economic Behavior, 11*, 111–145.

Blume, L., & Durlauf, S. (2003). Equilibrium concepts for social interaction models. *International Game Theory Review, 5*, 193–209.

Brock, W. (1993). Pathways to randomness in the economy: Emergent nonlinearity and chaos in economics and finance. *Estudios Economicos, 8*, 3–55.

Brock, W., & Durlauf, S. (2001a). Discrete choice with social interactions. *Review of Economic Studies, 68,* 235–260.

Brock, W., & Durlauf, S. (2001b). Interactions-based models. In J. Heckman & E. Leamer (Eds.), *Handbook of econometrics* (Vol. 5). Amsterdam: North Holland.

Brock, W., & Durlauf, S. (2001c). Growth empirics and reality. *World Bank Economic Review, 15,* 229–272.

Brock, W., & Durlauf, S. (2005 [forthcoming]). Identification of binary choice models with social interactions. *Journal of Econometrics.*

Brock, W., & Durlauf, S. (2006 [forthcoming]). A multinomial choice model with social interactions. In L. Blume & S. Durlauf (Eds.), *The economy as an evolving complex system III.* New York: Oxford University Press.

Brock, W., Durlauf S., & West, K. (2003). Policy analysis in uncertain economic environments (with discussion), with W. Brock and K. West. *Brookings Papers on Economic Activity, 1,* 235–322.

Burke, M., Fournier, G., & Prasad, K. (2004). *Physician social networks and geographical variation in medical care* (mimeo). Florida State University.

Cameron, A. C., & Trivedi, P. (2005). *Microeconometrics: Methods and applications.* New York: Cambridge University Press.

Conley, T., & Topa, G. (2002). Socio-economic distance and spatial patterns in unemployment. *Journal of Applied Econometrics, 17,* 303–327.

Durlauf, S. (1993). Nonergodic economic growth. *Review of Economic Studies, 60,* 349–366.

Durlauf, S. (1996). A theory of persistent income inequality. *Journal of Economic Growth, 1,* 75–93.

Durlauf, S. (2002a). On the empirics of social capital. *Economic Journal, 112,* 459–479.

Durlauf, S. (2002b). Bowling alone: A review essay. *Journal of Economic Behavior and Organization, 47,* 259–273.

Durlauf, S. (2004). Neighborhood effects. In J. V. Henderson & J.-F. Thisse (Eds.), *Handbook of regional and urban economics* (Vol. 4). Amsterdam: North Holland.

Durlauf, S. (2006 [forthcoming]). Groups, social influences, and inequality: A memberships theory perspective on poverty traps. In S. Bowles, S. Durlauf, & K. Hoff (Eds.), *Poverty traps.* Princeton, NJ: Princeton University Press.

Durlauf, S., & Fafchamps, M. (2004). Social capital. In P. Aghion & S. Durlauf (Eds.), *Handbook of economic growth.* Amsterdam: North Holland.

Ekeland, I., Heckman J., & Nesheim, L. (2002). Identifying hedonic models. *American Economic Review, 92,* 304–309.

Ekeland, I. Heckman J., & Nesheim, L. (2004). Identification and estimation of hedonic models. *Journal of Political Economy, 112,* S60–S109.

Evans, W., Oates, W., & Schwab, R. (1992). Measuring peer group effects: A study of teenage behavior. *Journal of Political Economy, 100,* 966–991.

Föllmer, H. (1974). Random economies with many interacting agents. *Journal of Mathematical Economics, 1,* 51–62.

Glaeser, E., Sacerdote, B., & Scheinkman, J. (1996). Crime and social interactions. *Quarterly Journal of Economics, 111,* 507–548.

Graham, B. (2005). *Identifying social interactions through excess variance contrasts* (mimeo). Harvard University.

Graham. B., & Hahn, J. (2004). *Identification and estimation of linear-in-means model of social interactions* (mimeo). Department of Economics, Harvard University.

Heckman, J. (1979). Sample selection bias as a specification error. *Econometrica, 47,* 153–161.

Heckman, J. (1996). Identification of causal effects using instrumental variables: Comment. *Journal of the American Statistical Association, 91,* 459–462.

Heckman, J. (1997). Instrumental variables. *Journal of Human Resources, 32,* 441–462.

Heckman, J. (2001). Micro data, heterogeneity, and the evaluation of public policy: Nobel lecture. *Journal of Political Economy, 109,* 673–748.

Hoff, K., & Sen, A. (2005). Home-ownership, community interactions, and segregation. *American Economic Review, 95,* 1167–1189.

Horst, U., & Scheinkman, J. (2004). *Equilibria in systems of social interactions* (mimeo). Princeton University.

Hoxby, C. (2000a). The effects of classroom size on student achievement: New evidence from population variation. *Quarterly Journal of Economics, 115,* 1239–1285.

Hoxby, C. (2000b). Peer effects in the classroom: Learning from gender and race variation. *National Bureau of Economic Research Working Paper No. 7867.*

Ioannides, Y., & Zabel, J. (2003a). Neighborhood effects and housing demand. *Journal of Applied Econometrics, 18,* 563–584.

Ioannides, Y., & Zabel, J. (2003b). *Interactions, neighborhood selection, and housing demand* (mimeo). Department of Economics, Tufts University.

Irwin, E., & Bockstaed, N. (2002). Interacting agents, spatial externalities, and the evolution of residential land use patterns. *Journal of Economic Geography, 2,* 31–54.

Kawachi, I., Kennedy, B., Lochner, K., & Prothrow-Stith, D. (1997). Social capital, income inequality, and mortality. *American Journal of Public Health, 87,* 1491–1498.

Kelly, M. (1997). The dynamics of Smithian growth. *Quarterly Journal of Economics, 112,* 939–964.

Kirman, A. (1997). The economy as an interactive system. In W. B. Arthur, S. Durlauf, & D. Lane (Eds.), *The economy as an evolving complex system II.* Redwood City, CA: Addison-Wesley.

Krauth, B. (2003). *Peer effects and selection effects on youth smoking in California* (mimeo). Simon Fraser University.

Krauth, B. (2004). *Simulation-based estimation of peer effects* (mimeo). Simon Fraser University.

Lindbeck, A., Nyberg, S., & Weibull, J. (1999). Social norms and economic incentives in the welfare state. *Quarterly Journal of Economics, 114,* 1–35.

Lochner, K., Kawachi, I., Brennan, R., & Buka, S. (2003). Social capital and neighborhood mortality rates in Chicago. *Social Science and Medicine, 56,* 1797–1805.

Manski, C. (1993). Identification of endogenous social effects: The reflection problem. *Review of Economic Studies, 60,* 531–542.

Manski, C. (2000). Economic analysis of social interactions. *Journal of Economic Perspectives, 14,* 115–136.

Manski, C. (2003). *Partial identification of probability distributions.* New York: Springer-Verlag.

Moffitt, R. (2001). Policy interventions, low-level equilibria, and social interactions. In S. Durlauf & H. P. Young (Eds.), *Social dynamics.* Cambridge, MA: MIT Press.

Nesheim, L. (2002). Equilibrium sorting of heterogeneous consumers across locations: Theory and implications. *Centre for Microdata Methods and Practice Working paper No. CWP08/02.*

Oakes, J. M. (2004). The (mis)estimation of neighborhood effects: Causal inference for a practicable social epidemiology. *Social Science and Medicine, 58,* 1929–1952.

Oomes, N. (2003). Local network trades and spatially persistent unemployment. *Journal of Economic Dynamics and Control, 27,* 2115–2149.

Portes, A. (1998). Social capital: Its origins and application in modern sociology. *Annual Review of Sociology, 24,* 1–24.

Portes, A. (2000). The two meanings of social capital. *Sociological Forum, 15,* 1–12.

Raudenbush, S., & Sampson, R. (1999). Ecometrics: Towards a science of assessing ecological settings, with application to the systematic social observation of neighborhoods. *Sociological Methodology, 29,* 1–41.

Rivkin, S. (2001). Tiebout sorting, aggregation, and the estimation of peer group effects. *Economics of Education Review, 20,* 201–209.

Sampson, R., Morenoff, J., & Gannon-Rowley, T. (2004). Assessing neighborhood effects: Social processes and new directions in research. *Annual Review of Sociology, 28,* 443–478.

Sirakaya, S. (2004). *Recidivism and social interactions* (mimeo). Department of Economics, University of Washington.

Soetevent, A., & Kooreman, P. (2004). *A discrete choice model with social interactions; with an application to high school teen behavior* (mimeo). University of Groningen.

Subramanian, S. (2004). The relevance of multilevel statistical methods for identifying causal neighborhood effects. *Social Science and Medicine, 58,* 1961–1967.

Topa, G. (2001). Social interactions, local spillovers, and unemployment. *Review of Economic Studies, 68,* 261–295.

Weinberg, B., Reagan, P., & Yankow, J. (2004). Do neighborhoods affect hours worked? Evidence from longitudinal data. *Journal of Labor Economics, 22,* 891–924.

Young, H. P., & Burke, M. (2001). Competition and custom in economic contracts: A case study of Illinois agriculture. *American Economic Review, 91,* 559–573.

CHAPTER THIRTEEN

MULTILEVEL STUDIES

Tony Blakely and S. V. Subramanian

Describing area-based differences in health outcomes has a long history (Macintyre and Ellaway 2003). We know that the average health of places differ, but do places make a difference to health? This question has received a systematic attention in the last decade or so (Diez-Roux, 2001; Duncan et al. 1993; Kawachi and Berkman 2003; Lynch et al. 2004; Macintyre et al. 1993; Pickett and Pearl 2001; Subramanian and Kawachi 2004). Besides its resonance with the move to look at "upstream" determinants of health and the recognition that health behaviors and outcomes need to be understood within their socioeconomic context (Beaglehole and Bonita 1997; Berkman and Kawachi 2000; Pearce 1996; Susser and Susser 1996), a major impetus for examining the role of contexts in explaining health variations comes from the advances in quantitative methods, in particular those related to multilevel statistical methods (Bryk and Radenbush 1992; Goldstein 1995). The term *multilevel* typically refers to the different, and distinct, levels or units of analysis.

Multilevel methods consist of statistical procedures that are pertinent in one or more of the following circumstances: (1) the observations that are being analyzed are correlated or clustered along spatial, non-spatial, or temporal dimensions; (2) the causal processes are thought to operate simultaneously at more than one level; or (3) there is an intrinsic interest in describing the variability and heterogeneity in the population, over and above the focus on average relationships (Diez-Roux 2002; Subramanian 2004a, 2004b; Subramanian et al. 2003). It is clear that individuals are organized within a nearly infinite number of levels of organization, from the individual up (for example, families, neighborhoods, counties, states), from the individual down (body organs, cellular matrices, DNA), and for overlapping units (area of residence and work environment). Therefore it is necessary that links should be made between these possible levels of analysis (McKinlay and Marceau 2000; Susser 1998).

The advent and advances in multilevel statistical methods offer substantive advantages, but traditional epidemiologic concerns relating to sources of error may become more pronounced. For example, such issues as the inclusion of a covariate as a putative confounder (either at the individual or neighborhood level) when it may also be on the causal pathway between a neighborhood property and health outcomes become critical (Blakely and Woodward 2000). Thus, it is important to note that "multilevel models are not a panacea" and like all statistical methods need to be used "with care and understanding" (Goldstein 2003). The application of multilevel statistical methods is now being considered more critically and carefully (Bingenheimer and Raudenbush 2004; Diez-Roux 2004; Oakes 2004; Subramanian 2004a). In addition to emphasizing the substantive and statistical properties of multilevel models, this chapter will also bring epidemiological issues to the fore.

Levels of Analysis and Inference

Until recently, much research has conflated levels of analysis and inference (Jones and Moon 1993). For example, the question of whether the aggregate or ecological association of average income with average health status across groups points to ecological and individual-level associations of income with health is often blurred. The ecological fallacy is well documented in epidemiology (Greenland 1992; Greenland and Morgenstern 1989; Morgenstern 1995), being a false inference of the association of individual-level variables on the basis of the observed association of the parallel ecological variables. For example, national gross domestic product (GDP) may be positively associated with motor vehicle fatality rates by country, but within countries the highest death rate from motor vehicle crashes may be for the low-income groups. But more crucially for social epidemiologists interested in possible contextual health effects, such aggregate analysis cannot distinguish the "contextual" (the difference a place makes) from the "compositional" (what or who is in a place) (Jones and Moon 1993). This conundrum has elsewhere been termed the "sociologistic fallacy" (Diez-Roux 1998). For example, national GDP may still have some association with death rates from motor vehicle crashes even after allowing for the individual-level association of income with crashes. Conversely, it is also important to avoid the "atomistic fallacy" (Alker 1969) that can occur by focusing exclusively at the individual level and thus missing the context in which individual action occurs. The need, therefore, is to simultaneously examine the circumstances of individuals at one level as well as the contexts or ecologies in which they are located at another level (Subramanian 2004a, 2004b; Subramanian et al. 2003).

Classifying and Measuring Ecological Variables

Broadly speaking, there are two ways of measuring ecological variables. First, we can use individual-level data and aggregate up (or otherwise summarize) to give average characteristics of groups. Second, we can directly measure properties of groups. Various authors have categorized this high-level bifurcation in different ways. For example, Macintyre (1997) refers to collective and contextual variables and Diez-Roux (1998) to derived and integral variables. And these two categories can be further subdivided—a summary classification of ecological variables is provided in Table 13.1, including the different terms for the same (or similar) variable used by different authors.

   Does the type of ecological variable matter? Macintyre has long argued that understanding what it is about neighborhoods that determines health will require the greater use of integral variables, not just derived variables (including deprivation indices) (Macintyre and Ellaway 2003; Macintyre et al. 1993). For example, five aspects of neighborhoods might be either health-promoting or health-damaging:

1. Physical features of the environment shared by all residents (for example, air and water quality; similar to Morgensterns's environmental variable in Table 13.1)
2. Availability of healthy environments at home, work, and play (for example, housing quality)
3. Services provided to support people in their daily lives (for example, education, transportation)
4. The sociocultural features of a locality (for example, political and economic history of areas)
5. The reputation of an area (for example, stigmatization of neighborhoods)

Such an approach to characterizing neighborhoods requires more than just deriving measures from census or survey data on individuals. It requires directly observing and measuring the neighborhood or groups themselves (Raudenbush 2003; Raudenbush and Sampson 1999). Unfortunately, such characterization is costly, time consuming, and difficult—but is nevertheless probably necessary to advance our understanding of why places or other contexts impact upon health.

TABLE 13.1. A CLASSIFICATION OF ECOLOGICAL VARIABLES.

Ecological Variable		Description	Examples
Derived Aggregate Contextual Analytical	(DR) (Morg) (Susser) (LM)	Aggregate of attributes measured at the individual-level. It is often expressed as a measure of central tendency (e.g., mean, median) but may be extended to include measures of variation of individual-level variables (e.g., SD).	• Mean income • Median social class • Proportion smoking • Area-based composite indices of need/ deprivation • Income inequality
Contagion Endogenous Peer	(Susser) (Manski) (Dietz)	Aggregate of the individual-level outcome, rather than exposure(s), that in turn affects the probability of the same outcome in individuals in the same population who are not yet affected.	• Prevalence of infectious disease • Suicide rate
Environmental	(Morg)	Physical characteristics of a place, with an individual-level analogue that usually varies between individuals (though it may remain unmeasured at the individual-level).	• Hours of sunlight • Environmental pollutant • Latitude and longitude • Weather
Structural	(LM)	Measure the pattern of relationships and interactions between individuals belonging to the group.	• Social networks
Integral Global	(Susser, DR) (Morg, LM)	Measure attributes of groups, organizations, or places and are not reducible to the individual-level. They are fixed for all, or nearly all, individual group members.	• Social (dis)organization • Social capital • Legislation or regulation

Susser = (Susser 1994); LM = (Lazarfeld and Menzel 1961); Morg = (Morgenstern 1998); Manski = (Manski 1993); DR = (Diez-Roux 2002); Dietz = (Dietz 2002).

Source: Adapted from Table 1 of Blakely and Woodward (2000).

A Typology of Ecological Effects

A two-level model includes three types of variables: the ecological exposure(s), X; the individual-level exposure(s), x; and the individual-level outcome, y. It is possible to conceptualize three ways that X can have an ecological effect on y: by directly affecting y (direct ecological effect); by modifying the relationship between *x* and *y* (cross-level effect modification or interaction); and by affecting *x* which in turn affects *y* (indirect ecological effect). These ecological effects are presented in Table 13.2. Effect modification may also occur between ecological variables, but is not shown in Table 13.2 as it is a step removed from the impact of one ecological exposure on a health outcome—nevertheless it is important when two or more ecological exposures are considered simultaneously.

In a reductionist sense, ecological variables cannot impact "directly" on individuals; instead, their effect must be mediated by intermediate variables at the individual level. For example, possible mechanisms linking income distribution to health include: variations in individual's access to life opportunities and material resources (for example, health care, education); social cohesion, whereby mutual support and co-operation secure better health outcomes; and possible direct psychosocial processes related to relative perceptions of position on the socioeconomic hierarchy (Kawachi and Kennedy 1999). Therefore, it may be argued that neither direct ecological effects nor cross-level effect modification are complete causal chains but require reduction to the myriad possible indirect ecological effects as shown in Table 13.2. To do so, however, would require perfect information on all possible variables. Such reductionism is helpful to understand etiologically how ecological exposures affect health but is often unnecessary and may even be counterproductive for the identification of intervention points for public health policy and action (Duncan et al. 1996; Mackenbach 1995; Pearce 1996; Rose 1992).

Sources of Error Estimating Ecological Effects on Individual Health—An Epidemiological Perspective

In this section we systematically consider the range of errors or biases that may arise in the estimation of ecological effects on health.

Insufficient Variation of the Ecological Variable of Interest

It is a *sine qua non* of any field of study that to detect an effect there must be variation in the independent variable (and dependent variable) under study. This essential prerequisite may be problematic for ecological exposures. Often macro-level socioeconomic exposures (for example, income inequality) do not vary within the eligible study population (for example, state or country or, more pragmatically, the available data set) at one point in time. The identification of small differences in the individual-level outcome variable by the observed levels of the ecological variable may, therefore, not fully reflect the potential magnitude of an ecological effect. When

TABLE 13.2. THREE TYPES OF ECOLOGICAL EFFECT.

Ecological Effect	Example	Possible Graphical Representation
1. Cross-level effect modification X_E - - - - ↓ - - - - $x \longrightarrow y$	*Example:* Income inequality (X_E) modifies the effect of personal income (x) on individual health (y).	 Legend: ■ Population with ecological exposure X; ◆ Population without ecological exposure X y axis, x [individual-level]
2. Direct ecological effect X_E - - - - ↘ - - - - $x \longrightarrow y$	*Example:* Income inequality (X_E) directly affects individual health (y).	 Legend: ■ Population with ecological exposure X; ◆ Population without ecological exposure X y axis, x [individual-level]
3. Indirect ecological effect a) X_E - - ↓ - - - - - $x \longrightarrow y$	*Example a:* Community tobacco control policies (X_E) may affect individual smoking (x), which in turn affects individual health (y).	Regression lines for individual-level outcome (y) on individual-level exposure (x) will not vary by population with varying ecological exposures (X), as any apparent effect of the ecological exposure(s) is explained away by including the relevant individual-level exposures (x).
b) X_E - - - - ↓ - - - - x_1 ↓ $x_2 \longrightarrow y$	*Example b:* Workplace organizational structure (X_E) may affect individual worker's decision latitude (x_1), which modifies the association of individual work demand (x_2) on coronary heart disease (y).	

Source: Table 2 of Blakely and Woodward (2000).

there is insufficient observed variation in the ecological exposure, extension of the study design across time or populations may provide the necessary variation. First, additional populations with different levels of the ecological exposure may be added to the analysis (for example, cross-national studies). A likely drawback, however, is a lack of comparability of unmeasured covariates between populations or data sets, or both. For example, "culture" may vary between countries and be independently associated with health. Second, a times-series study of one population may capture variation in the ecological exposure, but controlling for secular trends is difficult. Third, data for both multiple populations—or data sets—and different time periods may be combined in a mixed study design (Morgenstern 1995), thus combining the two former study designs. This mixed study design allows a simultaneous analysis of within-group changes over time in ecological exposure and outcome and between-group variation in ecological exposure and outcome. Unfortunately, data sets of this richness are likely to be rare.

Selection Bias

Selection bias in multilevel studies may arise at either the individual-level (level-1) or the group level (level-2). Considering ecological effects on individual health, selection bias at the group-level is the greatest concern. This may arise, for example, if in the taking of a random sample of neighborhoods one fails to achieve representativeness of all neighborhoods in the total population *and* the association of an ecological variable with individual health in these selected neighborhoods varies from that in the total population of neighborhoods. Selection bias may also arise at the individual-level if the effect of the ecological variable on individual health among those included in the study differs from that among the total population of individuals. As with traditional epidemiology, any selection bias may be accounted for by adjusting for covariates that are associated with selection probability and with both the ecological exposure and the health outcome. That is, adjusting for confounders may also adjust for selection bias. (It should be noted that selection bias is not the same as selection effects, whereby, for example, people with poor health may be more likely to live in exposed areas.)

Confounding

Confounding is a mixing of effects, whereby the association of an exposure with an outcome is distorted owing to an extraneous factor. In general, there are two types of confounding of ecological exposures: within ecological-level confounding by ecological covariates and cross-level confounding by individual-level covariates (Table 13.3). Within ecological-level confounding is conceptually the

TABLE 13.3. CONFOUNDING AS A SOURCE OF ERROR FOR ESTIMATED ECOLOGICAL EFFECTS.

Sources of Error	Description, Examples, and Comments
Cross-level confounding	An apparent direct ecological effect is due to cross-level confounding by an individual-level exposure (diagram a).
a) X_E $x \longrightarrow y$	*Example:* The association of neighborhood social capital (X_E) with individual health (y) is due to confounding by individual income (x).
	Comment: Diagram b) illustrates confounding by an ecological exposure of the association of an individual-level exposure and outcome. Using the framework of Diez-Roux (1998), diagram b) is an example of a "psychologistic fallacy," whereas diagram a) is an example of an "sociologistic fallacy."
b) X_E $x \dashrightarrow y$	
Within ecological-level confounding	An apparent direct ecological effect is due to confounding by an ecological covariate.
$X_{E1} = X_{E2}$ y	*Example:* The apparent association of neighborhood social capital (X_{E1}) with individual health (y) may be due to uncontrolled confounding by neighborhood resources (e.g., recreational facilities; X_{E2}).
$\longrightarrow$ $\longrightarrow$ $\dashrightarrow$ $=$	Solid thin arrows represent causal effects of individual-level covariates. Solid thick arrows represent causal effects of ecological exposures. Dashed arrows represent apparent, but false, observed associations. Double lines represent correlation generating confounding.

same as confounding in single-level epidemiology—both the exposure and confounders are at the same level of analysis. A major problem in multilevel studies, though, is that ecological variables are often strongly correlated, making it statistically difficult to include many ecological variables in any one model.

Cross-level confounding may be more conceptually challenging. A commonly cited example is individual-level income as a confounder of the association of income inequality with health (Gravelle 1998). As the association of individual income with health is non-linear (Backlund et al. 1996; Blakely et al. 2004), it is possible that the average income by ecological unit is not associated with income inequality by ecological unit, yet individual income could still be confounding the association of income inequality with health. To control for this cross-level confounding, individual income must be included in the model as well as specified as a categorical variable or some appropriate transformation of absolute income (for example, the natural logarithm) (Subramanian and Kawachi 2004).

It should be noted that if cross-level confounding by an individual-level variable of an association of an ecologic variable with individual health occurs, one might still be substantively interested in *why* individuals cluster by neighborhoods. That is, we should not always just dismiss the importance of context when an individual-level exposure is *systematically* distributed across neighborhoods (that is, some clustering of individuals' by personal exposures); rather, it may tell us something about the extent to which people are spatially sorted in the first place, disclosing spatiality or ecological patterning of individuals. For example, people in poor health may be more likely to migrate to areas with health services or other resources—what is sometimes termed a selection effect that can be "explained" by individual-level variables.

As shown in the "Multilevel Models" section on page 321, one can argue for a special case of cross-level confounding if variability at the levels of analysis is not specifically accounted for with multilevel statistics.

An important issue in multilevel research is that it may be difficult to differentiate between individual-level covariates as confounders and intermediary variables. If the latter, then "controlling" for the individual-level covariate will lead to overlooking indirect ecological effects. For example, the association of state-level income inequality with self-rated health in the United States is reduced when education is included at the individual-level (Blakely and Kawachi 2002; Subramanian and Kawachi 2004). Should education here be considered a confounder or an intervening variable between income inequality and health? It is suggested that less egalitarian states (that is, states with high income inequality) tend to underinvest in education, (Kaplan et al. 1996) thus placing individual education, at least in part, as an intermediary variable. Analyses with and without the individual-level covariate should be presented to give an upper and lower bound within which the reader may judge the "true" ecological effect.

Misclassification and Mismeasurement

We broadly differentiate information bias here into incorrect assignment of individuals to groups or ecological units and misclassification or mismeasurement of the ecological exposure and covariates.

Incorrect Assignment of Individuals to Ecological Units

An important issue is the grouping of individuals into ecological units, yet the implications of grouping strategies are often overlooked (Boyle and Willms 1999; Iversen 1991). As an example, consider an individual assigned to the wrong neighborhood in a study of the association between neighborhood cohesiveness and individual health. A first bias is that the level of cohesiveness for the assigned neighborhood may not be the same as the individual's true neighborhood, resulting in misclassification of the ecological exposure for that individual.

A second bias may arise if the measurement of cohesiveness was based on aggregated individual-level responses including incorrectly assigned individuals, thus biasing the observed level of cohesiveness for the given neighborhood.

These types of bias are likely to be magnified when grouping is not conducted specifically for the given study, but instead existent administrative groups (for example, census tracts) are used with likely incorrect assignment of both individuals and group "boundaries" (Boyle and Willms 1999; Duncan et al. 1993). The likely effect of using convenient rather than theoretically pre-determined ecological units is a reduced ability to detect any ecological effect, although one Canadian study that attempted to create natural neighborhoods found similar fixed effects for various ecological effects compared with an analysis using administrative census tracts as neighborhoods (Ross et al. 2004).

The lag time between an ecological exposure and individual-level health outcome is a form of misclassification bias that deserves specific mention. Many multilevel studies that consider ecological socioeconomic exposures have used cross-sectional survey data (Boyle and Willms 1999; Duncan et al. 1993, 1996). Not only does this introduce the possibility of reverse causation (health status affecting the ecological exposure) but it also implies a zero lag time between exposure and outcome. It is usually implausible for the effect of an exposure to be instantaneous, particularly in social epidemiology. If the ecological exposure is stable over time, then specification of a lag time may not be necessary—otherwise incorrect specification of lag time is another source of misclassification bias. Investigation of lag times between socioeconomic ecological exposures and individual outcomes is required (Blakely et al. 2000a).

Misclassification or Measurement Error of the Ecological Exposure. Nondifferential misclassification bias of exposure usually causes a bias to the null in single-level epidemiology (Rothman and Greenland 1998) but may cause bias in either direction in multilevel research dependent on the nature of the exposure (binary or continuous) and the level of measurement (ecological or individual-level)

(Brenner et al. 1992b). First, consider a binary individual-level exposure (home ownership as a proxy for wealth) nondifferentially misclassified during measurement at the individual-level and then represented as a derived ecological variable. Assume that the "unexposed" regions have 85 percent home ownership, the "exposed" regions 15 percent home ownership, and that there is a direct ecological effect of home ownership on health. If home ownership was nondifferentially misclassified at the individual-level, then those regions with 85 percent home ownership would have a *lower* observed home ownership: if 10 percent of all home ownership was recorded incorrectly by individuals, then ([85% $\times$ 0.90] + [15% $\times$ 0.10]) = 78% [rather than 85%]) 78 percent will be observed as homeowners in the "unexposed" regions. The reverse will happen for the exposed region: 22 percent of individuals will be observed as homeowners. If one then extrapolates any direct ecological effect for home ownership to the hypothetical instance of regions with full home ownership versus those with none, the ecological effect will be overestimated by (1/[0.78−0.22]) / (1/[0.85−0.15] = 1.25) 1.25, a bias *away* from the null. Note that such bias applies to derived variables where the interpretative meaning is accorded to the actual value (that is, neighborhoods with nil compared with full home ownership). If the derived variable is just used to rank neighborhoods into, say, quintiles, the observed difference between quintiles will not be biased.

Second, consider a continuous individual-level variable randomly mismeasured (that is, independent of true value) at the individual-level and then represented as a mean derived ecological exposure. Here, there may be no bias in the estimated ecological effect: the random mismeasurements for all individual within groups should sum to zero, meaning that there is no bias in the summary mean for the group.

Third, consider nondifferential misclassification and mismeasurement of ecological exposures measured directly at the ecological-level (for example, integral and environmental ecological exposures). Here measurement is at the same level as representation of the exposure, and effect measures will be biased to the null as for single-level epidemiology generally.

Misclassification or Measurement Error of Covariates. Regarding nondifferential misclassification of confounders, misclassification of individual-level confounders and ecological-level confounders (measured directly at the ecological-level) will generally reduce the ability to control for confounding. For ecological confounders that are first measured at the individual-level and then aggregated up, however, nondifferential misclassification during measurement at the individual-level may not reduce the ability to control for confounding (Brenner et al. 1992a).

Multilevel Models

Multilevel statistical models are also known as hierarchical, mixed, random-effects, covariance components, or random-coefficient regression models (Dempster et al. 1981; Goldstein 2003; Laird and Ware 1982; Longford 1993; Raudenbush and Bryk 2002). Fundamental to multilevel modeling is the recognition of data structures, which typically consist of individuals at the lower level and spatial (for example, areas) or non-spatial (for example, schools, hospitals) groupings at the higher level.

The importance of identifying and specifying the "higher" levels has been overlooked in social epidemiologic research. Researchers must *a priori* specify why they think that there will be variation in the outcome at these levels over and above variation at the individual level. Such thinking naturally leads to considerations of which levels to include in the model. For example, do we expect variation at the level of small neighborhoods (for example, census blocks) or larger neighborhoods (for example, census tracts)? The most common multilevel model is a two-level hierarchic nested modeling with many level-1 units within a smaller number of level-2 units. Such structures arise commonly in social epidemiology (for instance, individuals in neighborhoods, workers in organizations, patients in hospitals, and children within schools). Importantly, this multilevel structure can be recast, with remarkable advantage, to capture a wide range of data structures (Subramanian et al. 2003), and a brief overview is provided here.

Besides extending the two-level structure to a three-level structure of, for example, individuals (level-1) within neighborhoods (level-2) within counties (level-3), a number of other data structures can be thought to be a special case of multilevel. For instance, the well-known *repeated cross-sectional* design within a multilevel perspective could be individuals at level-1 being nested within time at level-2 and neighborhoods at level-3. The classic *panel* design, with its longitudinal structure, can also be considered a special case of multilevel design, with neighborhoods at level-3, individuals at level-2, and repeated measurement occasions at level-1. Another extension of a multilevel structure is the *multivariate* design, with multiple response outcomes (at level-1) nested within individuals (at level-2) who are in turn nested within neighborhoods (at level-3).

All of the previous examples are strictly hierarchical in that all level-1 units can belong to one and only one level-2 unit; however, data structures could be "non-hierarchical." An example of non-hierarchic nesting would be individuals at level-1 nested within *both* residential neighborhoods and workplaces at level-2 creating a *cross-classified* structure, because workplaces and neighborhoods do not nest within each other. Another instance of a non-hierarchical nesting occurs where level-1 units (for example, individuals) are simultaneously nested within

FIGURE 13.1.   MULTILEVEL STRUCTURE OF REPEATED MEASUREMENTS OF INDIVIDUALS OVER TIME ACROSS NEIGHBORHOODS WITH INDIVIDUALS HAVING MULTIPLE MEMBERSHIP TO DIFFERENT NEIGHBORHOODS ACROSS THE TIME SPAN.

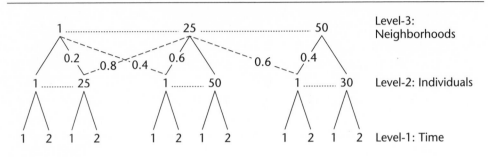

Source: Subramanian (2004b).

more than one level-2 grouping (for example, neighborhoods), leading to a *multiple membership* structure. The substantive rationale to consider such complex structures have been discussed elsewhere (Goldstein 2003; Subramanian et al. 2003).

Indeed, a structure can be a combination of more than one of the designs discussed earlier, as shown in Figure 13.1. Time measurements (level-1) are nested within individuals (level-2) who are in turn nested in neighborhoods (level-3). Importantly, individuals are assigned different weights for the time spent in each neighborhood. Thus, individual No. 25 moved from neighborhood No. 1 to neighborhood No. 25 during the study time-period, $t_1 - t_2$, spending 20 percent of her time in neighborhood No. 1 and 80 percent in her new neighborhood. This *multiple-membership panel* design could allow control of changing context as well as changing composition, besides enabling a consideration of weighted effects of proximate contexts (Langford et al. 1998). So, for example, the geographical distribution of disease can be seen not only as a matter of composition and the immediate context in which an outcome occurs, but also a consequence of the impact of nearby contexts with nearer areas being more influential than more distant ones. Goldstein (2003) presents an elegant and comprehensive *classification schema*.

The Distinction Between Levels and Variables

Each of the levels that were discussed in the previous section (for example, neighborhoods) can be considered as variables in a regression equation with an indicator variable specified for each neighborhood. Conversely, why are such variables as gender, ethnicity or race, and social class *not* a level? Treating neighborhoods, for example, as a level is critical because neighborhoods are treated as a *population* of units from which we have observed a random sample. This enables us to draw generalizations for a particular level (for example, neighborhoods) based on an observed sample of neighborhoods. In contrast, gender, for instance, is not a level because it is not a sample out of all possible gender categories. Rather, it is an attribute of individuals. Thus, male or female in our gender example are "fixed" discrete categories of a variable with the specific categories only contributing to their respective means. They are not a random sample of gender categories from a population of gender groupings.

The situation becomes less clear when the study includes all individuals in the population, and hence all neighborhoods, ethnic or race, gender, and social class groups are included. Such a study design arises when census data are linked to mortality data, for example (Blakely et al. 2000b). Why might we still consider neighborhoods here as levels, but not ethnicity or race? First, it is more efficient to model neighborhoods as a random variable given the (likely) large number of neighborhoods. Second, we would usually wish to ascribe a fixed effect to each ethnic group, but not each neighborhood. Rather, we wish to model an ecologic variable such as social capital at the neighborhood-level.

It is possible to consider "levels" as "variables." Thus, when neighborhoods are considered as a variable, they are typically reflective of a *fixed* classification. Although this may be useful in certain circumstances, doing so robs the researcher of the ability to generalize to all neighborhoods (or "population" of schools), and inferences are only possible for the specific neighborhoods observed in the sample.

Multilevel Models: A Basic Statistical Outline

Suppose we are interested in studying the variation in a health score, as a function of certain individual and neighborhood predictors. Let us assume that the researcher collected data on a sample of fifty neighborhoods and, for each of these neighborhoods, a random sample of individuals. We then have a two-level structure where the outcome is a health score (with higher score indicating better health), y, for individual i in neighborhood j. We will restrict this example to one individual-level predictor, poverty, x_{1ij}, coded as zero if not poor and one if poor, for every individual i in neighborhood j; and one neighborhood predictor, w_{1j}, a socioeconomic deprivation index in neighborhood j.

Multilevel models operate by developing regression equations at each level of analysis. In the illustration considered here, models would have to be specified at two levels, level-1 and level-2. The model at level-1 can be formally expressed as:

$$y_{ij} = \beta_{0j} + \beta_1 x_{1ij} + e_{0ij} \tag{1}$$

In this level-1 model, β_{0j} (associated with a constant, x_{0ij}, which is a set of 1s, and therefore, not written) is the mean health score for the jth neighborhood for the non-poor group; β_1 is the average differential in health score associated with individual poverty status (x_{1ij}) across all neighborhoods. Meanwhile, e_{0ij} is the individual or the level-1 residual term. To make this a genuine two-level model, we let β_{0j} become a random variable, with an assumption that:

$$\beta_{0j} = \beta_0 + u_{0j} \qquad (2)$$

where u_{0j} is the random neighborhood-specific displacement associated with the overall mean health score (β_0) for the non-poor group. Because we do not allow, at this stage, the average differential for the poor and non-poor group (β_1) to vary across neighborhoods, u_{0j} is assumed to be same for both groups. The equation (2) is then the level-2 between-neighborhood model.

It is worth emphasizing that the "neighborhood effect", u_{0j}, can be treated in one of the two ways. One can estimate each one separately as a fixed effect (that is, treat them as a variable, with fifty neighborhoods there will be forty-nine additional parameters to be estimated). Such a strategy may be appropriate if the interest is in making inferences about just those neighborhoods. In contrast, neighborhoods are treated as a (random) sample from a population of neighborhoods (which might include neighborhoods in future studies) if one has complete population data and the interest is in making inferences about the variation between neighborhoods in general. Adopting this multilevel statistical approach makes u_{0j} a random variable at level-2 in a two-level statistical model.

Substituting the level-2 model (equation 2) for the level-1 model (equation 1) and grouping them into fixed- and random-part components (the latter shown in parentheses) yields the following combined (also referred to as *random-intercepts* or *variance components*) model:

$$y_{ij} = \beta_0 + \beta_1 x_{1ij} + (u_{0j} + e_{0ij}) \qquad (3)$$

We have now expressed the response y_{ij} as the sum of a fixed part and a random part. Assuming a normal distribution with a zero mean, we can estimate a variance at level-1 (σ_{e0}^2: the between-individual within-neighborhood variation) and level-2 (σ_{u0}^2: the between-neighborhood variation), both conditional on fixed poverty differences in health score. It is the presence of more than one residual term (or the structure of the random part more generally) that distinguishes the multilevel model from the standard linear regression models or analysis-of-variance–type analysis. The underlying random structure (variance-covariance) of the model specified in equation (3) is: $Var[u_{0j}] \sim \mathcal{N}(0,\sigma_{u0}^2)$; $Var[e_{0ij}] \sim \mathcal{N}(0,\sigma_{e0}^2)$; and $Cov[u_{0j}, e_{0ij}] = 0$. It is this aspect of the regression model that requires special estimation procedures to obtain satisfactory parameter estimates (Goldstein 2003).

The model specified in equation (3) with the aforementioned random structure is typically used to partition variation according to the different levels, with the variance in y_{ij} being the sum of σ_{u0}^2 and σ_{e0}^2. This leads to a statistic known as *intra-class correlation*, or *intra-unit correlation*, or more generally *variance partitioning coefficient*, (Goldstein 2003) representing the degree of similarity between two randomly chosen individuals within a neighborhood. This can be expressed as:

$$\rho = \frac{\sigma_{u0}^2}{\sigma_{u0}^2 + \sigma_{e0}^2}.$$

We can expand the *random structure* in equation (3) by allowing the fixed effect of individual poverty (β_1) to randomly vary across neighborhoods in the following manner:

$$y_{ij} = \beta_{0j} + \beta_{1j}x_{1ij} + e_{0ij} \tag{4}$$

At level-2, there will now be two models:

$$\beta_{0j} = \beta_0 + u_{0j} \tag{5}$$

$$\beta_{1j} = \beta_1 + u_{1j} \tag{6}$$

Substituting the level-2 models in equations (5) and (6) into the level-1 model in equation (4) gives:

$$y_{ij} = \beta_0 + \beta_1 x_{1ij} + (u_{0j} + u_{1j}x_{1ij} + e_{0ij}) \tag{7}$$

Across neighborhoods, the mean health score for non-poor is β_0, and $\beta_0 + \beta_1$ is the mean health score for the poor, and the mean "poverty-differential" is β_1. The poverty differential is no longer constant across neighborhoods, but varies by the amount u_{1j} around the mean, β_1. Such models are also referred to as *random-slopes* or *random coefficient models*. These models have a much more complex variance-covariance structure than before:

$$Var\begin{bmatrix} u_{0j} \\ u_{1j} \end{bmatrix} \sim \mathcal{N}\left(0, \begin{bmatrix} \sigma_{u0}^2 \\ \sigma_{u0u1}\sigma_{u1}^2 \end{bmatrix}\right); \quad \text{and} \quad Var[e_{0ij}] \sim \mathcal{N}(0, \sigma_{e0}^2).$$

With this formulation, it is no longer straightforward to think in terms of a summary intraclass correlation statistic ρ, as the level-2 variation is now a function of an individual predictor variable, x_{1ij}. In our example, when x_{1ij} is a dummy variable, we will have two variances estimated at level-2: one for non-poor, which is σ_{u0}^2; and one for poor, which is $\sigma_{u0}^2 + 2\sigma_{u0u1}x_{1ij} + \sigma_{u1}^2 x_{1ij}^2$. That is, level-2 variation will be a quadratic function of the individual predictor variable when x_{ij} is a continuous predictor. Thus the notion of "random intercepts and slopes," while intuitive, is not entirely appropriate. Rather, what these models are really doing is modeling variance as some function (constant, quadratic, or linear) of a predictor variable (Goldstein 2003).

Building on this perspective of modeling the variance-covariance function (as opposed to "random intercepts and slopes"), we can extend the concept to modeling variance function at level-1. It is extremely common to assume that the variance is "homoskedastic" in the random part at level-1 (σ_{e0}^2; equation [7]), and indeed researchers seldom report whether this assumption was tested or not. One strategy would be to model the different variances for poor and non-poor of the following form:

$$y_{ij} = \beta_0 + \beta_1 x_{1ij} + (u_{0j} + u_{1j} x_{1ij} + e_{1ij} x_{1ij} + e_{2ij} x_{2ij}) \qquad (8)$$

where, $x_{1ij} = 0$ for non-poor, 1 for poor, and the new variable $x_{2ij} = 1$ for non-poor, 0 for poor, with $Var[e_{1ij}] = \sigma_{e1}^2$ giving the variance for poor, and $Var[e_{2ij}] = \sigma_{e2}^2$ giving the variance for non-poor, and $Cov[e_{1ij}, e_{2ij}] = 0$. There are other parsimonious ways to model level-1 variation in the presence of a number of predictor variables (Goldstein 2003; Subramanian et al. 2003). With this specification, we do not have an interpretation of the random level-1 coefficients as "random slopes" as we did at level-2. The level-1 parameters σ_{e1}^2 and σ_{e2}^2 describe the complexity of level-1 variation, which is no longer homoskedastic (Goldstein 2003). Anticipating and modeling heteroskedasticity or heterogeneity at the individual level may be important in multilevel analysis, as there may be cross-level confounding—what may seem to be neighborhood heterogeneity (level-2) to be explained by some ecological variable could be due to a failure to take account of the between-individual (within-neighborhood) heterogeneity (level-1). An attractive feature of multilevel models—one that is perhaps most commonly used in social epidemiologic research—is their utility in modeling neighborhood and individual characteristics, and any interaction between them, simultaneously. We will consider the underlying level-2 model related to equation (8), which is exactly the same as specified in equations (5) and (6) but now including a level-2 predictor: w_{1j}, the deprivation index for neighborhood j:

$$\beta_{0j} = \beta_0 + \alpha_1 w_{1j} + u_{0j} \qquad (9)$$

$$\beta_{1j} = \beta_1 + \alpha_2 w_{1j} + u_{1j} \qquad (10)$$

Note that the separate specification of micro and macro models correctly recognizes that the contextual variables (w_{1j}) are predictors of between-neighborhood differences. The extension of micro model (8) will now be:

$$y_{ij} = \beta_0 + \beta_1 x_{1ij} + \alpha_1 w_{1j} + \alpha_2 w_{1j} x_{1ij} + (u_{0j} + u_{1j} x_{1ij} + e_{1ij} x_{1ij} + e_{2ij} x_{2ij}) \qquad (11)$$

The combined formulation in equation (11) highlights an important feature, the presence of an interaction between a level-2 and level-1 predictor ($w_{1j} \cdot x_{1ij}$), represented by the fixed parameter, α_2. Now, α_1 estimates the marginal change in health score for a unit change in the neighborhood deprivation index for the non-poor, and α_2 estimates the extent to which the marginal change in health score for unit change in the neighborhood deprivation index is *different* for the poor.

More generally, this formulation has a direct translation to the assessment of social inequalities in health (Subramanian et al. 2003). For instance, evidence for an interaction between an ecologic predictor and individual predictor suggest that the effect of the ecologic predictor on the individual outcome is different at different levels of the individual predictor variable. Vice versa, it would also mean that the individual-based inequalities in health would be different at different levels of ecologic disparities. This multilevel statistical formulation allows *cross-level effect modification or interaction* between individual and neighborhood characteristics to be robustly specified and estimated.

Multilevel models are concerned with modeling both the average and the variation around the average, at different levels. To accomplish this they consist of two sets of parameters: those summarizing the average relationships(s), and those summarizing the variation around the average at both the level of individuals and neighborhoods. Models presented in equations (1–11) can be easily adapted to other structures with nesting of level-1 units within level-2 units. Additionally, these models can be extended to three or more levels. Whereas the preceding discussion considered a single, normally distributed response variable for illustration, multilevel models are capable of handling a wide range of responses. These include: *binary* outcomes, *proportions* (as logit, log-log, and probit models); *multiple categories* (as ordered and unordered multinomial models); and *counts* (as poisson and negative binomial distribution models). In essence, these models work by assuming a specific, "non-Gaussian" distribution for the random part at level-1 while maintaining the Normality assumptions for random parts at higher levels. Consequently, the discussion presented in this entry focusing at the neighborhood level would continue to hold regardless of the nature of the response variable, with some exceptions. For instance, determining intraclass correlation or partitioning variances across individual and neighborhood levels in complex *non-linear multilevel logistic models* is not straightforward (see for example, Browne et al., 2005; Goldstein et al., 2002.).

Context Versus Composition: Study Design, Analytical, and Inferential Issues

A common practice in social epidemiology has been to demonstrate differences in health by neighborhood socioeconomic position, adjust for (some) individual-level socioeconomic factors, find a remaining statistically significant association of neighborhood socioeconomic position with individual health, and then to declare that there truly is an independent association of neighborhood socioeconomic position with personal health over and above personal socioeconomic position; however, just as "declaring independence" in traditional epidemiology is prone to error (Davey Smith and Phillips 1990, 1992; Phillips and Davey Smith 1991, 1992), so too it is in multilevel studies.

Consider the example of a hypothetical study that finds an association of neighborhood deprivation with mortality after: (1) adjusting for personal income and then (2) adjusting for all individual-level variables used in the deprivation index. The measure of neighborhood deprivation is constructed from individual-level variables for all or a sample of members of the group to calculate a composite index such as the Carstairs index (Carstairs 1995), using statistical methods such as principal components analysis. The individual-level variables that are used to build the index typically include variables such as the proportion of unemployed and solo parents in the neighborhood, average income, and so on.

A multilevel model approach to this scenario would typically first use a model of the type specified in equation (3), with an explicit interest in the level-2 variance. The question of interest is: Are there statistically significant health variations between neighborhoods (σ_{u0}^2) after accounting for the observed characteristics of the individuals residing in these neighborhoods? The next step (having modeled individual-level variables and confounders at level-1) would be to introduce a fixed effect for neighborhood deprivation (equivalent to w_{1j} in equation [9]) at level 2 and interpret the size and statistical significance of its coefficient (equivalent to α_1 in equation [9]).

Although the variance parameter at the neighborhood level σ_{u0}^2, the variance partitioning coefficient ρ, and the fixed effect of neighborhood deprivation α_1 are all useful to establish assessment of the potential importance of neighborhoods, drawing substantive inferences are not straightforward. The following is a checklist to consider.

Were the Neighborhoods Specified Correctly?

Researchers have to make sure that the level-2 units are clearly defined and motivated in addition to constituting a random sample (with exchangeable properties) of all level-2 units (to avoid selection bias). In educational research, with schools or classes serving as level-2 units, the definition of level-2 units is usually straightforward. Similarly, institutional settings such as hospitals and clinics are more clearly defined than neighborhoods. It is also clear that all of the observed variation (net of individual characteristics) need not be systematically related to the (unobserved) neighborhood predictor. Rather, a part of it could be simply due to sampling variation due to the sample of neighborhoods. Epidemiologically, incorrect specification of neighborhood boundaries would probably cause an underestimation of neighborhood effects due to the introduction of nondifferential misclassification bias. So, whilst a potential (and inevitable) source of error, it is unlikely to give rise to a spurious positive finding.

Was Personal Socioeconomic Position Adequately Controlled For?

Any substantive interpretation of σ_{u0}^2 or α_1 is entirely dependent on the "appropriate" specification of the other parts of the model, specifically, the fixed part of the model (that is, individual-level and ecological-level confounders) as well as the random part specification of level-1. Returning to our preceding hypothetical example and a substantive interpretation of the fixed effect of neighborhood deprivation, the model that controlled just for personal income was probably inadequate. Personal socioeconomic position is a complex and multidimensional construct that is often viewed as including income, educational attainment, social class, and (more recently) some measure of personal deprivation of hardship. Therefore, controlling for just one socioeconomic factor is unlikely to fully adjust for personal socioeconomic position. That is, residual confounding would remain. Nevertheless, the practice of adjusting for just one socioeconomic factor before declaring neighborhood effects is not uncommon.

Even the model that fully adjusts for all the parallel individual-level variables that went into the construction of the neighborhood deprivation index may still be prone to residual confounding. First, for a fluctuating variable such as income, the average neighborhood income may be a better measure of your likely average income than personally declared (including reporting errors) income for the last year. Second, a measure or a personal socioeconomic factor at one point in time does not capture dynamics over the life course. Although just one study, it is interesting to note that there was no association of neighborhood deprivation with mortality among a cohort of Scottish men after adjustment for social class at multiple points in the life course (Davey Smith et al. 1997). Third, even if a satisfactorily full set of socioeconomic factors across the life course can be included in the analysis, the issue of (inevitable) measurement error of these covariates and resulting "resonant confounding" of the neighborhood deprivation-mortality association remains (Marshall and Hastrup 1996).

What About the Interpretation of Between-Neighborhood Variation, σ_{u0}^2?

It is a common finding that such variation is small in social epidemiology studies and often not statistically significant—be it before or after the adjustment for individual-level covariates; however, direct interpretation of these variations for neighborhood-health research must be done cautiously, especially when the outcome is not linear (for example, binary). Rather, the major utility of σ_{u0}^2 lies statistically in allowing robust and reliable fixed-effect estimates of level-2 exposures on health (that is, estimating the size and precision of direct ecological effects and cross-level effect modification). Within the framework of the "context versus composition" question, undue focus on the random variation, especially in non-linear models, may be problematic. Importantly, moderately strong and statistically significant ecological effects are often found in the absence of statistically significant between-neighborhood variation (Merlo 2003).

Were Other Individual-Level Confounders Adequately Controlled For?

This is a difficult, if not unanswerable, question for any observational study. By including further covariates, we gain from adjusting for further potential confounding. But, we risk including variables that are also on the causal pathway from neighborhood deprivation to health. For example, smoking may be patterned by one's context, meaning that adjusting for smoking is actually an attempt at quantifying the indirect ecological effect of neighborhood deprivation mediated by smoking. This problem of variables that are both likely to be confounders and mediating variables in the association of an exposure with outcome is a perplexing problem in all observational studies. Short of conducting intervention studies on neighborhood deprivation, a longitudinal study with repeated measures of individual histories of changing neighborhood deprivation is one study design that may assist; however, data-sets with both repeated measures and ecological-level variables are uncommon.

Do I Need To Use Multilevel Statistical Methods?

This chapter has attempted to illustrate that multilevel statistical modeling meshes well with multilevel thinking. But there are other approaches to modeling clustered data (for example, Generalized Estimating Equation [GEE]); however, it is beyond the scope of this chapter to canvas these options in detail. Briefly however, the GEE approach will often deliver the same result. The key difference between the GEE and multilevel approach is that the latter models the random variation as being of intrinsic interest rather than a nuisance to overcome. As such, the choice of strategy is really dependent upon the conceptual motivation of the researcher (Heagerty and Zeger 2000).

Conclusion

In addition to careful study design, thorough analysis, and careful interpretation, there are some other pointers that we would suggest to social epidemiologists trying to identify true casual associations of ecologic exposures with health. First, rely less on interpreting residual associations, and model directly the ecological exposure. The preceding example of a composite index of socioeconomic deprivation is a classic illustration. It is difficult to interpret a residual association of such an index with individual health, for the reasons listed above and because it is not actually clear what properties of neighborhoods the index is actually capturing. Following the longstanding exhortations of Macintyre and others (Cummins et al. 2005; Macintyre and Ellaway 2003; Macintyre et al. 1993, 2002), conceptualizing and directly measuring those characteristics of neighborhoods that are hypothesized to effect health are likely to be more rewarding in the long-run, albeit more difficult.

Second, although often impossible to conduct, intervention studies that actually change ecological or neighborhood characteristics should be seized upon by social epidemiologists whenever possible (Oakes 2004). Third, longitudinal studies with repeated measurements of neighborhood characteristics over peoples' life courses should also be sought out.

Finally, we need to be cognizant of the limits of quantitative multilevel analysis and empiricism more generally. There is a deep, complex, and dynamic interrelationship between people and context. Where you live influences who you are (for example, employment opportunities), and who you are influences your neighborhood. It will not always be possible, nor correct, to decompose health variations to personal and contextual characteristics. Rather, we will also need qualitative and other social science approaches.

References

Alker, H., Jr. (1969). A typology of ecological fallacies. In M. Dogan & S. Rokkan (Eds.), *Quantitative ecological analysis* (pp. 69–86). Cambridge, MA: Massachusetts Institute of Technology.

Backlund, E., Sorlie, P. D., & Johnson, N. J. (1996). The shape of the relationship between income and mortality in the United States: Evidence from the National Longitudinal Mortality Study. *Annals of Epidemiology, 6*(1), 12–20.

Beaglehole, R., & Bonita, R. (1997). *Public health at the crossroads: Achievements and prospects.* Cambridge: Cambridge University Press.

Berkman, L., & Kawachi, I. (2000). *Social epidemiology.* New York: Oxford University Press.

Bingenheimer, J., & Raudenbush, S. (2004). Statistical and substantive inferences in public health: Issues in the application of multi-level models. *Annual Review of Public Health, 25,* 53–77.

Blakely, T., & Kawachi, I. (2002). Education does not explain association between income inequality and health. *BMJ, 324,* 1336.

Blakely, T., & Woodward, A. (2000). Ecological effects in multi-level studies. *Journal of Epidemiology and Community Health, 54,* 367–374.

Blakely, T., Kawachi, I., Atkinson, J., & Fawcett, J. (2004). Income and mortality: The shape of the association and confounding New Zealand Census-Mortality Study, 1981–1999. *International Journal of Epidemiology, 33,* 874–883.

Blakely, T., Kennedy, B., Glass, R., & Kawachi, I. (2000a). What is the lag time between income inequality and health status? *Journal of Epidemiology and Community Health, 54,* 318–319.

Blakely, T., Salmond, C., & Woodward, A. (2000b). Anonymous linkage of New Zealand mortality and Census data. *Australian and New Zealand Journal of Public Health, 24,* 92–95.

Boyle, M., & Willms, J. (1999). Place effects for areas defined by administrative boundaries. *American Journal of Epidemiology, 149,* 577–585.

Brenner, H., Greenland, S., & Savitz, D. (1992a). The effects of non-differential confounder misclassification in ecologic studies. *Epidemiology, 3*(5), 456–459.

Brenner, H., Greenland, S., Jockel, K.-H., & Savitz, D. (1992b). Effects of non-differential exposure misclassification in ecologic studies. *American Journal of Epidemiology, 135*(1), 85–95.

Browne, W. J., Subramanian. S. V., Jones, K., & Goldstein, H. (2005). Variance partitioning in multilevel logistic models that exhibit overdispersion. *Journal of Royal Statistical Society A 168,* 599–613.

Bryk, A., & Radenbush, S. (1992). *Hierarchical linear models: Applications and data analysis methods.* Newbury Park, CA: Sage.

Carstairs, V. (1995). Deprivation indices: Their interpretation and use in relation to health. *Journal of Epidemiology and Community Health, 49*(Suppl. 2), S3–S8.

Cummins, S., Macintyre, S., Davidson, S., & Ellaway, A. (2005). Measuring neighborhood social and material context: Generation and interpretation of ecological data from routine and non-routine sources. *Health & Place, 11*(3), 249–260.

Davey Smith, G., & Phillips, A. (1990). Declaring independence: Why we should be cautious. *Journal of Epidemiology and Community Health, 44,* 257–258.

Davey Smith, G., & Phillips, A. (1992). Confounding in epidemiological studies: Why "independent" effects may not be all they seem. *British Medical Journal, 305,* 757–759.

Davey Smith, G., Hart, C., Blane, D., Gillis, C., & Hawthorne, V. (1997). Lifetime socioeconomic position and mortality: Prospective observational epidemiology. *British Medical Journal, 314,* 547–552.

Dempster, A. P., Rubin, D. B., & Tsutakawa, R. K. (1981). Estimation in covariance components models. *Journal of the American Statistical Association, 76,* 341–353.

Dietz, R. (2002). The estimation of neighborhood effects in the social sciences: An interdisciplinary approach. *Social Science Research, 31,* 539–575.

Diez-Roux, A. (1998). Bringing context back into epidemiology: Variables and fallacies in multilevel analysis. *American Journal of Public Health, 88,* 216–222.

Diez-Roux, A. V. (2001). Investigating neighborhood and area effects on health. *American Journal of Public Health, 91*(11), 1783–1789.

Diez-Roux, A. V. (2002). A glossary for multilevel analysis. *Journal of Epidemiology and Community Health, 56*(8), 588–594.

Diez-Roux, A. V. (2004). Estimating neighborhood health effects: The challenges of causal inference in a complex world. *Social Science & Medicine, 58*(10), 1953–1960.

Duncan, C., Jones, K., & Moon, G. (1993). Do places matter? A multi-level analysis of regional variations in health-related behavior in Britain. *Social Science & Medicine, 37*(6), 725–733.

Duncan, C., Jones, K., & Moon, G. (1996). Health-related behavior in context: A multilevel modelling approach. *Social Science & Medicine, 42*(6), 817–830.

Goldstein, H. (1995). *Multilevel statistical models.* London: Edward Arnold.

Goldstein, H. (2003). *Multilevel statistical models.* London: Edward Arnold.

Goldstein, H., Browne, W. J., & Rasbash, J. (2002) Partitioning variation in multilevel models. *Understanding Statistics 1,* 223–232.

Gravelle, H. (1998). How much of the relation between population mortality and unequal distribution of income is a statistical artefact? *BMJ, 316,* 382–385.

Greenland, S. (1992). Divergent biases in ecologic and individual-level studies. *Stat Med, 11,* 1209–1223.

Greenland, S., & Morgenstern, H. (1989). Ecological bias, confounding, and effect modification. *Int J Epidemiol, 18*(1), 269–274.

Heagerty, P., & Zeger, S. (2000). Marginalized multilevel models and likelihood inference (with discussion). *Statistical Science, 15,* 1–26.

Iversen, G. (1991). *Contextual analysis.* Newbury Park, CA: Sage.

Jones, K., & Moon, G. (1993). Medical geography: Taking space seriously. *Progress in Human Geography, 17*(4), 515–524.

Kaplan, G., Pamuk, E., Lynch, J., Cohen, R., & Balfour, J. (1996). Inequality in income and mortality in the United States: Analysis of mortality and potential pathways. *British Medical Journal, 312,* 999–1003.

Kawachi, I., & Berkman, L. (2003). *Neighborhoods and Health* (p. 352). New York: Oxford Press.

Kawachi, I., & Kennedy, B. (1999). Income inequality and health: Pathways and mechanisms. *Health Services Research, 34,* 215–227.

Laird, N., & Ware, J. H. (1982). Random-effects models for longitudinal data. *Biometrics, 38,* 963–974.

Langford, I. H., Bentham, G., & McDonald, A. L. (1998). Multilevel modelling of geographically aggregated health data: A case study on malignant melanoma mortality and UV exposure in the European Community. *Statistical Medicine, 17,* 41–57.

Lazarfeld, P., & Menzel, H. (1961). On the relation between individual and collective properties. In A. Etzioni (Ed.), *Complex organization* (pp. 422–440). New York: Holt, Reinhart and Winston.

Longford, N. (1993). *Random coefficient models.* Oxford: Clarendon Press.

Lynch, J., Davey Smith, G., Harper, S., Hillemeier, M., Ross, N., Kaplan, G., et al. (2004). Is income inequality a determinant of population health? Part 1. A systematic review. *Milbank Quarterly, 82*(1), 5–99.

Macintyre, S. (1997). What are the spatial effects and how can we measure them? In A. Dale (Ed.), *Exploiting national surveys and census data: The role of locality and spatial effects* (pp. 1–28). Manchester: Center for Census and Survey Research, University of Manchester.

Macintyre, S., & Ellaway, A. (2003). Neighborhoods and Health: An overview. In I. Kawachi & L. Berkman (Eds.), *Neighborhoods and health* (pp. 20–42). New York: Oxford Press.

Macintyre, S., Ellaway, A., & Cummins, S. (2002). Place effects on health: How can we conceptualise, operationalise and measure them? *Social Science & Medicine, 55,* 125–139.

Macintyre, S., Maciver, S., & Sooman, A. (1993). Area, class and health: Should we be focusing on places or people? *Journal of Social Policy, 22*(2), 213–234.

Mackenbach, J. (1995). Public health epidemiology. *Journal of Epidemiology and Community Health, 49,* 333–334.

Manski, C. (1993). Identification problems in the social sciences. *Sociological Methodology, 23,* 1–56.

Marshall, J., & Hastrup, J. (1996). Mismeasurement and the resonance of strong confounders: Uncorrelated errors. *American Journal of Epidemiology, 143*(10), 1069–1078.

McKinlay, J. B., & Marceau, L. D. (2000). To boldly go. *American Journal of Public Health, 90*(1), 25–33.

Merlo, J. (2003). Multilevel analytical approaches in social epidemiology: Measures of health variation compared with traditional measures of association. *Journal of Epidemiology and Community Health, 57,* 550–552.

Morgenstern, H. (1995). Ecologic studies in epidemiology: Concepts, principles, and methods. *Am Review Public Health, 16,* 61–81.

Morgenstern, H. (1998). Ecologic studies. In K. Rothman & S. Greenland (Eds.), *Modern epidemiology* (pp. 459–480). Philadelphia: Lippincott-Raven.

Oakes, J. M. (2004). The (mis)estimation of neighborhood effects: Causal inference for a practicable social epidemiology. *Social Science & Medicine, 58*(10), 1929–1952.

Pearce, N. (1996). Traditional epidemiology, modern epidemiology, and public health. *American Journal of Public Health, 86*(2), 678–683.

Phillips, A., & Davey Smith, G. (1991). How independent are "independent" effects? Relative risk estimation when correlated exposures are measured imprecisely. *Journal of Clinical Epidemiology, 44,* 1223–1231.

Phillips, A., & Davey Smith, G. (1992). Bias in relative odds estimation owing to imprecise measurement of correlated exposures. *Statistical Medicine, 11,* 953–961.

Pickett, K., & Pearl, M. (2001). Multilevel analyses of neighborhood socioeconomic context and health outcomes: A critical review. *Journal of Epidemiology and Community Health, 55,* 11–122.

Raudenbush, S., & Bryk, A. (2002). *Hierarchical linear models: Applications and data analysis methods.* Thousand Oaks, CA: Sage Publications.

Raudenbush, S., & Sampson, R. (1999). Ecometrics: Toward a science of assessing ecological settings, with application to the systematic social observation of neighborhoods. *Social Methodology, 29,* 1–41.

Raudenbush, S. W. (2003). The quantitative assessment of neighborhood social environment. In I. Kawachi & L. F. Berkman (Eds.), *Neighborhoods and health.* New York: Oxford University Press.

Rose (1992). *The strategy of preventive medicine.* Oxford: Oxford University Press.

Ross, N., Tremblay, S., & Graham, K. (2004). Neighborhood influences on health in Montreal, Canada. *Social Science & Medicine, 59*(7), 1485–1494.

Rothman, K., & Greenland, S. (1998). *Modern epidemiology.* Philadelphia: Lippincott-Raven.

Subramanian, S. (2004a). Multilevel methods, theory and analysis. In N. Anderson (Ed.), *Encyclopedia on health and behavior.* (pp. 602–608). Thousand Oaks, CA: Sage Publications.

Subramanian, S., Jones, K., & Duncan, C. (2003). Multilevel methods for public health research. In I. Kawachi & L. Berkman (Eds.), *Neighborhoods and health* (pp. 65–111). New York: Oxford Press.

Subramanian, S. V. (2004b). The relevance of multilevel statistical methods for identifying causal neighborhood effects. *Social Science & Medicine, 58*(10), 1961–1967.

Subramanian, S. V., & Kawachi, I. (2004). Income inequality and health: What have we learned so far? *Epidemiologic Reviews, 26,* 78–91.

Susser, M. (1994). The logic in ecological: I. The logic of analysis. *American Journal of Public Health, 84*(5), 825–829.

Susser, M. (1998). Does risk-factor epidemiology put epidemiology at risk? Peering into the future. *J Epidemiol Community Health, 52,* 608–611.

Susser, M., & Susser, E. (1996). Choosing a future for Epidemiology: I. Eras and paradigms. *American Journal of Public Health, 86*(5), 668–673.

CHAPTER FOURTEEN

EXPERIMENTAL SOCIAL EPIDEMIOLOGY—CONTROLLED COMMUNITY TRIALS

Peter J. Hannan

"Randomization by cluster accompanied by an analysis appropriate to randomization by individual is an exercise in self-deception, however, and should be discouraged"

CORNFIELD (1978) PP. 101

Origins and History

Disease is individual but also social, in the sense that a common environment may contribute to illness, as probably best exemplified by the waves (epidemics) of colds passing through close-knit communities each winter. Social epidemiology has as its object the investigation of the connection between the social environment and the health of individuals. Consequently, social epidemiology deals with at least two levels of data, those relating to the environment and those relating to the individual. If all exposed individuals succumbed to disease, individual characteristics would be irrelevant, and individual level data could not explain differences in disease between different environments. But not all exposed individuals exhibit disease, so the data of social epidemiology is necessarily multilevel.

One way to deal with hierarchical data is to collapse over the lower level, resulting in simple correlational analysis at the community level relating prevalence of disease to exposure. By observing the patterns of cholera, Dr. John Snow published in 1849 his hypothesis that, in contrast to the commonly held "miasma" theory, water from one of two suppliers in London was contaminated and was the source of exposure to some causal agent (Snow 1849; see www.csiss.org/classics/content/8). In perhaps

341

the earliest social epidemiological experiment, when a second cholera outbreak occurred in 1854, he was able to test his argument through an experiment in which the handle of the Broad Street pump was removed as a way to prevent exposure if the hypothesis were true; the cholera epidemic was contained. But one might argue that the epidemic was going to decline for other reasons and the intervention just happened to coincide. It was not a randomized, controlled trial. For another example, see a study of the control of tuberculosis (Frost 1937).

Hierarchical statistical models have been in use in statistics (under the name of mixed models) from Fisher's pioneering work on nested models for split-plot designs (Fisher 1935). The essential ingredient in hierarchical models is that more than a single error variance exists. The simplest example is that of repeated measures, in which a within-component of variance is realized on each measurement occasion and a between-component of variance is realized for each individual (here, individual = unit). Now move up a level to having communities as the units and the "inhabitants" as the repeated measures within the unit; an error-component of variance is realized for each individual measurement, and a between-component of variance takes on a realized value for each community. In a cohort community study design, each of the individual- and the unit-components of variance can themselves be modeled as having two components, one for level of the measurement (whether individual or unit) and one for the time-varying component of variance (whether individual or unit). Thus we can have repeated measures on the individual as well as repeated measures on the community, each showing a correlation over time.

Experimental hierarchical designs occurred commonly in educational research, where interventions were applied to all the students in the classroom; these experiments were analyzed ignoring the clustering in classrooms (Goldstein 1987). In the late 1970s (for example, Corbeil and Searle 1976; Wedderburn 1974, 1976) and early 1980s (for example, Laird and Ware 1982), statistical progress in the analysis of mixed models allowed these concepts to enter the educational field as a debate of the statistical issue of the unit of analysis (Hopkins 1982). Educationists have continued to contribute to the topic as witnessed by the work, for example, of Bryk and Raudenbush (1992).

Epidemiology began using observational clustered studies, such as physiologist Keys's ground-breaking Seven Countries Study (Keys et al. 1967), which followed cohorts of male participants in sixteen centers in seven different countries. The concentration on males was because males were primarily affected by the epidemic of heart disease in western society. Because this was an observational study and data were collapsed to the level of country for comparisons, the term "ecological fallacy" reared its head; that is, other characteristics, like the specific gene pools, may explain the differences. As a result of the finding, Finland labeled with the dishonor of having the highest heart attack rates of the sixteen cohorts, Finnish researchers under Puska (Puska et al. 1983) instituted a controlled trial (that is, an experiment) in which the province of North Karelia was chosen to receive an intervention aimed at reducing the risk factors for heart disease, whereas the companion province of Kuopio was monitored as a control. Absent randomization, this is called a "quasi-experiment" (Cook and Campbell 1979). Despite the control, might an alternative explanation exist for the outcome of the experiment? Might structural or environmental differences (or both) exist between North Karelia and Kuopio that could equally explain the observed result? With only one province in each condition, the alternative explanation is at least tenable. Blackburn's visit in 1971 to the organizing meeting under the aegis of the World Health Organization (WHO) for the North Karelia Project helped crystallize his ideas on the prevention of heart disease in whole populations. The ideas that were circulating were published in a report from the WHO Expert Committee on the prevention of coronary heart disease, held in Geneva in late 1981, which presented the population approach to reducing the burden of heart disease (see WHO Expert Committee 1982). The whole U.S. population had elevated risk factors for heart disease, with the distribution of cholesterol levels in the United States having almost no overlap with cholesterol levels in the Japanese cohorts of the Seven Countries Study. Blackburn inferred from this that intervention efforts should not focus on only high-risk individuals. In the United States in the early 1970s, Farquhar had set up the quasi-experimental Stanford Three-Community Study, with one intervention and two control communities with the same aims as the North Karelia Project but with increased attention to the use of the media (Farquhar 1978; Farquhar et al. 1977; Williams et al. 1981). In the late 1970s and early 1980s came three controlled community quasi-experiments—an expanded Stanford Five-City Study (Farquhar et al. 1985), the Minnesota Heart Health Program (MHHP) under Blackburn (Jacobs et al. 1986), and the Pawtucket Heart Health Program under Carleton (Carleton et al. 1995). For an interesting reflection on the history of these community-based studies for prevention of cardiovascular disease, see Blackburn (2004, pp. 24–38).

The first three to four years of data in MHHP were troubling the researchers at the University of Minnesota's Division of Epidemiology because city-wide means were showing more variability than was expected. Leslie Kish, who was on the MHHP Scientific Advisory Board, introduced the group to the design effect (DEFF) already well known in survey sampling when sampling is by clusters (Kish 1965). When asked his suggested remedy, the reply was "recruit fifty cities"! The Stanford Five-Cities Study had five communities, MHHP six communities, and the Pawtucket Heart Health Program two communities. Cornfield's (1978) discouragement quoted at the start of this chapter began to make sense. In

Canada, Donner et al. heeded the message early, and Donner as a consultant to MHHP helped us in Minnesota understand the problem (see Donner 1982, 1985; Donner and Koval 1982; Donner et al. 1981). The publication of *Generalized Linear Models* (McCullagh and Nelder 1983, 1989) crystallized the statistical research conveniently. The statistical implications of the group randomized trials, or GRTs as they are now affectionately known, had direct impact on the design of a number of studies, including the Healthy Worker Project (Jeffery et al. 1993), the Community Intervention Trial for Smoking Cessation (COMMIT) Trial (Gail et al. 1992), Communities Mobilizing for Change on Alcohol (CMCA) (Wagenaar et al. 1994), and Child and Adolescent Trial for Cardiovascular Disease (CATCH) (Zucker et al. 1995). Since then, a plethora of GRTs have been implemented and, over time, an increasing fraction has been analyzed correctly (see Donner et al. 1990; Simpson et al. 1995; Varnell et al. 2004). The article by Zucker (1990) laid out clearly the proper analysis for GRTs. Summaries of the status of GRTs in the mid 1990s are given in Koepsell et al. (1995); more recent summaries are provided by Murray et al. (1994); Donner and Klar (1996, 2000) and Murray et al. (2004). Sorenson et al. (1998) provides a view of where group randomized trials were situated by the mid 1990s.

The characteristic of clustered data is the presence of more than one component of error variance, inducing correlation between measurements repeated within the cluster, hence the term multilevel data. Just as collapsing data may introduce the "ecological fallacy" in which associations between groups are assumed to reflect individual associations (Alker 1969; Krieger 1992; Robinson 1950), so too may ignoring clusters introduce the "individualistic fallacy" (Alker 1969; Krieger 1992, 1994). In relating the occurrence of disease to environmental context, both individual and contextual data are needed. Strong inference requires randomized experiments, and epidemiologic investigation in a social context requires multilevel data. Thus the importance to social epidemiology of the proper design and analysis of randomized trials.

Randomization and Dependence

Randomization promises that, at least in the long run (statistical expectation), there is no selection bias and unmeasured (and indeed, even unthought-of) confounders are balanced. Unfortunately, statistical expectation is an asymptotic property (a large number of repetitions would be required) whereas the actual randomization is carried out once to give the *realized* randomization. The single realization is more likely to be balanced if a sufficiently large number of entities are randomized.

The randomized controlled clinical trial (RCT) is largely regarded as the ideal experimental design, involving as it does two elements—experimental intervention and randomization to either experimental or control condition (but see Senn 2004). As detailed in Chapter One in this volume, the strongest inference for an effect of an intervention would be to evaluate the state of a unit in the absence of, and in the presence of, the intervention being tested with the evaluations being under identical conditions. This may be possible in physics, but hardly possible in social contexts. In lieu of the ideal, multiple "comparable" units are selected and randomized to represent either the intervention experience or the control experience. Intervention (read "experimentation") and randomization are crucial to the strength of the inference.

Experimentation and Inference

In science using the experimental method, the acceptance of new theories is based largely on prediction, temporal sequence, and replicability of the experiment by others. A prediction is made and an experiment is carried out to see if the prediction holds. To strengthen the connection between theory and reality, and to help exclude alternative explanations, the experimental method looks for the appearance of the predicted phenomenon when the posited "cause" is introduced and the disappearance of the phenomenon when the posited "cause" is removed and the original situation is restored. Finally, to help exclude the possibility that it was not some other contemporaneous influence, the experiment must be replicated, preferably by others.

Experimentation is important. The deliberate introduction of change, which is followed by the predicted effect and the deliberate removal of the change followed by the disappearance of the effect, is cogent. Replication strengthens the inference by excluding the likelihood of other chance possibilities being responsible. What is possible in physics is infeasible in social epidemiology. The pre/post randomized controlled trial captures the aspect of the introduction of change via the pre/post design and approximates the "off-on-off" aspect via the controls. Internal replication is approximated by the multiple units, coupled with the statistical methods that generate estimates of what the range of outcomes might be if the sample were retaken under the same conditions: thus the importance in the study of human and societal behavior of the *trial*.

Importance of Randomization

By the Law of Large Numbers (see, for example, Mood 1950), randomization guarantees in the probabilistic sense that the two groups will be comparable; measured, unmeasured, and indeed even unthought-of confounders are guaranteed *asymptotically* to be balanced between the two groups. Thus the group of units randomized to the control experience can be considered *as if they were* the group of units randomized to the experimental experience, the only difference being the experimental manipulation. The guarantee, however, requires an infinity of units or, equally but conceptually, an infinity of randomizations, making for an infinity of replicated experiments. That is what asymptotically means. In practice, we have a finite number of units to be randomized, and we can do only one randomization—called a single realization. We need to craft the selection process for these units to be already as comparable as possible—in other words, we need to assist chance to achieve approximate balance in the single realization effected. This can be done in the design phase by the use of matching or of stratification of units to be randomized and, in the analysis phase, by appropriate covariate adjustment. Nevertheless, randomization of a sufficiently large number of carefully selected units is essential for a strong inference.

Effect of Dependence

The units we have been talking about could be individuals, as in an RCT, or social groups, as in a group randomized trial (GRT). In the latter, intact social groups are randomized so that the members within a social group are assigned to the same experimental condition, be it intervention or control. Individuals are not randomized, and all individuals in the unit are in the same experimental condition. How, if possible, can the uniqueness of the unit be separated from the experimental condition, since the unit is nested in the condition? In fact, if we have only one unit per condition, the uniqueness of the unit and the effect of condition are completely confounded. If we have multiple units per condition, we can impose a statistical model to account for the uniqueness of each unit by assuming that the units come with "bumps" or "shifts" realized from a common probabilistic distribution. The usual statistical model assumes that the outcome measure for each member of a unit has a common bump, establishing a correlation between measures of members within a unit. Members within a unit tend to be more like other members in the unit than to be like members from other units. If your friend smokes, your friend's spouse is more likely also to smoke.

The implication of the statistical model is that pooling information over members within a unit carries redundancy. The second member of a group may add only 0.95 units of information about the measure instead of a full unit of information. Let Y_k represent the measure for member k, $k = 1, 2, 3 \ldots m$. Y is made up of a member specific contribution, v_k, and common "bump" u, so that $Y_k = v_k + u$. Assume that the v_k is drawn from a distribution with mean μ and variance σ^2 and that u is a realization from a distribution with mean zero and variance τ^2. The expectation of each Y_k is μ and the variance of each Y_k is $(\sigma^2 + \tau^2)$. The mean of Y in the group is $Y_{avg} = \Sigma Y_k / m$.

The *statistical expectation* of Y_{avg} is:

$$E(Y_{avg}) = E(\Sigma Y_k/m) = \Sigma E(Y_k)/m = \Sigma E(v_k + u)/m = \Sigma(\mu + 0)/m = \mu.$$

The *variance* of Y_{avg} is more intriguing:

$$\begin{aligned}
V(Y_{avg}) &= V(\Sigma Y_k/m) = V(Y_1 + Y_2 + \cdots + Y_m)/m^2 \\
&= m \, Var(Y)/m^2 + \Sigma_k \Sigma_j \, Cov(Y_k, Y_j) \quad (j \neq k) \\
&= (\sigma^2 + \tau^2)/m + m(m-1)\,\tau^2/m^2 \\
&= (\sigma^2/m) \times [1 + m \, VCR]) \quad OR \quad = ([\sigma^2 + \tau^2]/m) \times (1 + [m-1]ICC)
\end{aligned}$$

where $VCR = \tau^2/\sigma^2$ is the variance components ratio, and $ICC = \tau^2/(\sigma^2 + \tau^2)$ is the intraclass correlation coefficient.

Note:

1. If $\tau^2 = 0$, we have the familiar result for the variance of the mean of m independent observations from a common distribution.
2. σ^2 is the variance *within* member, but $(\sigma^2 + \tau^2)$ is the *total* variance of Y.
3. The covariance between Y_k and Y_j arises through the common "bump," u.
4. $ICC = VCR/(1 + VCR)$ and if VCR is small, $ICC \approx VCR$.
5. Clustering implies that the variance of a mean is inflated by factor $(1 + [m-1]ICC)$, called the Design Effect, DEFF, by Kish (1965), and the Variance Inflation Factor, VIF, by Donner et al. (1981).
6. The factor $(1 + mVCR)$ inflates the *residual* variance component, as would be estimated in an analysis of variance (ANOVA), and defines the residual variance inflation factor, $RVIF = (1 + mVCR)$.
7. If the size of the cluster is $m = 1$, no inflation of the variance of the mean exists.
8. For large unit size, m, the inflation may be serious even for seemingly small ICC.
9. Estimates of σ^2 and of τ^2 will differ according to different analytic models, even for the same outcome (Y), especially as covariates are used in the analysis with varying success in "explaining" between- or within-variance (or both)—hence there is no single value for the ICC, but a value for an ICC depending on the analytic model used.
10. The estimated ICC also is liable to sampling (replication) error—the estimate comes with an implicit uncertainty, capturing the variation likely to be encountered if the experiment were to be done again (replicated).

For example, in the Minnesota Heart Health Program, for community clusters of average size $m = 410$, we found an ICC estimate for the prevalence of smoking equal to 0.00272 based on 31 degrees of freedom (Hannan et al. 1994, Table 4). The individual (binomial) variance for current smoking can be estimated by $p(1 - p)$ where p is the average prevalence of smoking (0.22, or 22 percent prevalence); estimated $\sigma^2 = 0.1716$. The estimate of τ^2 is $VCR_x\sigma^2 = 0.00047$, so $(\sigma^2 + \tau^2) = 0.1716 + 0.0005 = 0.1721$. If there were no clustering, the sampling variance of a mean over 410 persons would be σ^2/m giving a standard error ± 0.02 ($= \sqrt{0.1716/410}$). The Design Effect from the seemingly small ICC is DEFF $= (1 + 409 \times 0.00272) = 2.1125$, effectively doubling the variance of the estimated community prevalence of smoking based on a large survey of 410 persons randomly selected from within a socially intact cluster. The inflated variance of an estimated smoking prevalence is $0.1721/410 \times 2.1125 = 0.000887$, for an estimated standard error 0.03. Hence, instead of reporting the prevalence (as percents) as 22 ± 2 percent, clustering leads to a prevalence estimate reported as 22 ± 3 percent.

Implications of Clustering: Proper Inference in Community Trials

Community trials are characterized by having correlated observations, which implies more than a single source of variability. The statistical terminology for data having more than a single source of error is varied: mixed models (Laird and Ware 1982), hierarchical linear models (Bryk and Raudenbush 1992; Raudenbush and Bryk 2002), or random coefficients (RC) models (Longford 1993). The ANOVA is a useful method for laying out the relationships between the variability at different levels—the individual and the community levels (Murray 1998). The simplest case of ANOVA is for measurements in a single cross-section of individuals in communities.

Suppose there are $r = 1 \ldots m$ members in each of $j = 1 \ldots g$ communities or social units per condition, randomized into $i = 1 \ldots c$ experimental conditions, commonly just two, intervention ($i = 1$) or control ($i = 2$). The ANOVA table presents the sources of variability, the degrees of freedom available for estimating a level of variance (df), the partitioned sums of squared deviations (SSQ), the mean sum of squares (MS) being the SSQ divided by the corresponding df, and the expected mean sum of squares, E(MS), on the basis of the model (see Table 14.1). We use a colon (:) to represent nesting of one effect within another; for example, *unit:Cond* represents the fact that each social unit occurs in one and only one condition, not crossed with Cond. The statistical model for a continuous outcome measure, $y_{r:j:i}$, taken on person r within unit j within condition i, may be written

$$Y_{r:j:i} = \mu + C_i + u_{j:i} + e_{r:j:i}$$

TABLE 14.1. ANOVA PARTITION OF THE SUMS OF SQUARES IN A SINGLE CROSS-SECTION GROUP RANDOMIZED TRIAL HAVING UNIT AS A RANDOM EFFECT.

Source	df	Sum Sq	Mean Sq	E(MS)
Intercept	1	—	—	—
Condition	$c - 1$	SSQcond	MScond	$\sigma^2 + m\tau^2 + mg\,\Sigma(C_i - \mu)^2/(c - 1)$
unit:Cond	$c(g - 1)$	SSQunits	MSunit	$\sigma^2 + m\tau^2$
member:unit:Cond	$cg(m - 1)$	SSQres	MSerror	σ^2
Total $df =$	cgm			

Cond = condition

where μ and C_i are fixed effects representing the overall mean and the shift in the mean attributable to the ith intervention; $u_{j:i}$ represents a "bump" common to all members in the jth unit, and the multiple-valued $u_{j:i}$ are assumed to be Gaussian distributed across units, $u \sim \mathcal{N}(0, \tau^2)$, and $e_{r:j:i}$ represents residual error at the member level, assumed to be a realization from a Gaussian distribution, $e \sim \mathcal{N}(0, \sigma^2)$. Statistical theory of mixed models generates the ANOVA table, which indicates that, under the null hypothesis that the C_i are equal, MScond and MSunit have the same expectation and consequently the ratio MScond/MSunit is distributed as an F-statistic based on numerator $df = (c - 1)$ and denominator $df = c(g - 1)$. Under the alternative hypothesis that the C_i are not equal, the F-statistic has a non-centrality parameter $\Sigma(C_i - \mu)^2/(c - 1)$. Although the non-centrality parameter is not a random variable, it is commonly represented as if it were a variance component, ϕ. Of course, under the null hypothesis, $\phi = 0$.

The important point of the ANOVA is that the test of the hypothesis that the intervention had an effect must compare the variation at the condition level against the variation at the unit level—not against the variation at the member level. Zucker (1990) makes this point most cogently; however, the message is frequently ignored in the analyses of published papers as shown by the review articles of Donner et al. (1990), Simpson et al. (1995), and Varnell et al. (2004). Testing the MScond against the residual error will produce erroneously larger F-statistics and erroneously smaller p-values. Ineffective interventions will be more likely to be declared worthwhile, and even effective interventions will be over-interpreted. Thus the integrity of the inferential process would be jeopardized if the nesting of units within interventions were ignored. The MSunit in the ANOVA table is easily related to the variance of the mean merely by dividing by m and later by g. Recall in the "Effect of Dependence" section that $V(Y_{\text{avg}}) = \sigma^2/m$ $(1 + m\text{VCR})$, that is, $V(Y_{\text{avg}}) = \sigma^2/m + \tau^2$; the variance of a condition-mean made up of g independent unit-means is $[\sigma^2/m + \tau^2]/g$, and the variance of the difference between two condition-means will be $2[\sigma^2/m + \tau^2]/g$. With just two conditions, the non-centrality parameter measuring the separation between the conditions is $\Sigma(C_i - \mu)^2/(2 - 1) = \Sigma (C_i - (C_1 + C_2)/2)^2 = (C_1 - C_2)^2/2$. At a hypothesized separation between the two condition means, $\Delta = (C_1 - C_2)$, the "official" F-test ($F = \text{MScond}/\text{MSunit}$) based on 1 and $2(g - 1)$ df is equivalent to testing the difference between the condition means against the standard error of that difference with a t test based on $2(g - 1)$ df. Hence the fundamental test statistic is

$$t = \Delta/\sqrt{\{2[\sigma^2/m + \tau^2]/g\}} \sim t_{2(g-1)} \tag{1}$$

Efficient Allocation of Resources Subject to Constraints

Improving statistical efficiency refers to achieving smaller variance for the target statistic. For the moment we focus on only the balance of the number of members within unit and the number of units in reducing variance, while remaining within a budget cap. Later, in the section on Statistical Implications of Clustering, we will see that the number of units chosen has a further impact on the statistical power through the number of degrees of freedom for estimating variance components internally to the study. From equation (1) we have the variance of a condition mean, $[\sigma^2/m + \tau^2]/g$. Increasing m will control the member contribution to variation of the mean. But increasing m brings diminishing returns in reducing the variance, because increased m does not control the between-unit contribution to the variance of the mean. Increasing the number of units controls both the member and the unit contributions to the variance of a condition mean. The limited value of increasing m can be seen by plotting the variance of a unit-mean against m, that is, plotting $\sigma^2/m + \tau^2 = \sigma^2(1/m + \text{VCR})$ as a function of m. In fact, it suffices to plot $(1/m + \text{VCR})$ against m, because the σ^2 is inherent member variability (see Figure 14.1).

It looks as if there is little gain in efficiency by increasing sample size, m, within-unit beyond about fifty when the VCR in the range encountered in many community trials is $(0.01, 0.05)$. When the VCR (or, equivalently, ICC) is non-zero, measurements on each additional member within the same unit carry some information redundant to that already collected. The returns diminish with larger within-unit sample size; what is needed is more information about the variation *between* units; however, given budgetary or other feasibility constraints, the number of units selected for study cannot be increased indefinitely.

FIGURE 14.1.   VARIANCE OF A UNIT-MEAN AS A FRACTION OF WITHIN-UNIT VARIANCE, σ^2, PLOTTED AGAINST THE NUMBER OF MEMBERS PER UNIT, AT DIFFERENT LEVELS OF THE CLUSTER EFFECT, VCR.

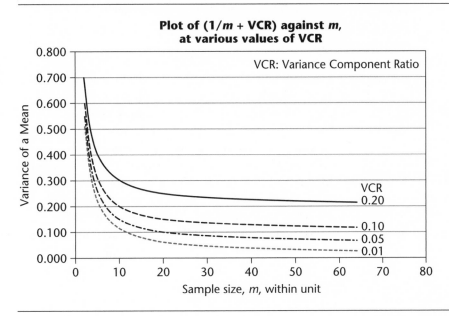

We can balance allocation of resources within and between units by considering the minimization of the variance subject to the budgetary constraints of overhead cost of recruiting units, of the intervention, and of collecting member data. A simple example: you intend to apply for a grant of $200,000 and estimate the cost of recruiting units will be $800, whereas for those units randomized to intervention, the overhead costs of the intervention will be about $1,000 more. The cost of recruiting a member and collecting data is estimated to be $100. An extremely simple model for a post-test only design with g units per condition and m members per unit would have the constraint

$$g\,\$800 + g\,\$1800 + 2gm\$100 = \$200,000$$
$$g\,(2,600 + 200\ m) = 200,000$$
$$g\,(13 + m\,) = 1,000.$$

Suppose we expect the VCR to be 0.05, which might suggest on the basis of Figure 14.1, taking m somewhere between forty and eighty. Let's choose $m = 50$, so $g = 15.87$. We will have to use integral numbers, so fix $g = 16$, and $m = 50$. The variance of the difference in condition means as a multiple of σ^2 is $2(1/m +$ VCR$)/g = 0.00875$. But suppose we instead decided to increase the number of units per condition (g) to 25, for which we could afford only $m = 27$. The variance of the difference in condition means becomes 0.00696. The second design has a relative efficiency of 126 percent ($= 0.00875/0.00696$). Of course, it may be impossible to recruit fifty units, but at least we have some guidance as to where to put our resources.

The g and m parameters that minimize variance for a given design and budget depend on the VCR and the various costs. Typically the principal investigator has in mind a range of possibilities to fit within the proposed budget and the statistician makes explicit the implications for power or detectable difference for various choices of numbers of members and units. Some have developed formulae and/or programs which bring costs and overall budget constraints into the statistical design. See, for example, McKinlay (1994), using estimated VCR parameters from Feldman and McKinlay (1994) and Raudenbush (1997).

The major message is that the more units the better in a GRT. We remind the reader that maximization of statistical power goes further than minimizing variance. Maximization of power requires consideration be given to the available degrees of freedom that govern the spread of the reference distributions under both the null and alternative hypotheses. The point is taken up in the Statistical Implications of Clustering section.

Example of Designing a GRT and Some Further Issues

How does one design a group randomized trial, plan analyses, calculate expected power, and implement the trial? Consider the study "Communities Mobilizing for Change on Alcohol" or CMCA as it is commonly named. This study was conducted out of the Alcohol Epidemiology Program in the Division of Epidemiology, School of Public Health at the University of Minnesota, under the Principal Investigator Dr. Alex Wagenaar in the period 1992 to 1998. Conceptualization, design, grant writing, and funding all preceded the beginning of implementation in 1992. The study aims were to test:

> (1) whether local political and social changes can be achieved using developing theories of citizen politics and public action, and (2) whether community changes brought about by such organized action lead to reduced sales of alcohol to underage persons by commercial outlets, reduced provision of alcohol to underage persons by community residents, reduced youth drinking, and reduced alcohol-related problems among youth.

> (Wagenaar et al. 1994, p. 99)

The statistical design involved a number of interesting elements. By very reason of the hypotheses to be tested, the social intact units of communities are the objects of intervention—behavior in persons and sales practice in alcohol outlets being sampled representatives of the community in which they exist. From a frame of twenty-four eligible communities surviving explicit exclusion criteria, fifteen communities agreed to randomization to control or intervention status. The CMCA design carefully matched these communities into "similar" pairs (one triplet) based on criteria thought to have a possible influence on the communities' present norms and practice and on readiness to work for change. Although randomization will balance confounders *in expectation,* that is, under many replications, the randomization of a limited number of communities will not assure balance in the single realized randomization. Stratification, or the stronger matching, of communities prior to randomization will improve baseline comparability. Randomization is a prime requisite for inference, whereas stratification or matching (or both) prior to randomization is a useful technique to help randomization achieve balance in a limited number of units; statistical adjustment can be used to address residual confounding associated with measured covariates as well as for reducing residual variance. Although communities are matched in the design, a matched analysis will have about one-half the degrees of freedom for estimating the community variance component compared with an unmatched analysis. In most community trials the number of units is not large and the unmatched analysis of the matched design will have more degrees of freedom for the error term and will be preferred (Diehr et al. 1995a; Martin 1993; Proschan 1996).

The design used both "nested cross-sectional" and "nested cohort" designs (Murray and Hannan 1990). In a "nested cross-sectional" design, different members are sampled at different times from within the intact social units as the units are followed over time. In a "nested cohort" design the same members are followed at different times as the units are followed. In CMCA, the surveys of 18-to 20-year-olds in 1992 and 1995 were of different young adults (cross-sectional data) at the two times, whereas the surveys of ninth-graders in 1992 followed the cohort and re-surveyed the same students as twelfth-graders in 1995 (cohort). The article points out some of the advantages and disadvantages of each of these designs; see also Diehr et al. (1995b) and Murray (1998). In contrast to clinical trials in which a cohort offers the advantage of reduced variance because of correlated outcomes, in group randomized trials this advantage is less important because of the unit component of variance and the fact that one deals with a "cohort" of units, that is, repeated measures on the units. Other issues to be considered in selecting a cohort or a cross-sectional design are the length of the study and possible attrition, the mobility and consequent tracking of members, and any perceived threat to anonymity in a cohort data collection that may introduce bias in response to sensitive items. A fundamental issue is whether the study-aim for the intervention is to change individuals or to change infrastructures (which will have an impact on individuals). If the former, only the cohort design is cogent; if the latter, a cross-section is more appropriate. The design paper for CMCA detailed analysis procedures and expected detectable differences using methods appropriate to a group randomized trial. Further, Murray and Short (1995) publish ICCs for many alcohol-related outcomes in nine areas; they present crude ICCs and then changes in ICCs and residual error as adjustment is made for (1) age and gender, (2) one to three personal characteristics, and (3) for zero to two community-level covariates, depending on the outcome. Such estimates are valuable in power estimation in the planning of studies. The paper also gives two examples of the use of these ICCs. Power estimation uses design effects (DEFF) (Kish 1965) or, equivalently, variance inflation factors (Donner et al. 1981, 1992) on the basis of ANOVA tables of expected means squares. We turn to these methods in the next section.

Statistical Implications of Clustering: Power, Sample Sizes, and Detectable Differences

In group randomized trials, estimates of power, sample sizes, and detectable differences are complicated by having to allow for more than the usual single residual component of variance. The two major statistical models applied to group randomized trials are (1) analysis of covariance (ANCOVA) and 2) random coefficients (RC), leading to some differences in power calculations. A third nonparametric method relies on permutation distributions.

The ANCOVA Model

The post-test only design, while weak inferentially, has the simplest model specification on which we can build. Refer to "Implications of Clustering" section for the notation and the ANOVA table (Table 14.1) for the post-test only design. A person may have covariates $x_{r:j:i}$ in which case the regression model with mean μ is:

$$y_{r:j:i} = \mu + C_i + G_{j:i} + b \cdot x_{r:j:i} + e_{r:j:i}$$

where b is the regression coefficient for the covariate (which could be a vector of covariates). For simplicity we will omit covariates from the model so we have

$$y_{r:j:i} = \mu + C_i + G_{j:i} + e_{r:j:i} \tag{2}$$

Note that because of the nesting within unit and condition, both the $G_{j;i}$ and the error term are necessarily modeled as random effects (Zucker 1990). Table 14.1 for the post-test only design also applies to the baseline-adjusted analysis of a nested cohort design. Consequently, referring back to equation (1), the ratio of the baseline-adjusted difference between the conditions at follow-up to its standard error follows the t-distribution based on $2(g - 1)$ df, but the components of variance are adjusted-components of variance:

$$\Delta / \sqrt{\{2[\sigma^2_{\text{adj}}/m + \tau^2_{\text{adj}}]/g\}} \sim t_{2(g-1)}$$

The effect of the regression adjustment for the baseline value of the outcome (and any other covariates) is to reduce the variance by a factor $(1 - R^2)$. Here we have two adjustments coming out of the regression, so we have two factors, $(1 - R^2_m)$ on the member-variability and $(1 - R^2_u)$ on the unit-variability. The variance of Δ can then also be written $\text{Var}(\Delta) = 2[\sigma^2(1 - R^2_m)/m + \tau^2(1 - R^2_u)]/g$. In a cohort of members $R^2_m \approx \rho^2_m$, the square of the member repeat correlation; approximate values of ρ_m are usually readily available. Knowledge of likely values of R_u is not common. In our experience with outcomes mainly in schools, R_u has often been about 0.2, but in a recent (unpublished) study of physical activity in the elderly living in communities, the unit repeat correlation was estimated in a pilot wave of data collection to be about 0.6.

Under the null hypothesis (Ho: $\Delta = 0$) the t-distribution is centered on 0, while under the alternative hypothesis that the actual effect is $\Delta \neq 0$, it is centered on the value Δ. Figure 14.2 shows two Gaussian distributions, the Rejection Region for the null hypothesis for two-sided 5 percent Type I error (outside the vertical lines at ± 1.96 on the horizontal scale), and the Power when the separation between the Null and the Alternative Hypotheses is Δ. Power is the amount of the alternative distribution that lies in the Rejection Region. It is apparent that if the separation were just 1.96 standard errors of Δ, the power would be only 50 percent. To generate power of 85 percent, the separation between the hypotheses must exceed the boundary of the Rejection Region by enough to pull 85 percent of the distribution under the alternative into the Rejection Region. Suppose we have a GRT with six units per condition. Let $t_{d,p}$ represent the value of the p-percentile point on the t-distribution based on d df. In a GRT with six units per condition for example, $t_{10,0.025} = 2.23$ defines the Rejection Region for a two-sided test with Type I error of 5 percent. For 85 percent power we have $t_{10,0.85} = 1.09$ indicating that the separation that is detectable with 85 percent power is 3.32 (2.23 + 1.09) standard errors of Δ. In general, $\Delta \geq (t_{d,1-a/2} + t_{d,\text{power}})$ SE(Δ) and in particular for the *nested cohort baseline-adjusted* analysis

$$\Delta \geq (t_{2(g-1),1-a/2} + t_{2(g-1),\text{power}}) \sqrt{\{2[\sigma^2(1 - R^2_m)/m + \tau^2(1 - R^2_u)]/g\}} \quad (3)$$

FIGURE 14.2. RELATIONSHIP BETWEEN THE DETECTABLE DIFFERENCE (Δ) AND POWER.

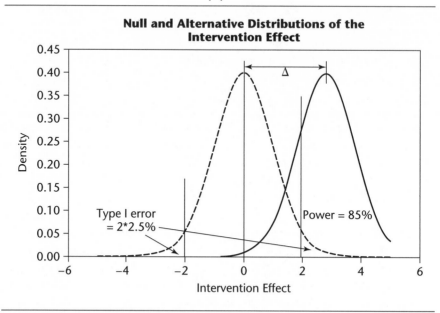

Using *repeated measures* instead of baseline adjustment would involve comparing four means instead of two, but the full effect of member-correlation would be felt, so

$$\Delta \geq (t_{2(g-1),1-a/2} + t_{2(g-1),\text{power}}) \sqrt{\{4[\sigma^2(1 - \rho_m)/m + \tau^2(1 - \rho_u)]/g\}} \quad (4)$$

Formulation (3) uses the actual components of variance, and σ^2 is the within-person variance, not the total variance of a single observation, which is $(\sigma^2 + \tau^2)$. Many authors use the ICC as a standardized and portable measure of clustering effect; in formulae, I prefer the VCR $(= \tau^2/\sigma^2)$, but the two are readily interconvertible. We can re-write (3) parsing out the factor $\sigma^2(1 - R_m^2)$ to give

$$\Delta \geq (t_{2(g-1),1-a/2} + t_{2(g-1),\text{power}}) \sqrt{\{2\sigma^2(1 - R_m^2)}$$
$$\times [1 + m(\tau^2/\sigma^2)(1 - R_u^2)/(1 - R_m^2)]]/mg\} \quad (5)$$

Note that VCR is different depending on the adjustments. Without adjustments $\text{VCR}_{\text{unadj}} = \tau^2/\sigma^2$, whereas with adjustments $\text{VCR}_{\text{adj}} = (\tau^2/\sigma^2)(1 - R_u^2)/(1 - R_m^2)$. When there is more than one occasion of measurement, an important adjustment is adjustment for change (as in 4) or adjustment for baseline values (as in 3, implying that VCR (and ICC) for change will most likely differ from VCR (and ICC) for level. Another consequence of differing R_u and R_m is that adjustment for personal characteristics may increase the VCR_{adj} over VCR_{unadj}, depending on the relative impact of explaining personal level variance and the reduction in unit level variance. The lesson is that, in choosing from published estimated values of ICCs, the onus is on the user to ensure that the circumstances of the estimation fit the usage being made of them and, in particular, the analysis planned for the data.

Often we have a good idea of the residual error, σ^2, and knowledge is accumulating for the likely values of the ICC, which would give an estimate of τ^2 as $\sigma^2 \, ICC/(1 - ICC)$. Even better is to conduct a pilot study to generate good estimates of the components of variance for use in revising previously made power or detectable difference estimates. A useful variant on (5) is to express the minimal detectable difference, Δ, as a fraction of the total standard deviation, $S = \sqrt{\sigma^2 + \tau^2} = \sigma\sqrt{1 + VCR}$. This standardized difference, the difference as a fraction of the standard deviation in the population, is called by Cohen (1988, 1992) the Effect Size ($ES = \Delta/S = \Delta/\sigma\sqrt{1 + VCR}$). An extremely powerful experiment may be able to detect minute effects, but are the experimentally induced shifts worthwhile on the practical scale? The experiment could be a waste of resources. In contrast, an underpowered experiment is able to detect only massive and unrealistic differences, for example, a whole standard deviation; again, the experiment is a waste of resources as it is unlikely to achieve any improvement in knowledge. A good experiment is designed to be fairly sure (power 80 percent or more) to detect feasible (not too large) yet worthwhile (that is, of practical import) differences. For primary outcomes, Effect Sizes between 0.2 and 0.3 (at adequate power) are usually both feasible and worthwhile, making for an excellent experiment; Effect Sizes between 0.3 and 0.4 may be adequate in some contexts; those between 0.4 and 0.5 are weak for primary outcomes but may be useful for pilot studies or for the exploration of the impact of the intervention on secondary outcomes in order to generate hypotheses.

We now extend the post-test only—or equally the baseline adjusted nested cohort—design by crossing the design with a factor T (for time). The model (2) in shorthand can be written

$$y = \mu + C + G:C + e$$

By adding in the effect of crossing ("expanding") the right-hand side by T we get

$$y = \mu + C + G:C + e + T + TC + TG:C + Te \qquad (6)$$

in which we have used the facts that (1) the interaction of T with a constant, $T\mu$, is just the main effect of T; (2) the interaction of two fixed effects is a fixed effect,

TABLE 14.2. ANOVA TABLE FOR THE REPEATED MEASURES ANALYSIS IN A NESTED COHORT DESIGN, OR THE PRE/POST-TEST ANALYSIS IN A NESTED CROSS-SECTION DESIGN.

Line	Source	df	Mean Square	Expected (MS)†
8	Intercept	1		
7	Cond	$c - 1$	MScond	$\sigma^2 + t\eta^2 + mt\omega^2 + mtg\,\phi_c$
6	u : C	$c(g - 1)$	MSunits	$\sigma^2 + t\eta^2 + mt\omega^2$
5	m:u:C	$cg(m - 1)$	MSmember	$\sigma^2 + t\eta^2$
4	Time	$t - 1$	MStime	$\sigma^2 + m\tau^2 + mgc\,\phi_t$
3	TC	$(t - 1)(c - 1)$	MStime*cond	$\sigma^2 + m\tau^2 + mg\,\phi_{tc}$
2	TG : C	$c(t - 1)(g - 1)$	MStime*unit	$\sigma^2 + m\tau^2$
1	Tm : u : C	$cg(t - 1)(m - 1)$	MSerror	σ^2
	Total df =	$cgtm$		

Note : Line 5 must be dropped down to line 1 for the nested cross-sectional design.

†The ϕ_c, ϕ_t, and ϕt_c are non-centrality parameters for the main effects of condition, time, and their interaction respectively. Under null hypotheses they are 0.

but the interaction of a fixed effect with a random effect is random; and (3) a main effect for member (e) is estimable in a cohort, that is, member is crossed with T in a cohort, as each member of a cohort is observed at each time. On this last point, in a nested cross-section with multiple times of observation, the main effect for member (e) would be dropped from the model and its *df* go to error. The separation of the member variability into e and *Te* is exactly the usual separation of variability in repeated measures into between-person variability (e) and within-person variability (*Te*). In the corresponding ANOVA Table 14.2, each entry on the right-hand side of (6) must have a line in the ANOVA. The expected mean squares can be determined with the method proposed in Hopkins (1976), which is much simpler than that of the Cornfield-Tukey algorithm described in Winer (1971).

The question of interest is whether the experiment changed the differences of the intervention means away from the control means. The null hypothesis is Ho : $\phi_{tc} = 0$ and is tested by the ratio of MStime*cond/MStime*unit, where, under the null hypothesis, numerator and denominator would have the same expected values, though based on different *df*. The ratio under Ho is distributed as an *F*-statistic based on $(t - 1)(c - 1)$ and $c(t - 1)(g - 1)$ *df*. This overall test for *any* differences is very non-specific and, if significant, would always be followed by an investigation of a specific difference, for example, between intervention and control ($c = 2$) conditions comparing baseline to a specific time point ($t = 2$). Then the *F*-statistic has 1 and $2(g - 1)$ *df*. The square root of an *F*-statistic with $1, 2(g - 1)$ *df* is distributed as a *t*-statistic based on $2(g - 1)$ *df*.

For the *nested cross-section* line 5 is dropped and its $cg(m-1)$ df fall down to line 1 to make the error $df = cg(t-1)(m-1) + cg(m-1) = cgt(m-1)$. The form of this df term is $(m-1)$ df in every cell and is another indicator that in the nested cross-section, member is nested in the time $\times$ unit cell, that is, the member observation occurs only in a specific time in a specific unit. The repeat correlation for the units is $\rho_u = \omega^2/(\tau^2 + \omega^2)$. In the nested cohort, the within member repeat correlation is $\rho_m = \eta^2/(\sigma^2 + \eta^2)$. In the nested cross-section, we would be comparing four means instead of the two, just as in equation (4) but with $\rho_m = 0$; however, member-level covariates may be introduced to form adjusted means, reducing the member-level residual variance by a factor $(1 - R_m^2)$. The R_u^2 still includes a unit repeat correlation as long as the repeat design returns to the same units.

Let us duplicate with the VCR the calculation with the ICC of the detectable difference given in Wagenaar et al. (1994, pp. 97–98). Note that σ^2 in their notation is the total variance, which we symbolize $\sigma_w^2 + \tau^2$, although previously we have omitted the subscript w (for within). The design calls for 200 persons per community. For thirty-day alcohol use, the within-person variance estimate is $\sigma_w^2 = 0.2331$, which must be divided by $(1 - \text{ICC})$ to produce the total variance; the CMCA paper did not quite get this right. The ICC = 0.02 implies VCR = 0.02/0.98; VIF = $(1 + 199 \times 0.02) = 4.98$, whereas the RVIF = $(1 + 200 * 0.02/0.98) = 5.0816$. Calculations will differ in having $4.98 \times (\sigma_w^2/0.98)$ versus $5.0816 \times \sigma_w^2$ under the square-root sign; however these quantities are numerically equivalent, so the detectable difference calculated using VCR or ICC will be the same. Also note that the assumption is being made that the between-unit component of variance will have the same 50-percent variance reduction from the use of baseline drinking, age, and gender as covariates. The VCR formulation keeps the components separated and allows separate fractions for variance reduction of the within-unit and the between-unit components of variance.

The ANOVA model based on Table 14.2 makes a strong assumption. It assumes that each unit is expected to respond equally to the intervention or lack of it. With only two time points, one cannot separate variability of unit-response from inherent variability of units—the difference and the response "slope" are measured by the same subtraction. If the number of occasions is three or more, then a more realistic model relaxing this assumption is that each unit has its own response-slope, but the average response slopes differ between the intervention and control conditions (Murray et al. 1998). This is the random coefficients (RC) model.

The Random Coefficients Model

When the design calls for more than two time points and interest lies in response to time on a parametric rather than categorical scale, a more robust model making weaker assumptions than the ANOVA model is possible and preferred. The RC model assumes that the units in a condition have trajectories that exhibit random variation around the mean trajectory in that condition, whereas in the ANOVA model it is assumed that each unit in a condition has a common trajectory. For a comparison of the models by simulation, see Murray et al. (1998); for practical applications, see Brown and Prescott (1999) and Twisk (2003); for theory, see Longford (1993). Many other references would be possible, especially in the educational sphere, for example, Bryk and Raudenbush (1992), Raudenbush and Bryk (2002). Estimates of components of variance for slopes are not as yet available in the literature; for two outcomes in a single context, see Murray et al. (2000).

The Impact on Power From a Limited Number of Units

Whether in the ANOVA or the RC model for analyzing a GRT with t time-points, the degrees of freedom of the test statistic are governed by the number of units per condition (g), in the ANOVA model ($t - 1)2(g - 1)$ or in the RC model $2(g - 1)$, indexing the precision with which the variability between the units is assessed. As a consequence, a design with few units has double penalties—the means per condition are less precise because of being divided by a smaller g, and the Rejection Region is wider because the precision for estimating the standard error of the intervention effect is less. This is a good reason to reread Cornfield's statement quoted at the head of this chapter. We have already examined how power and detectable difference depend on the choices of the number of units (g) per condition and on the number of members (m). What is the impact of the degrees of freedom on the term $(t_{d, 1 - a/2} + t_{d, \text{Power}})$ and consequently on the increased value of detectable Δ? Assuming typical values for Type I error at 5 percent (two-sided) and power at 85 percent, Table 14.3 shows the value required for $\Delta/\text{SE}(\Delta)$ in power formulae and the percent increase (penalty) in the separation between the null and alternative hypotheses. Having six units per condition ($df = 10$) may be sustainable, but the penalty increases rapidly if fewer units per condition are in the design. The comparison is against the Gaussian distribution (equivalent to $df = $ infinity)

Permutation Distributions and Significance Tests

How reliable are the distributional assumptions underlying the model-based analyses typified by the ANOVA and RC models? Fisher (1935) introduced the randomization approach to testing, which he considered the gold-standard; indeed, Fisher has said that ANOVA is good only so far as its results approximate those of the randomization test. Application of the permutation test to randomized community trials especially belongs to Gail et al. (1992, 1996). Under the null

TABLE 14.3.   IMPACT ON THE FACTOR ($t_{1-a/2} + t_{Power}$) IN POWER CALCULATIONS AS A FUNCTION OF *df* AVAILABLE.

t-dist *df*	$t_{1-a/2}$	t_{Power}	$t_{1-a/2} + t_{Power}$	Penalty
Gaussian	1.96	1.04	3.00	—
100	1.98	1.04	3.03	1%
50	2.01	1.05	3.06	2%
20	2.09	1.06	3.15	5%
16	2.12	1.07	3.19	6%
10	2.23	1.09	3.32	11%
6	2.45	1.13	3.58	20%
4	2.78	1.19	3.97	32%
2	4.30	1.39	5.69	90%

Type I error=a=5% (two-sided) and Power=85%.

hypothesis, the designation of a unit as intervention or control is irrelevant, so arbitrary re-assignment of one-half the units into "intervention" and the other half into "control" status generates an equally possible (under Ho) experimental result. All possible re-assignment permutations are enumerated and the corresponding experimental results generated. These theoretically equi-possible results (under Ho) constitute the distribution against which the actual observed result is assessed. If the observed result lies far in the tail, it has a low probability of being observed under Ho, raising suspicion against Ho—a true significance test. Given that community trials typically have small numbers of units, the permutation or randomization test procedure may have appeal. It is possible to adjust the unit statistic, commonly the mean, for covariates before permuting (Murray et al., 2006). An entry to the extensive literature may be gained from Braun and Feng (2001), Berger (2000), Ludbrook (1994), Ludbrook and Dudley (1998), Good (1994), Edgington (1995), and Manly (1997). Power calculations for the permutation test are difficult and may best be done with simulation methods (Brookmeyer and Chen 1998).

Power Calculations Require Compromises

Power and sample size calculations have quite a few parameters to be set or to be estimated. Usually straight-forward are the Type I error rate (5 percent two-sided) and the power (80 percent or 85 percent). Less standard are the detectable difference and, in GRTs, the combination of members (whether cross-sectional or cohort) and the number of units. Add in estimated ICCs, estimated reductions in variance achievable by covariate adjustment, and how any multiple comparisons are handled (in the case of more than one *primary* outcome), and the mix is, to say the least, "interesting." How all these parameters are juggled to make a cogent package is the art of grant writing; the scenarios presented need to be meaningful, realistic, and almost invariably a reasonable compromise showing that according to good estimates the study is neither too powerful nor too weak—both a waste of resources.

Some studies try to boost power by resorting to a one-sided test, which indeed does require less separation between the null and alternative hypotheses for a given power. Unless a solid argument can be made that the intervention can in no way have a deleterious (if unexpected) outcome, such a strategy is suspect. Furthermore, in a well-designed study with adequate power, little is gained by using a one-sided test. A study with an adequate sixteen units ($df = 14$) and 85 percent power using a two-tailed 5 percent test to detect a realistic outcome— in other words, a good study—would push the power up to 91 percent at the cost of the assumption underlying the use of the one-sided test. In contrast, a weak study having eight units ($df = 6$) with power 70 percent under the two-sided 5 percent test would increase the power to about 83 percent if the switch was made to a one-sided test. Good study designs gain little from using a one-sided test; invoking a one-sided test is indicative of a weak study struggling to increase power at the expense of a strong assumption, which ignores the possibility of unintended consequences.

Thus the statistician and the principal investigator need to work together in an iterative pattern to arrive at a reasonable place "in the ball park." Specification of the expected intervention effect, that is, the detectable difference, is the province of the principal investigator. In the Trial of Activity in Adolescent Girls (TAAG) with its six centers, the principal investigators at each site were polled for what they would expect as a likely intervention effect—indeed, for those exposed to two years of intervention, and a different amount for those girls exposed to only the second year of intervention. Finally a consensus compromise was achieved and those values in the TAAG power calculations (Stevens and others 2005). Other areas of discussion between the researchers and the statistician involve the variability and correlation of the outcome measures, including which survey instrument(s) will be used, which measure(s) is (are) primary, and general ideas about the budget constraint making certain scenarios unrealistic. Finally, the study design comes together into a cogent whole that is in the ball park from all perspectives. That is why it is a game, involving compromise and diplomacy.

Power is calculated on a statistical model, and we need always to keep in mind the dictum of G.E.P. Box (1979): "All models are wrong, but some are useful." Albert Einstein said, "Models should be simple, but not too simple." The hypotheses to be tested in a group randomized trial in social epidemiology are relatively simple, so the methods used for power can be relatively simple.

Finally, power is calculated based on the assumption that the intervention achieves such an effect. An exaggerated estimate by an overly optimistic researcher of the likely magnitude of the effect achievable by the intervention will lead to optimistic power estimates. Power needs to be calculated for realistic detectable differences, neither too small to be worthwhile substantively, nor too big to be "pie in the sky." Cohen's effect size helps keep magnitudes of detectable differences in perspective. Ultimately, the experiment relies on a strong, well-applied intervention.

Implementation of Randomized Community Trials

We have seen that design of GRTs is complicated. Implementation of design is complicated also. An experiment starts as a germ in the head of the principal investigator, based on some theoretical model of how things work, and ends with inferences based on the observed results. In between, attention must be given to many details and solutions found to many difficulties that arise. Experts in subject matter, in statistics, in public relations, in management, in planning and coordination, in intervention, and in evaluation each have parts to play. Attention must be given to areas such as:

- Deciding on a "frame" of units
- Deciding primary and secondary outcome measures
- Dealing with institutional review boards, both local and in the communities
- Securing agreement to randomization—from units, from members
- Getting the units interested and motivated
- Agreement from units to participate, even if randomized to control status
- Data for matching or stratification in the design
- Baseline before randomization, and extended baseline for maturational history
- Actual randomization
- Implementation of the intervention
- Measuring fidelity to intervention program
- Process measures

Some idea can be gained of the nitty-gritty difficulties of actually setting up a community randomized trial from the report by Watson et al. (2004). Not often does the readership of the scientific journals become acquainted with the picky details of implementing a cluster randomized trial. More on the statistical aspects but, again, laying out some of the items that call for attention are to be found in the reports from, for example, Tobacco Policy Options for Prevention (TPOP) (Forster and Wolfson 1998) or Allina Medical Systems (Roski 2003).

Summary

Why do GRTs? The arguments against GRTs are strong—they are expensive, difficult to implement, fraught with problems along the way, tend to be weak in power, and some of the audience question what the GRT means for individual behavior or health.

So, why do GRTs? The T (trial) and the R (randomization) of GRT are crucial for inference whether group randomized or not, so the question simplifies to: Why use groups? From the theoretic perspective, when interest focuses on contextual effects, the GRT is the most feasible way to manipulate contexts by having the control groups act as surrogates for the (unobservable) counterfactual experience. Second, from the practical perspective, the only way to implement a truly contextual intervention is by acting on whole groups. Sometimes an individually directed intervention may be implemented as a GRT to avoid contamination between control and intervention participants, but in this case it is well worth asking the question, "Can the intervention be crossed with the units in which the experiment will be carried out?" For example, a doctor in a clinic may be blinded to the status of a patient and unknowingly prescribe an active drug or placebo to the patient. This would be unlikely to pass institutional review board review, but at least it is a conceivable design! The Teachable Moment Study TEAM (Hennrikus et al. 2005) did indeed have four hospitals, but both intervention and control participants occurred in each hospital, so that intervention was crossed with hospital. In that case, because intervention is not nested in the hospital, the analyst has the option of considering hospital as a fixed or as a random effect. The contrast of intervention effect with control effect effectively removes the "bump" associated with any realized hospital component of variance; however, a true contextual intervention must apply to the whole unit and, hence, must be a group randomized trial. And be warned that not all collaborators, nor all reviewers, will understand that a contextual study is not just an individual level intervention applied in a group.

Social epidemiology is concerned with contextual effects. In lieu of observational studies that are inherently weak inferentially (Oakes 2004a, 2004b), the GRT offers the inferential benefits of the RCT (randomized controlled clinical trial) to researchers concerned with the impact of social contexts on health of people in communities.

References

Alker, H. R., Jr. (1969). A typology of ecological fallacies. In M. Doggan & S. Rokkan (Eds.), *Social ecology* (pp. 69–81). Cambridge, MA: MIT Press.

Berger, V. W. (2000). Pros and cons of permutation tests in clinical trials. *Statistics in Medicine, 19*, 1319–1328.

Blackburn, H. (2004). *It isn't always fun . . . .* (privately published) Library of Congress: ISBN 1–887268–05–7.

Box, G.E.P. (1979). Robustness in the strategy of scientific model building. In R.L. Launer & G. N. Wilkinson (Eds.), *Robustness in statistics* (P. 201). New York: Academic Press.

Brookmeyer, R., & Chen, Y.-Q. (1998). Person-time analysis of paired community intervention trials when the number of communities is small. *Statistics in Medicine, 17*(18), 2121–2132.

Braun, T., & Feng, Z. (2001). Optimal permutation tests for the analysis of group randomized trials. *Journal of the American Statistical Association, 96*(456), 1424–1432.

Brown, H., & Prescott, R. (1999). *Applied mixed models in medicine.* New York: John Wiley and Sons.

Bryk, A. S., & Raudenbush, S. W. (1992). *Hierarchical linear models: Applications and data analysis methods* (1st ed.). Newbury Park: Sage Publications.

Carleton, R. A., Lasater, T. M., Assaf, A. R., Feldman, H. A., McKinlay, S., & The Pawtucket Heart Health Program Writing Group. (1995). The Pawtucket Heart Health Program: Community changes in cardiovascular risk factors and projected disease risk. *American Journal of Public Health, 85*(6), 777–785.

Cohen, J. (1988). *Statistical power analysis for the behavioral sciences* (2nd ed.). Hillsdale, NJ: Lawrence Erlbaum.

Cohen, J. (1992). A primer on power. *Psychological Bulletin, 112*(1), 155–159.

Cook, T. D., & Campbell, D. T. (1979). *Quasi-experimentation: Design and analysis issues for field settings.* Boston: Houghton Mifflin Company.

Corbeil, R. R., & Searle, S. R. (1976). Restricted maximum likelihood (REML) estimation of variance components in the mixed model. *Technometrics, 18,* 31–38.

Cornfield, J. (1978). Randomization by group: A formal analysis. *American Journal of Epidemiology, 108*(2), 100–102.

Diehr, P., Martin, D. C., Koepsell, T., & Cheadle, A. (1995a). Breaking the matches in a paired *t*-test for community interventions when the number *o* pairs is small. *Statistics in Medicine, 14,* 1491–1504.

Diehr, P., Martin, D. C., Koepsell, T., Cheadle, A., Psaty, B. M., & Wagern, E. H. (1995b). Optimal survey design for community intervention evaluations: Cohort or cross-sectional? *Journal of Clinical Epidemiology, 48*(12), 1461–1472.

Donner, A. (1982). An empirical study of cluster randomization. *International Journal of Epidemiology, 11*(3), 283–286.

Donner, A. (1985). A regression approach to the analysis of data arising from cluster randomization. *International Journal of Epidemiology, 14*(2), 322–326.

Donner, A. (1992). Sample size requirements for stratified cluster randomization designs. *Statistics in Medicine, 11,* 743–750.

Donner, A., Birkett, N., & Buck, C. (1981). Randomization by cluster: Sample size requirements and analysis. *American Journal of Epidemiology, 114*(6), 906–914.

Donner, A., Brown, K. S., & Brasher, P. (1990). A methodological review of non-therapeutic intervention trials employing cluster randomization, 1979–1989. *International Journal of Epidemiology, 19,* 795–800.

Donner, A. & Klar, N. (1996). Statistical considerations in the design and analysis of community intervention trials. *Journal of Clinical Epidemiology, 49*(4), 435–439.

Donner. A., & Klar, N. (2000). *Design and analysis of cluster randomization trials in health research.* London: Arnold.

Donner, A., & Koval, J. J. (1982). Design considerations in the estimation of intraclass corre-lation. *Annals of Human Genetics 46,* 271–277.

Edgington, E. S. (1995). *Randomization tests* (3rd ed.). New York: Marcel Dekker.

Farquhar, J. W., McCoby, N., Wood, P. D., et al. (1977). Community education for cardiovas-cular health. *Lancet, 1,* 1192–1195.

Farquhar, J. W. (1978). The community-based model of life style intervention trials. *American Journal of Epidemiology, 108*(2), 103–111.

Farquhar, J. W., Fortman, S. P., Maccoby, N., Haskell, W. L., Williams, P. T., et al. (1985). The Stanford Five-City Project: Design and methods. *American Journal of Epidemiology, 122,* 323–334.

Feldman, H. A., & McKinlay, S. M. (1994). Cohort versus cross-sectional design in large field trials: Precision, sample size, and a unifying model. *Statistics in Medicine, 13,* 61–78.

Fisher, R. A. (1935). *The design of experiments.* Edinburgh: Oliver and Boyd, reprinted New York: Hafner Publishing Company, 1971 (8th ed.) and re-issued in *Statistical Methods, Exper-imental Design, and Scientific Inference* (1990). Oxford: Oxford University Press.

Forster, J. L., & Wolfson, M. (1998). Youth access to tobacco: Policies and politics. *Annual Review Public Health, 19,* 203–235.

Frost, W. H. (1937). How much control of tuberculosis? *AJPH, 27,* 759–766.

Gail, M. H., Pechacek, T., & Corle, D. (1992). Aspects of statistical design for the community intervention trial for smoking cessation (COMMIT). *Controlled Clinical Trials, 13,* 6–21.

Gail, M. H., Mark, S. D., Carroll, R. J., Green, S. B., & Pee, D. (1996). On design considera-tions and randomization-based inference for community intervention trials. *Statistics in Medicine, 15,* 1069–1092.

Goldstein, H. (1987). *Multilevel models in educational and social research.* New York: Oxford Uni-versity Press.

Good, P. I. (1994). *Permutation tests. A practical guide to resampling methods for testing hypotheses.* New York: Springer-Verlag.

Hannan, P. J., Murray, D. M., Jacobs, D. R., Jr., McGovern, P. G. (1994). Parameters to aid in the design and analysis of community trials: Intraclass correlations from the Minnesota Heart Health Program. *Epidemiology, 5,* 88–95.

Hennrikus, D. J., Lando, H. A., McCarty, M. C., et al. (2005). The TEAM Project: The effectiveness of smoking cessation intervention with hospital patients. *Preventive Medicine, 40,* 249–258.

Hopkins, K. D. (1976). A simplified method for determining expected mean squares and error terms in the analysis of variance. *Journal of Experimental Education, 45*(2), 13–18.

Hopkins, K. D. (1982). The unit of analysis: Group means versus individual observations. *American Education Research Journal, 19*(1)5–18.

Jacobs, D. R., Luepker, R. V., Mittelmark, M., Folsom, A. R., Pirie, P. L., Mascoli, S. R., et al. (1986). Community-wide prevention strategies: Evaluation design of the Minnesota Heart Health Program. *Journal of Chronic Diseases, 39*(10), 775–788.

Jeffery, R. W., Forster, J. L., French, S. A., Kelder, S. H., Lando, H. A., McGovern, P. G., et al. (1993). The Healthy Worker Project: A worksite intervention for weight control and smoking cessation. *American Journal of Public Health, 83*(3), 395–401.

Keys, A., Blackburn, H. W., Van Buchem, F. S. P., Buzina, R., Djordjevic, B. S., Dontas, A. S., et al. (1967). Epidemiological studies related to coronary heart disease: Characteristics of men aged 40–59 in seven countries. *Acta Med Scand, 460*(Suppl. 180), 1–392.

Kish, L. (1965). *Survey sampling.* New York: John Wiley and Sons.

Koepsell, T. D., Diehr, P. H., Cheadle, A., & Kristal, A. (1995). Invited commentary: Symposium on community intervention trials. *American Journal of Epidemiology, 142*(6), 594–599.

Krieger, N. (1992). Overcoming the absence of socioeconomic data in medical records: Validation and application of a census-based methodology. *American Journal of Public Health 82,* 703–310.

Krieger, N. (1994). Epidemiology and the web of causation: Has anyone seen the spider? *Social Science & Medicine 39*(7), 887–903.

Laird, N. M., Ware, J. H. (1982). Random-effects models for longitudinal data. *Biometrics 38,* 963–74.

Longford, N. T. (1993). *Random coefficients models.* New York: Oxford University Press.

Ludbrook, J. (1994). Special article: Advantages of permutation (randomization) tests in clinical and experimental pharmacology and physiology. *Clinical and Experimental Pharmacology and Physiology, 21,* 673–686.

Ludbrook, J., & Dudley, H. (1998). Why permutation tests are superior to *t* and *F* tests in biomedical research. *The American Statistician 52,* 127–132.

Manly, B.F.J. (1997). *Randomization, bootstrap and Monte Carlo methods in biology* (2nd ed.). London: Chapman & Hall.

Martin, D. C., Diehr, P., Perrin, E. B., & Koepsell, T. (1993). The effect of matching on the power of randomized community intervention studies. *Statistics in Medicine, 12,* 329–338.

McCullagh, P., & Nelder, J. A. (1983). *Generalized linear models* (1st ed.). New York: Chapman and Hall.

McCullagh, P., & Nelder, J. A. (1989). *Generalized linear models* (2nd ed.). New York: Chapman and Hall.

McKinlay, S. M. (1994). Cost-efficient designs of cluster unit trials. *Preventive Medicine, 23,* 606–611.

Mood, A. (1950). *Introduction to the theory of statistics* (Sec.7.5, pp.133–136). New York: McGraw-Hill Book Company.

Murray, D. M. (1998). *Design and analysis of group randomized trials.* New York: Oxford University Press.

Murray, D. M., Feldman, H. A., McGovern, P. G. (2000). Components of variance in a group-randomized trial analyzed via a random-coefficients model: The REACT Trial. *Statistical Methods in Medical Research, 9,* 117–133.

Murray, D. M., & Hannan, P. J. (1990). Planning for the appropriate analysis in school-based drug-use prevention studies. *Journal of Consulting and Clinical Psychology, 58*(4), 458–468.

Murray, D. M., Hannan, P. J., Wolfinger, R. D., Baker, W. L., & Dwyer, J. H. (1998). Analysis of data from group-randomized trials with repeat observations on the same groups. *Statistics in Medicine, 17,* 1581–1600.

Murray, D. M., McKinlay, S. M., Martin, D., Donner, A. P., Dwyer, J. H., Raudenbush, S. W., et al. (1994). Design and analysis issues in community trials. *Evaluation Review 18,* 493–514.

Murray, D. M., & Short, B. (1995). Intraclass correlation among measures related to alcohol use by young adults: Estimates, correlates and applications in intervention studies. *Journal of Studies on Alcohol, 56*(6), 681–694.

Murray, D. M., Varnell, S. P., Blitstein, J. L. (2004). Design and analysis of group-randomized trials: A review of recent methodological developments. *American Journal of Public Health, 94*(3), 423–432.

Murray, D. M., Hannan, P. J., Varnell, S. P., McGowan, R. G., Baker, W. L., & Blitstein, J. L. (2006). A comparison of mixed-model regression and permutation methods using simulated data from a group trial with or without randomization. *Statistics in Medicine, 25,* 375–388.

Oakes, J. M. (2004a). The (mis)estimation of neighborhood effects: Causal inference in a practicable social epidemiology. *Social Science & Medicine, 58,* 1929–1952 (with discussion).

Oakes, J. M. (2004b). Causal inference and the relevance of social epidemiology. *Social Science & Medicine, 58,* 1969–1971.

Proschan, M. A. (1996). On the distribution of the unpaired *t*-statistic with paired data. *Statistics in Medicine, 15,* 1059–1063.

Puska, P., Salonen, J. T., Nissenen, A., Tuomilehto, J., Vartiainen, E., Korhonen, H., et al. (1983). Change in risk factors for coronary heart disease during 10 years of community intervention programme (North Karelia Project). *British Medical Journal Clinical Research Edition, 287*(6408), 1840–1844.

Raudenbush, S. W. (1997). Statistical analysis and optimal design in cluster randomized trials. *Psychological Methods, 2*(2), 173–185.

Raudenbush, S. W., & Bryk, A. S. (2002). *Hierarchical linear models: Applications and data analysis methods* (2nd ed.). Thousand Oaks, CA: Sage Publications.

Robinson, W. S. (1950). Ecological correlations and the behavior of individuals. *American Sociological Review, 15,* 351–357.

Roski, J., Jeddeloh, R., An, L., Lando, H., Hannan, P. J., Hall, C., & Zhu, S.-H. (2003). The impact of financial incentives and a patient registry on health quality: Targeting smoking cessation clinical practice patterns and patient outcomes. *Preventive Medicine, 36,* 291–299.

Senn, S. (2004). Added values: Controversies concerning randomization and additivity in clinical trials. *Statistics in Medicine, 23*(24), 3729–3753.

Simpson, J. M., Klar, N., & Donner, A. (1995). Accounting for cluster randomization: A review of primary prevention trials, 1990 through 1993. *American Journal of Epidemiology, 85*(10), 1378–1383.

Snow, J. (1849). *On the mode of communication of cholera* (2nd ed. [1955]). London. Retrieved from http://www.csiss.org/classics/content/8

Sorenson, G., Emmons, K., Hunt, M. K., & Johnston, D. (1998). Implications of the results of community intervention trials. *Annual Review of Public Health 19,* 379–416.

Stevens, J., Murray, D. M., Catellier, D. J., Hannan, P. J., Lytle, L. A., Elder, J. P., Young, D. R., Simons-Morton, D. G., & Webber, L. S., (2005). Design of the Trial of Activity in Adolescent Girls (TAAG). *Controlled Clinical Trials, 26,* 223–233.

Twisk, J.W.R. (2003). *Applied longitudinal data analysis in epidemiology: A practical guide.* New York: Cambridge.

Varnell, S. P., Murray, D. M., Janega, J. B., Blitstein, J. L. (2004). Design and analysis of group-randomized trials: A review of recent practices. *American Journal of Public Health, 94*(3), 393–399.

Wagenaar, A. C., Murray, D. M., Wolfson, M., Forster, J. L., & Finnegan, J. R. (1994). Communities mobilizing for change on alcohol: Design of a randomized community trial. *Journal of Community Psychology CSAP, Special Issue,* 79–101.

Watson, L., Small, R., Brown, S., Dawson, W., & Lumley, J. (2004). Mounting a community-randomized trial: Sample size, matching, selection and randomization issues in PRISM. *Controlled Clinical Trials, 25*(3), 235–250.

Wedderburn, R.W.M. (1974). Quasilikelihood functions, generalized linear models and the Gauss-Newton method. *Biometrika, 61,* 439–447.

Wedderburn, R.W.M. (1976). On the existence and uniqueness of the maximum likelihood estimates for certain generalized linear models. *Biometrika, 63,* 27–32.

WHO Expert Committee (1982). *Prevention of coronary heart disease. Technical Report Series 678.* Geneva: World Health Organization.

Williams, P. T., Fortmann, S. P., Farquhar, J. W., Varady, A., & Mellen, S. (1981). A comparison of statistical methods for evaluating risk factor changes in community-based studies: An example from the Stanford Three-Community Study. *Journal of Chronic Diseases 34*(11), 565–571.

Winer, B. J. (1971). *Statistical principles in experimental design* (2nd ed., pp. 371–375). New York: McGraw-Hill Book Company.

Zucker, D. M. (1990). An analysis of variance pitfall: The fixed effects analysis in a nested design. *Educational and Psychological Measurement, 50,* 731–738.

Zucker, D. M., Lakatos, E., Webber, L. S., Murray, D. M., McKinlay, S. M., Feldman, H. A., et al. (1995). Statistical design of the Child and Adolescent Trial for Cardiovascular Health (CATCH): Implication of cluster randomization. *Controlled Clinical Trials, 16,* 96–118.

CHAPTER FIFTEEN

PROPENSITY SCORE MATCHING FOR SOCIAL EPIDEMIOLOGY

J. Michael Oakes and Pamela Jo Johnson

Every epidemiologist knows that observational studies are troublesome because of the potential for confounding, a condition that implies improper comparisons and potentially biased effect estimates. Although standardization is still used, covariance adjustment via regression has long been the principal tool through which investigators try to recover "proper" comparisons and unbiased estimates. Regression techniques are now remarkably easy to implement, owing to the availability of powerful yet inexpensive computers and user-friendly statistical software. But with such ease comes the potential for misuse or misunderstanding, be it intentional or accidental (Berk 2004). Too many contemporary analysts, it seems to us, fail to appreciate the assumptions inherent in regression methods, to say nothing of the hypothetical experiment their observational study surely aims to mimic. A key concern is that investigators alter their (often implicit) causal regression models based not on theory but on indicators of sampling variability (for example, p-values) or other aspects of the relationship between dependent and independent variables. Models end up capitalizing on chance and being overfit and otherwise misleading with respect to causal inference. The problem is not with regression technology itself, but with its application.

Though clearly no panacea, we believe that propensity score methods may allow social epidemiologists to (1) better appreciate and more closely mimic experimental study designs, (2) minimize approaches to model specification that rely on testing, and (3) increase the transparency of inference. Accordingly, we believe propensity score methods are important and worthy of both study and use.

Our goal here is to motivate, explain, and offer an example of how social epidemiologists might use the propensity score approach. Methodologically, we offer nothing especially new or ground-breaking. Instead we aim to synthesize and make accessible existing research and show that the combined use of a counterfactual framework for causal inference, an explicit causal contrast study design, and propensity score matching methods is a useful alternative approach to regression models. "Accessibility" is essential, because the relevant literature is both vast and often quite technical if not impenetrable for non-statisticians. Even some of the published tutorials (for example, D'Agostino 1998; Joffe and Rosenbaum 1999; Little and Rubin 2000) can present challenges, and none are tailored for social epidemiologists. Because social epidemiology is clearly interested in estimating the effect of neighborhood contexts on health outcomes (that is, neighborhood effects), we use such an investigation as an example and departure point for discussion. Accordingly, we divide this chapter into four sections: (1) the counterfactual framework, (2) propensity score-matching methods, (3) example, and (4) conclusion.

The Counterfactual Framework

We motivate our discussion of propensity score methods by considering the counterfactual framework, which is merely a tool for conducting thought experiments that often illuminate problems and prospects that analysts face in the "real" world. The genesis of the approach is often attributed to Hume, but many contemporary philosophers and scientists have extended, clarified, and refined it (Hausman 1998).

Within the framework, a causal effect is ascertained through a comparison of "potential outcomes" that would have been observed under different exposures for the same unit (Little and Rubin 2000). For example, to calculate the causal effect of neighborhood poverty on the health of Jane's new baby, we must simultaneously observe the baby's health under two conditions: one in which Jane resided in, say, a middle-class neighborhood, and another when Jane resided in an impoverished neighborhood. If it were possible to observe both of these situations (that is, all potential outcomes), then it would be easy to calculate the desired causal effect. As in the following discussion, the effect would be the difference (or any contrast) of the two outcomes under the two scenarios. Of course it is not possible to simultaneously observe Jane's birth outcome under both conditions: Jane either lived in poverty during her pregnancy or she didn't. This fact—that we are missing observable data for one of the potential outcomes—is so important that it has been called the "fundamental problem of causal inference" (Holland 1986). To be clear, the *unobservable* data in the above scenario is called the "counterfactual," because it is counter to fact (Winship and Morgan 1999).

FIGURE 15.1.   CONCEPTUAL DIAGRAM OF TARGET VALUES AND CAUSAL CONTRAST.

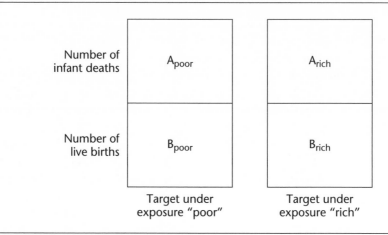

Maldonado and Greenland (2002a; 2002b) show that to estimate a valid causal effect in epidemiologic research, one must first specify an explicit causal contrast. Extending the counterfactual framework to groups (which entails several assumptions), they define a causal contrast as a comparison of the outcome frequency in *one* target population under *two* "exposure distributions." To see this, imagine that we now have a group of infants as our target population and we are interested in the effect of neighborhood poverty on infant death. Let two exposure distributions represent exposure to "poor" neighborhoods and exposure to "rich" neighborhoods for the very same group of infants. The following diagram (Figure 15.1) and discussion of a causal contrast is adapted from Maldonado and Greenland (2002a).

$R_{poor} = A_{poor}/B_{poor}$ such that R_{poor} represents the incidence proportion of deaths (for example, infant mortality rate) in the target population had they been exposed to "poor" neighborhoods. Similarly, $R_{rich} = A_{rich}/B_{rich}$, such that R_{rich} represents the ratio for that same group of infants had they instead been exposed to "rich" neighborhoods. A causal contrast ratio may then be represented by:

$$RR_{causal} = \frac{R_{poor}}{R_{rich}} = \frac{A_{poor}/B_{poor}}{A_{rich}/B_{rich}} \tag{1}$$

which is the familiar incidence proportion ratio or rate ratio. Similarly, a causal contrast *difference* (for example, rate difference) is represented by:

$$RD_{causal} = R_{poor} - R_{rich} \tag{2}$$

It is now easy to see the problem of the missing "potential outcomes" data. Specifically, our "target" group can only be observed under one exposure condition at a given point in time. Thus, *at least* one of the previously shown exposure conditions and subsequent outcome frequencies is unobservable or counterfactual. This means that in order to estimate a causal contrast we must obtain valid and observable *substitute* quantities for the desired counterfactual quantities (Maldonado and Greenland 2002a). This substitution step is the crux of the causal contrast, the counterfactual framework, and causal inference more generally. If substitutes are *exchangeable* with targets, we are in good shape; if not, we suffer confounded effects, which may be useless.

Exchangeability is a key concept that is related to confounding and elemental aspects of probability theory (De Fineti 1974; Greenland and Robins 1986). Technically, exchangeability is a property of a joint distribution of a sequence of random variables that are unchanged by an arbitrary permutation of the sequence (Dodge 2003). In simple terms, *exchangeability* is a term that connotes equality or substitution without penalty or change. As used here, groups are exchangeable if their substitution yields no impact on effect estimates. If substituting an observed control or comparison group for an unobservable counterfactual group (hypothetically!) yields the same effect estimate, then the observed and counterfactual groups are exchangeable. If the substitution yields a different effect estimate, then the groups are not exchangeable and estimated effects are confounded.

We believe it is critical for social epidemiologists to appreciate that exchangeability implies that an observed counterfactual substitute *could have been* treated or exposed (or both) just as the unobservable counterfactual could (theoretically) have been. Indeed, estimates of causal effects in observational studies presume that the exposure of interest *could have happened* to anyone in the data (Rosenbaum 2002). If this is not possible, the substitution is improper and no causal inference may follow. Because there is no way to empirically confirm whether or not the observed substitution is exchangeable with the unobservable counterfactual, careful thinking is a must.

Randomized controlled trials are typically viewed as the "gold standard" for inferring cause because, by dint of successful randomization, the treated and untreated groups are identical in expectation save for the treatment. The two groups are exchangeable because the group that received the treatment (for example, a pill) is identical to the control group. In other words, the treatments could have been reversed and the long-run effect estimate would be unchanged.

Returning to our motivating example, this means that the scientifically best way to answer the question about poverty and infant mortality is to randomize a large number of women to rich and poor neighborhoods and observe birth outcome distributions. Or better yet, as described by Oakes (2004), randomize aspects of poverty (for example, poor sidewalks or perhaps nutritional opportunities) to women through a cluster trial design. Anything short of intervention and randomization (with large numbers) and we must worry about exchangeability and confounded effects. It follows that one must try to overcome these issues in any observational design, which may now be understood as studies in which the investigator does not control the treatment assignment mechanism (for example, randomization) and thus cannot achieve exchangeability by design.

How do epidemiologists typically make observable substitutes exchangeable with unobservable counterfactuals in observational designs? They do it through the analytic techniques of regression and stratification, both of which are limited. For purposes here, the most pressing concerns with regression models are (1) omitted variable bias and (2) off-support inference. The former point is presumably obvious: if investigators fail to measure and adjust for all confounders, observed substitutes may not be exchangeable for unobserved counterfactuals and estimates may remain confounded. Because in practice confounding is often detected by examining the impact (for example, 10-percent reduction in magnitude) of including this or that potential confounder in a model, analysts have incentive to "play with" their data and model specifications for an indeterminate amount of time. This specification rule is inferentially suspect and may very often lead to model "over-fitting" and other problems related to chance and sampling variability (Berk 2004; Clogg and Haritou 1997; Leamer 1978). Again, this is not a criticism of regression technology per se but rather its application in practice—as least as we see it.

The problem of off-support inference—a term we attribute to Manski (1993), though Heckman (1997), Rubin (1977), and Lord (1967) make the point clear— is related but perhaps more subtle. At risk of being glib, the problem may best be internalized and appreciated by considering an old joke:

A statistician was asked to determine the temperature of the water in two buckets: one bucket's water was very cold, the other's was very hot. To do this, the statistician took off his socks and shoes and put one foot in each bucket. Although his left foot turned blue from the cold and his right blistering red from the heat, the statistician exclaimed that the water temperature was, on average, *just right.*

The point is that averages and other statistical procedures that summarize information may end up obscuring fundamental differences between considered objects. With respect to the joke, the statistic—average water temperature—is purely synthetic and without any empirical link, for there is no "just right" water in the statistician's world, at least until the two buckets are (experimentally) mixed. So although mathematically correct, the statistician's report is not only useless but misleading, if not dangerous: a caregiver should not rely on the statistic and bathe an infant child in one of the two buckets. Among other things, a concern about off-support inference is a concern about the ease with which statistical procedures may end up masking fundamental differences between treatment and control groups and thus the identification of effects through actual observations. Rosenbaum makes this point by considering efforts to assess the impact of the Head Start program by comparing low-income students treated by the program to wealthy students not treated by the program. He correctly insists that effects calculated from such comparisons rest on pure extrapolation and speculation (Rosenbaum 2004). Of course the issue of synthetic statistics masking facts is not at all new; we see similarities in the foundational debates between Quetelet and others contemplating the "law of binomial errors" and the "average man," circa 1840 (Desrosieres 1998).

Note well that the issue of off-support inference is not related to effect-modification or collapsibility as understood in epidemiology. These phenomena are concerned with different effects, if not causal forces, in different strata or perhaps populations (Greenland and Robins 1986; Greenland et al. 1999). By contrast, off-support inference is a concern about the ability to identify *any* effect, be it homogeneous or heterogeneous across strata. Effect modification presupposes the identification of (differential) effects and thus data to support such inference. Off-support inference is more fundamental; it is a nuts-and-bolts issue with one's actual data, not a formula or theory.

We believe the issue of off-support inference has especially important implications for social epidemiology, and such implications are germane to our example about the effect of being born into a poor neighborhood on infant death. Because we know that subjects in poor neighborhoods are sociodemographically (for example, financially and educationally) different than subjects in rich neighborhoods, we might be tempted to estimate a regression model that "adjusts" or "controls" for potential confounders such as age, income, education, marital status, and so forth. Yet common sense is stretched when systematic differences between those residing in low and high socioeconomic status neighborhoods are "controlled" in this fashion. It is not difficult to show that parameter estimates may be based not on comparisons between actual persons but rather on extrapolation, interpolation, regression smoothing, and imputation more generally. Again, the extent to which inferences are based on "imputed" data is the extent to which inferences are on- or off-support.

To assess "support" in this example, one should examine how many people across rich and poor neighborhoods share the same sociodemographic characteristics. Because of social stratification (at least in America), we doubt there will be many, because the wealthy will never live in poor neighborhoods and the poor cannot afford to live in rich ones. Indeed, such social sorting has long been recognized and even formalized in 1956 by economist Tiebout (1956).

We go so far as to use the term "structural confounding" to convey this problem. The confounding is structural because it cannot be overcome by better sampling methods or larger sample sizes. It can only be overcome by imagining a massive social revolution—what Lewis (1973) calls a "miracle" intervention. But employing such counterfactuals violates a hidden principle: counterfactuals should be reasonable. Hawthorn says we should consider only "plausible worlds," and Lewis states that we should focus on the "closest possible world" (Hawthorn 1991; Lewis 1973). Miracle revolutions also violate what Rossi calls "policy space"—alternative policies or remedies that appear within reach or politically possible (Rossi 1980). Whatever one calls it, the regression model does not care about it: the model will induce exchangeability through imputation, the veracity of which cannot be easily tested.

The upshot is that, in practice, regression adjustment is too easy to abuse. The technology does not force one to consider exchangeability or examine the "support" on which inferences may be based. The assumptions needed for one to reasonably leap from description to causal inference with regression are typically unrecognized and untestable, if not unwarranted (Berk 2004; Clogg and Haritou 1997). The problems appear not solved but amplified in "multilevel" regression models (Oakes 2004).

Besides regression, the other standard practice to account for observed differences between groups is subclassification or matching. Subclassification has been used for decades to "adjust" for differences between exposure groups on a single factor. The distinct advantage of subclassification over multiple regression is that in large data sets it is relatively easy to assess the degree of covariate overlap or balance (that is, support) between exposure groups. The disadvantage of subclassification is that it quickly becomes unwieldy when there are more than one or two classification factors under consideration. If we had five dichotomous covariates on which we needed to simultaneously subclassify, we would need 2^5 or 32 strata. If we had many continuous covariates or categorical covariates with many levels, subclassification would be impossible. This is called the dimensionality problem, a term dating back at least to Bellman (1961).

Matching is a special case of subclassification where each (un)exposed subject and its match creates a strata—in experimental design, this is called "blocking." There are many matching techniques, even some incorporating qualitative "thick description" (see Rosenbaum and Silber 2001). Because each matched pair represents an (un)exposed subject and its counterfactual substitute, causal contrasts are easily calculated. But matching suffers the dimensionality problem too. How can we mimic randomization by simultaneously matching persons on many observed covariates? Propensity score matching methods address this very problem.

Propensity Score-Matching Methods

Propensity score methods were introduced by Rosenbaum and Rubin in 1983. A propensity score is defined as the conditional probability of being exposed or treated (or both) (Rosenbaum and Rubin 1983, 1984). This might seem strange: because analysts know the exposure status of each subject, why do they need to estimate the probability of being exposed? The reason is because the propensity score is useful for reducing the dimensionality of a large set of potential confounders to unity, and this is conducive to simple matching or subclassification. In other words, once we have estimated the propensity score, we can match subjects in both exposed and unexposed conditions by their propensity scores. This matches subjects with the same probability of having been exposed when, in fact, one of them was exposed and the other was not. This is what randomization does, except it (typically) forces all subjects to have a true propensity of exposure equal to 0.50 and works on unmeasured confounders too. Subject to concern over unobserved variables and measurement error, which may be great, matching permits us to be more comfortable with the assumption that these two subjects are exchangeable (except for the exposure). And any observed difference in outcome between the two may be inferred to be due to the exposure alone, as in randomized experiments. It is in this way that propensity score matching methods force one to consider and mimic experimental designs.

Propensity Score Estimation

Just as in experiments, observational studies should be designed such that the outcome of interest plays no role in the probability of exposures or treatments. Accordingly, it is best to limit consideration of covariate information to that which predicts not the outcome but the *exposure* or treatment of interest. Unlike multiple regression procedures that, despite warnings from methodologists, tend to direct attention to the outcome variable and *p*-values of regressors, propensity score matching methods direct the analyst's attention to covariate imbalance across exposure groups.

Propensity scores can be estimated with a traditional logistic regression model—which is why the method is often considered semi-parametric instead of nonparametric. There is nothing magical about the procedure: presuming a social epidemiological analysis, the predicted value from a logistic regression model of the observed exposure (yes = 1; no = 0) on a set of covariates (or predictors) of the exposure is a person's propensity score. This means that each person in the analytic dataset gets a propensity score, unless of course they have missing values on covariates (discussed later in this chapter). Extreme instances notwithstanding, note that the method encourages the use of a rich set of covariates, including interaction and higher-order terms. The more the better, so long as the covariates are "proper"—that is, not themselves the effects or outcomes of the exposure of interest—which is often especially challenging to discern in social epidemiology. Further step-wise regression procedures or related techniques should never be used. Finally, it should be obvious that use of a set of covariates unrelated to exposure yields unacceptably imprecise propensity score values.

Often overlooked, the key to causal inference from observational studies using propensity score methods is to examine the overlap in propensity scores between the two exposure groups (exposed and unexposed). If there is no overlap, there is nothing more that can be done; the two groups are not comparable and subjects are not exchangeable (Lord 1967; Rubin 1977). This point stands in stark contrast to most conventional regression methods where overlap is hidden by model assumptions, linearities, and the like. Unless one is relying on an extremely inappropriate comparison group there will often be some overlap in propensity scores between exposure groups, which means that these are the subjects for whom there is "common support" in the data and for whom inferences can be made. To the dismay of those who think any data is good data, subjects that do not overlap cannot be used, at least in this simplified approach and discussion. Again, to see the importance of this, recall that in a simple randomized experiment all subjects have a propensity of 0.50, which means inference is perfectly supported by data, not model assumptions.

Figure 15.2 attempts to illustrate the importance of assessing overlap. This fictitious graph depicts the overlap (or lack of it) in propensity scores when all in the exposed group have a high estimated probability of being exposed and those in the unexposed group all have a low probability of being exposed. This might be the case in an observational study when some subjects come from exceedingly rich neighborhoods and others from poor ones. The point of the overly dramatic graph is that there are no subjects with similar propensity scores, and so if the propensity score model is correctly specified, then no subjects between groups are exchangeable. The upshot of this is that there is no common support and no possibility for causal inference. All inference with this data would be off-support of the data and uncomfortably model-dependent.

Propensity Score Matching

Estimated propensity scores can be used in three general ways: (1) matching, (2) subclassification, or (3) as a regression covariate or "sampling" weight; each has tradeoffs. If we use the propensity score for direct matching we can achieve more

FIGURE 15.2.   FICTITIOUS GRAPH OF OVERLAP IN PROPENSITY SCORES.

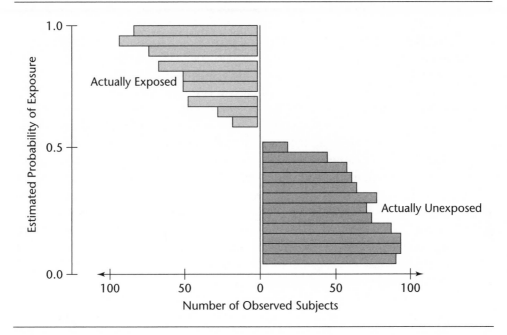

exactness in covariate balance, but it is possible that not all subjects will be matched and so we throw away some information or data. Using the propensity score for subclassification (for example, propensity score quintiles) permits retention of all data, but we may find that we have minor covariate imbalances as well as some support problems. Using a propensity score as a regression covariate or weight in social epidemiology can yield troubling off-support inference, and so we discourage the novice practitioner from such use.

We prefer to use the propensity scores for direct matching. Yes, this may result in the loss of subjects for whom adequate matches cannot be found, but matching will produce the most comparable comparison groups and thus it seems the "cleanest" inference, at least for the matched. There are several direct matching algorithms and each has benefits and pitfalls. Because it is most transparent, we prefer the "nearest neighbor within calipers" procedure in which each exposed subject is matched to an unexposed subject within a predetermined range of the exposed subject's estimated propensity score (Rosenbaum and Rubin 1985b). This predetermined range is set by the analyst and is called a "caliper." Because propensity scores are probabilities, they range in value from 0.0 to 1.0. Specified calipers represent a range of acceptability around each estimated propensity score. There is a trade-off between specifying tight calipers and loose calipers that is directly related to the trade-off between incomplete and inexact matching (Rosenbaum and Rubin 1985a). Caliper width should coincide with our (statistical) confidence in the predicted propensity score. Whereas guidance for selecting caliper width around propensity scores when using Mahalanobis matching has been established (Rosenbaum and Rubin 1985b), we are not aware of any "rules of thumb" for caliper width when matching directly on the propensity score; however, in practice many seem to use values between 0.01 and 0.05. Clearly, more applied research on this topic is needed. As in the following discussion, we recommend an analysis of the sensitivity of caliper-width on outcome estimates.

To understand the implications of caliper choice, consider an exposed subject with a propensity score of 0.794 that needs to be matched to a non-exposed subject. If we set the caliper at ±0.05, the range of acceptable propensity score values is 0.744 to 0.844. This means that we assume an unexposed subject with a propensity score inside the range is a suitable match for the exposed subject; that is, we *assume* the two subjects are exchangeable and any difference in their outcome is due to exposure or treatment.

After matching subjects on propensity scores within specified calipers, it is important to assess covariate balance across the two exposure groups. One way to do this is by using standardized differences (D'Agostino 1998; Rosenbaum and Rubin 1985a), which can be calculated with equation (3):

$$\text{standardized difference} = \frac{100(\bar{x}_{\text{exposed}} - \bar{x}_{\text{unexposed}})}{\sqrt{\dfrac{s^2_{\text{exposed}} + s^2_{\text{unexposed}}}{2}}} \tag{3}$$

where $\bar{x}_{\text{exposed}}$ and $\bar{x}_{\text{unexposed}}$ are the means of a given covariate for the exposed and unexposed groups, respectively. Likewise, s^2_{exposed} and $s^2_{\text{unexposed}}$ are the standard deviations of a given covariate for the exposed and the unexposed groups, respectively. It has been suggested that differences of greater than 10 percent are unacceptable (D'Agostino 1998). The objective, of course, is to achieve small differences or balance in observed covariates, just as we would expect if we had randomized subjects to conditions. We can further assess the adequacy of our matching by calculating the percent bias reduction, as shown in equation (4):

$$\% \text{ Bias Reduction} = 1 - \left(\frac{|\text{Standardized Difference}_{\text{matched}}|}{|\text{Standardized Difference}_{\text{unmatched}}|} \right) \tag{4}$$

where the absolute value of the standardized difference in means for the matched sample is divided by the absolute value of the standardized difference in means for the unmatched sample, which is then subtracted from one to represent the percent reduction.

Average Effect of the Treatment on the Treated and Standard Errors

Once satisfied that we have assembled appropriate exposed and unexposed (counterfactual) matched pairs, it is straightforward to estimate a causal effect of the exposure. Our interest is the average effect of the treatment on the treated (ATT). Again, there is nothing mysterious about the ATT; it is merely the average effect of the neighborhood exposure on those who are in fact exposed. Conceptually, and with respect to our example, the ATT is a comparison of the proportion of deaths among infants born into high-poverty neighborhoods (that is, exposed) with what the proportion would have been had these same infants been born into low-poverty neighborhoods (that is, unexposed). Unlike intention to treat (ITT) analyses, only the exposed (or compliant) are of interest here (Dehejia and Wahba 1999; Smith and Todd 2005).

Within an *applied* propensity score-matching framework, we literally substitute matched but unexposed outcomes for each target's unobservable counterfactual. Accordingly, a computational estimate of the ATT difference may be written,

$$\widehat{\text{ATT}} = \frac{\sum y_{e_i} - y_{u_i*}}{n_e} = \frac{\sum \Delta_e}{n_e} = \overline{\Delta}_e \tag{5}$$

where y_e is the outcome of an exposed (e) subject (i); y_{u_i*} is the outcome of the matched unexposed (counterfactual substitute) subject; n_e is the sample size of the pair-matches; and Δ_e is the pair-matched difference in outcomes. To the extent that observed matched controls are exchangeable with the unobservable counterfactuals our estimate approaches the true value; more technically, $\widehat{\text{ATT}} \rightarrow \text{ATT}$.

It is worth pointing out that ATT is often used interchangeably with the term "average treatment effect" (ATE) or "average causal effect" (ACE). But the two estimators are conceptually and mathematically different (Angrist et al. 1996; Kaufman et al. 2003). The ACE estimator does not condition or limit employed data to the treated (or compliant) and corresponding counterfactuals. Because the impact of this may be great in the presence of confounding or attrition, it is important to keep the difference in mind. Furthermore, there is an important (highly technical) literature on related kinds of "treatment effects" that motivated researchers should study; see especially Rosenbaum (2002, chap. 5).

Once we have calculated our ATT, we seek a satisfactory standard error (SE). Within a frequentist perspective, the SE represents the standard deviation of a sampling distribution of means (Barnett 1999). Because there are no closed form methods for calculation of the SE of propensity score-matched effect estimates, we use bootstrap resampling methods (Efron and Tibshirani 1986, 1993). Briefly, bootstrapping is a technique where a computer algorithm draws a specified number of random samples (with replacement) of the original data. An ATT is calculated for each drawn sample. After, say, 1,000 repetitions, we will have a sampling distribution of means (that is, ATTs) from which to calculate the SE of our observed ATT. It is relatively easy to bootstrap with modern statistical software programs (for example, SAS, Stata).

Worked Example

To fix ideas, we now apply the propensity score matching approach to a neighborhood effects question, simplified here for *method demonstration* purposes. See Johnson (2005) for a more comprehensive analysis. The research question is: What is the effect of being born into a high-poverty neighborhood compared with being born into a low-poverty neighborhood on American Indian infant death? In other words, what would be the number of deaths among American Indian infants born into high-poverty neighborhoods *if instead* they had been born into low-poverty neighborhoods?

Our analytic end point is infant death, which is traditionally defined as an infant that dies prior to its first birthday. We operationalize neighborhood poverty as the proportion of American Indians living below poverty level within a census tract. A dichotomous variable representing "high-poverty" neighborhood (≥ 50 percent poverty) compared with "low-poverty" neighborhood (<25 percent poverty) is used to classify our subjects as exposed or not. We have sample sizes of 1,994 and 762 subjects (that is, newborns) in high- and low-poverty neighborhoods, respectively.

As with any model, covariates should be chosen by the analyst based on scientific or theoretical criteria. Additionally for propensity score estimation, "proper" covariates are those that are predictive of the exposure of interest but not a result of it. In other words, we are interested in variables that are expected to differ across exposure categories. Because social stratification surely plays a role in where American Indians live, we selected all available parental sociodemographic variables available in our dataset as predictors of neighborhood exposure. These include maternal age, marital status, maternal education, paternal race, and paternal education. Other covariates expected to differ across exposure categories and that occurred prior to the infant being exposed to the neighborhood include maternal smoking status, prenatal care utilization, number of previous living children, and number of previous child deaths. It should be noted that maternal smoking, inadequate prenatal care utilization, and previous child deaths may be the effects of living in poverty rather than predictors of it; however, our intention here is to predict infant exposure to poverty, not maternal exposure (although clearly the two are inextricably linked).

Table 15.1 defines each covariate and shows the level of imbalance of each in the unmatched sample and the consequent need for matching. Specifically, we can see from Table 15.1 that most of the covariates are significantly different across exposure groups.

A propensity score for each infant–mother can be estimated with a logistic regression model such that the "high-poverty neighborhood" indicator variable (high poverty = 1; otherwise = 0) is the dependent variable, and the covariates listed in Table 15.1 and their interaction terms are the independent or predictor variables. Again, this is strictly a prediction model and no effort is made to assess statistical significance of regressors. A propensity score from this model is then calculated for each infant in the dataset representing that infant's conditional probability of being exposed to a high-poverty neighborhood given the observed covariates.

The next step is to match our infants using estimated propensity scores. Figure 15.3 provides a graphical display of the actual overlap in propensity scores by exposure group. This figure clearly shows sufficient overlap in the distribution of propensity scores, which means we are likely to find adequate matches for most of the exposed infants. This is not surprising because, to demonstrate good practice, we intentionally limited our investigation to infants born to American Indian women living in one geographic area instead of places known to be quite different, such as Appalachia and Beverly Hills. Actual exchangeability is enhanced because it seems plausible that relocation within our chosen urban area is actually possible for all subjects.

There is a problem in our data that affects our matching criteria. In Figure 15.3 there are many more exposed infants than unexposed infants—notice the longer bars to the left. If we attempt simple pair matching we will lose nearly two-thirds of our exposed infants, because there are not enough unexposed (that is, less impoverished) infants to go around. This would have the undesirable effect of inducing substantial selection bias. An alternative is to match *with replacement,* an idea akin to sampling with replacement. In other words, after an exposed infant is matched to an unexposed infant, the unexposed infant is returned to the pool for potential future matching. Although some of our exposed infants will be matched to the same unexposed infant, such procedures are consistent with counterfactual inference (Smith and Todd 2001).

The matching process can be aided by using statistical software such as Stata or SAS. We use Stata's PSMATCH2 module. We chose to match with a "nearest

TABLE 15.1. COVARIATE IMBALANCE ACROSS EXPOSURE GROUPS PRIOR TO MATCHING.

Covariate	Defined for Propensity Score Estimation	High Poverty (mean)	Low Poverty (mean)	Standardized Difference	t Statistic	p-Value
Maternal demographics						
Mother's age	Years 12–44	23.89	24.59	−11.6	−2.75	0.006
Unmarried	0, 1	0.874	0.743	33.7	8.43	0.000
Maternal education						
Education adequate for age	Referent	0.513	0.664	−31.0	−7.20	0.000
Education inadequate for age	0, 1	0.436	0.304	27.4	6.34	0.000
Missing data	0, 1	0.051	0.031	9.9	2.21	0.027
Previous live births						
Number of child deaths	Integers 0–3	0.06	0.04	7.3	1.70	0.088
Number of living children	Integers 0–12	1.93	1.37	33.0	7.46	0.000
Year of birth	1990–1999	1993.9	1994.2	−9.4	−2.21	0.028
Maternal smoking						
Non-smoking documented	Referent	0.457	0.564	−21.5	−5.04	0.000
Smoking documented	0, 1	0.466	0.335	27.0	6.27	0.000
Missing data	0, 1	0.077	0.101	−8.5	−2.07	0.039
Prenatal care utilization (ACOG)						
Intensive	Referent	0.026	0.045	−10.4	−2.59	0.010
Adequate	0, 1	0.087	0.151	−19.9	−4.94	0.000
Moderate	0, 1	0.387	0.450	−12.8	−3.02	0.003
Inadequate	0, 1	0.219	0.122	26.0	5.82	0.000
No PNC	0, 1	0.046	0.024	12.3	2.70	0.007
Missing data	0, 1	0.235	0.209	6.4	1.49	0.137
Paternal education						
Education adequate for age	Referent	0.172	0.339	−38.9	−9.63	0.000
Education inadequate for age	0, 1	0.082	0.070	4.6	1.06	0.287
Missing data	0, 1	0.746	0.592	33.2	8.03	0.000
Race of the father						
White	Referent	0.115	0.245	−34.3	−8.63	0.000
American Indian	0, 1	0.231	0.188	10.7	2.47	0.013
Other race	0, 1	0.046	0.077	−13.0	−3.23	0.001
Missing data	0, 1	0.607	0.490	23.8	5.63	0.000

FIGURE 15.3.   OVERLAP IN PROPENSITY SCORES BY NEIGHBORHOOD EXPOSURE GROUP.

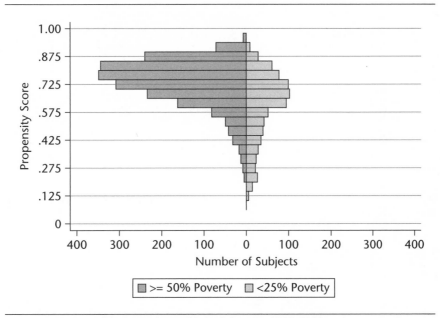

Source: MN Dept Health, Center for Health Statistics, LBD 1990–1999.

available neighbor" algorithm and a caliper of ± 0.01 on the probability scale. All but eleven exposed infants were matched to an unexposed infant with the largest propensity score difference between matched pairs being 0.009875; however, if we had chosen a different caliper, say, ± 0.001, 211 exposed infants would not be matched; a caliper of ± 0.0001 left us with 1,488 exposed infants not matched.

The next step is to reassess the covariate balance in the matched sample. Table 15.2 shows the effectiveness of the propensity score-matching procedures in reducing covariate imbalance between the two groups. Only one covariate became less balanced (inadequate education of the father), but the standardized difference was still less than the 10-percent threshold.

Once satisfied with the balance in covariate patterns, we can estimate the ATT. This may be done through hand-calculation (using equation [5]) or with a computer algorithm such as PSMATCH2 (Leuven and Sianesi 2004) available for use with Stata software (StataCorp 2003). The program also let us bootstrap SEs for this ATT estimate and calculate a 95-percent confidence interval (CI) using a bias-corrected CI (as recommended by Efron and Tibshirani 1993, p. 188).

TABLE 15.2. REDUCTION IN COVARIATE IMBALANCE AFTER MATCHING ON THE PROPENSITY SCORE.

	Matched Pairs		Standardized Difference	% Bias[a] Reduction	t	p-Value
	High Poverty (mean)	Low Poverty (mean)				
Maternal demographics						
Mother's age	23.87	23.90	−0.3	97.1	−0.02	0.98
Unmarried	0.873	0.891	−4.5	86.5	−1.32	0.19
Maternal education						
Education adequate for age	0.516	0.498	3.7	88.0	0.77	0.44
Education inadequate for age	0.437	0.468	−6.5	76.2	−1.62	0.11
Missing data	0.047	0.034	6.6	33.3	2.09	0.04
Previous live births						
Number of child deaths	0.057	0.057	−0.2	97.3	0.15	0.88
Number of living children	1.923	1.932	−0.6	98.3	0.03	0.98
Year	1993.9	1994.0	−3.9	59.0	−0.98	0.33
Maternal smoking						
Non-smoking documented	0.457	0.432	5.1	76.4	1.27	0.20
Smoking documented	0.466	0.507	−8.4	68.9	−2.06	0.04
Missing data	0.077	0.061	5.5	35.7	1.56	0.12
Prenatal care utilization (ACOG)						
Intensive	0.025	0.021	2.2	78.8	0.73	0.47
Adequate	0.085	0.075	3.0	85.1	1.07	0.29
Moderate	0.389	0.394	−1.1	91.2	−0.37	0.71
Inadequate	0.220	0.248	−7.4	71.4	−1.69	0.09
No PNC	0.046	0.044	1.1	91.0	0.21	0.83
Missing data	0.235	0.217	4.2	33.5	1.07	0.28
Paternal education						
Education adequate for age	0.173	0.161	2.8	92.7	0.75	0.45
Education inadequate for age	0.082	0.108	−9.9	−115.1	−2.29	0.02
Missing data	0.745	0.731	3.0	90.9	0.89	0.38
Race of the father						
White	0.116	0.119	−0.8	97.7	−0.29	0.78
American Indian	0.231	0.229	0.6	94.2	0.13	0.89
Other race	0.046	0.051	−2.1	83.9	−0.62	0.54
Missing data	0.606	0.601	1.1	95.3	0.34	0.73

[a]Percent reduction in bias is represented by the percent reduction in the standardized differences before and after matching.

These procedures yield an effect estimate (ATT difference) of 16.6 infant deaths per 1,000 births (95 percent CI = 9.9, 28.9). This is the estimated difference in the rate of deaths for infants born into high-poverty neighborhoods (24.1 deaths per 1,000) compared with what the rate of deaths would have been had these same infants instead been born into low-poverty neighborhoods (7.5 deaths per 1,000). Expressed as a rate ratio, we can infer that infants born into high-poverty neighborhoods are 3.2 times more likely to die than they would have been if instead they had been born into low-poverty neighborhoods (95 percent CI = 2.1, 23.5).

An important question is the degree to which caliper width affects estimates. Figure 15.4 presents results of this sensitivity analysis. It can be seen that increasing the caliper width for matching does impact our ATT results. Recalling that we (a priori) chose the value of 0.01, the figure shows that decreasing the caliper width impacts the ATT estimates inside of 0.005. The reason for this is the decreasing proportion of matches at these smaller caliper values (that is, selection bias). Increasing the width beyond 0.01 has little impact until very large values are used, and at this point one would have better success with subclassification procedures instead of matching procedures.

FIGURE 15.4.   EFFECT ESTIMATES AS A FUNCTION OF CALIPER WIDTH.

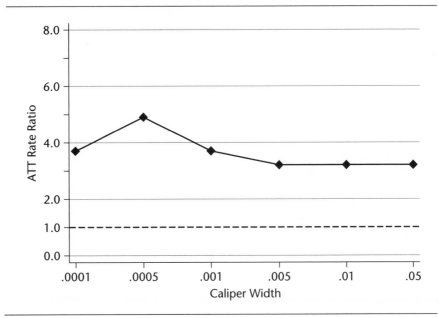

Because they are closer to ACE estimates, comparing our ATT estimates to regression model estimates and effects are technically inappropriate, but it seems natural to be interested anyway. It turns out that the crude odds ratio obtained from bivariate logistic regression of infant death on poverty status was 1.23 (95 percent CI = 0.68, 2.21). After adjustment for the same set of variables used in propensity score estimation, the model showed that the odds of high poverty compared with low poverty diminished to 1.13 (95 percent CI = 0.58, 2.22). Clearly, traditional logistic regression yields a much smaller neighborhood effect compared with our propensity score matched estimate *in this case.*

Why are these regression estimates different from those of the propensity score-matched approach? Because propensity score-matching methods weight the data differently, the key issue being propensity score's 1:1 matching where unexposed observations were matched with replacement. Applying such weights to the adjusted logistic regression yields an adjusted odds ratio of 3.76 (95 percent CI = 1.96, 7.20). What is more, adding the propensity score to the weighted model (in lieu of the many covariates) yields an odds ratio of 3.26 (95 percent CI = 1.82, 5.84), which was quite similar to the propensity score matched ATT estimate. Not surprisingly, the multilevel model analog of this approach is very similar too, because there is little within-neighborhood clustering.

But again we emphasize that comparison between the propensity score matched ATT estimates and logistic regression estimates are technically incorrect and akin to comparing apples with oranges. Because it tends to force one to consider off-support issues, we prefer the ATT estimate in these contexts and believe that neighborhood effect researchers do too, despite many failing to appreciate that regression models do not directly yield them. Finally, we emphasize that other data sets will likely yield different relationships from the ones presented here. Generalizations cannot be made because results will vary with data. Our methodological choice must therefore rely on logic and theory, preferably built up from first principles.

Conclusions

Propensity score-matching methods are an alternative approach to estimating causal effects with observational data, but they are no panacea. Several limitations merit careful attention. The first four are well known and surely apply to all applications; the last two limitations are discussed less frequently but may be especially relevant for social epidemiology.

First and perhaps most important, propensity score matching does not account for unobserved or unobservable characteristics (that is, "hidden bias").

Additional steps to quantify the amount of error in our effect estimates should be undertaken with some method of sensitivity or uncertainty analysis (Greenland 1996; Lash and Fink 2003; Phillips 2003).

Second, the method tends to limit investigations to binary treatment effects, such as exposed and unexposed. Propensity score methods have been extended to continuous treatments (Hirano and Imbens 2003); thus it is possible to incorporate more "treatment arms," but such a discussion is beyond the scope here. In any case, it is not clear that such an extension would be useful given the current state of social epidemiology.

Third, there is admittedly something fishy about a method that aims to overcome many of the limitations of regression model specification by using multiple logistic regression. Propensity score model misspecification (for example, improper or endogenous covariates) may impact effect estimates (Smith and Todd 2001). Fortunately, the impact appears no greater than misspecification in ordinary least squares (OLS) regression (Drake 1993); however, this remains an active area of research, and we urge caution.

Fourth and relatedly, if there are missing data on propensity-score predictors, the propensity score itself will be missing. Thus decisions regarding how to account for these missing data must be addressed. This, too, is an active area of research (D'Agostino and Rubin 2000).

Fifth and perhaps more relevant to social epidemiology, the method does not incorporate "clustering." This may be important because the central motivation for using multilevel regression models over conventional OLS models is that that multilevel models "deal" with the clustering and yield (more) proper SEs. Current propensity score models do not address clustering, though it is unclear if they should. Again, this is an active area of research.

Sixth, propensity score methods do not address the violations of Rubin's Stable-Unit-Treatment-Value-Assumption (SUTVA) (Rubin 1978, 1980) or other synergistic effects that complicate causal inference (Durlauf 2001). As with most other methods and models, propensity score methods ignore dynamics that are ubiquitous in social epidemiology.

Limitations notwithstanding, regression tends to obscure fundamental aspects of causal inference. Along with Berk (2004), we worry that such models often end up capitalizing on chance, being overfit, and otherwise misleading with respect to causal inference. Though clearly no panacea, we believe propensity score methods allow social epidemiologists to (1) better appreciate and more closely mimic experimental study designs, (2) minimize p-value and other arbitrary approaches to model specification, and (3) increase the transparency of inference. Not surprisingly, we believe propensity score methods are important and worthy of both study and use, if not advancement within social epidemiology.

References

Angrist, J. D., Imbens, G. W., & Rubin, D. B. (1996). Identification of causal effects using instrumental variables (with discussion). *Journal of the American Statistical Association, 91,* 444–472.

Barnett, V. (1999). *Comparative statistical inference.* New York: John Wiley & Sons.

Bellman, R. (1961). *Adaptive control processes.* Princeton, NJ: Princeton University Press.

Berk, R. (2004). *Regression analysis. A constructive critique.* Thousand Oaks, CA: Sage Publications.

Clogg, C., & Haritou, A. (1997). The regression method of causal inference and a dilemma confronting this method. In V. R. McKim & S. P. Turner (Eds.), *Causality in crisis? Statistical methods and the search for causal knowledge in the social sciences* (pp. 83–112). Notre Dame, IN: University of Notre Dame Press.

D'Agostino, R. B., Jr. (1998). Propensity score methods for bias reduction in the comparison of a treatment to a non-randomized control group. *Statistical Medicine* 17, 2265–81.

D'Agostino, R. B., Jr., & Rubin, D. B. (2000). Estimating and using propensity scores with partially missing data. *Journal of the American Statistical Association, 95,* 749–759.

De Fineti, B. (1974). *Theory of probability: A critical introductory treatment* (2 Vols, A. Smith, Trans.). London: John Wiley & Sons.

Dehejia, R. H., & Wahba, S. (1999). Causal effects in non-experimental studies: Re-evaluation of training programs. *Journal of the American Statistical Association, 94,* 1053–1062.

Desrosieres, A. (1998). *The politics of large numbers: A history of statistical reasoning* (C. Naish, Trans.). Cambridge, MA: Harvard University Press.

Dodge, Y. (2003). *The Oxford dictionary of statistical terms* (T.I.S. Institute, Ed.). London: Oxford University Press.

Drake, C. (1993). Effects of misspecification of the propensity score on estimators of treatment effect. *Biometrics, 49,* 1231–1236.

Durlauf, S. N. (2001). A framework for the study of individual behavior and social interactions (with comment). *Sociol Methodology, 31,* 47–87.

Efron, B., & Tibshirani, R. (1986). Bootstrap methods for standard errors, confidence intervals, and other measures of statistical accuracy. *Statistical Science, 1,* 54–77.

Efron, B., & Tibshirani, R. (1993). *An introduction to the bootstrap.* New York: Chapman & Hall.

Greenland, S. (1996). Basic methods for sensitivity analysis of biases. *International Journal of Epidemiology, 25,* 1107–1116.

Greenland, S., & Robins, J. M. (1986). Identifiability, exchangeability, and epidemiological confounding. *International Journal of Epidemiology, 15,* 413–419.

Greenland, S., Robins, J. M., & Pearl, J. (1999). Confounding and collapsibility in causal inference. *Statistical Science, 14,* 29–46.

Hausman, D. M. (1998). *Causal asymmetries.* New York: Cambridge.

Hawthorn, G. (1991). *Plausible worlds: Possibility and understanding in history and the social sciences.* New York: Cambridge University Press.

Heckman, J. (1997). Randomization as an instrumental variables estimator: A study of implicit behavioral assumptions in one widely-used estimator. *Journal of Human Resources, 32,* 442–462.

Hirano, K., & Imbens, G. W. (2003). The propensity score with continuous treatments. In A. Gelman & X.-L. Meng (Eds.), *Applied Bayesian modeling and causal inference from incomplete-data perspectives, Wiley series in probability and statistics.* Hoboken, NJ: John Wiley & Sons.

Holland, P. W. (1986). Statistics and causal inference. *Journal of the American Statistical Association, 81*, 945–960.

Joffe, M. M., & Rosenbaum, P. R. (1999). Invited commentary: Propensity scores. *American Journal of Epidemiology, 150*, 327–333.

Johnson, P. J. (2005). The effect of neighborhood poverty on American Indian infant death (Doctoral dissertation, University of Minnesota, 2004). *Dissertation Abstracts International-B, 65*, 3973.

Kaufman, J. S., Kaufman, S., & Poole, C. (2003). Causal inference from randomized trials in social epidemiology. *Social Science & Medicine, 57*, 397–409.

Lash, T. L., & Fink, A. K. (2003). Semi-automated sensitivity analysis to assess systematic errors in observational data. *Epidemiology, 14*, 451–458.

Leamer, E. (1978). *Specification searches: Ad hoc inference with nonexperimental data.* New York: John Wiley & Sons.

Leuven, E., & Sianesi, B. (2004). PSMATCH2: Stata module to perform full Mahalanobis and propensity score matching, common support graphing, and covariate imbalance testing.

Lewis, D. K. (1973). *Counterfactuals.* Malden, MA: Blackwell.

Little, R. J., & Rubin, D. B. (2000). Causal effects in clinical and epidemiological studies via potential outcomes: concepts and analytical approaches. *Annual Review of Public Health, 21*, 121–145.

Lord, F. M. (1967). A paradox in the interpretation of group comparisons. *Psychological Bulletin, 68*, 304–305.

Maldonado, G., & Greenland, S. (2002a). Estimating causal effects. *International Journal of Epidemiology, 31*, 422–429.

Maldonado, G., & Greenland, S. (2002b). Response: Defining and estimating causal effects. *International Journal of Epidemiology, 31*, 435–438.

Manski, C. F. (1993). *Identification problems in the social sciences* (P. V. Marsden, Ed.). San Francisco: Jossey-Bass.

Oakes, J. M. (2004). The (mis)estimation of neighborhood effects: Causal inference for a practicable social epidemiology. *Social Science & Medicine, 58*, 1929–1952.

Phillips, C. V. (2003). Quantifying and reporting uncertainty from systematic errors. *Epidemiology, 14*, 459–466.

Rosenbaum, P. R. (2002). *Observational studies.* New York: Springer-Verlag.

Rosenbaum, P. R. (2004). Matching in observational studies. In A. Gelman & X.-L. Meng (Eds.), *Applied Bayesian modeling and causal inference from incomplete-data perspectives, Wiley series in probability and statistics* (pp. 15–24). Hoboken, NJ: John Wiley & Sons.

Rosenbaum, P. R., & Rubin, D. B. (1983). The central role of the propensity score in observational studies for causal effects. *Biometrika, 70*, 41–55.

Rosenbaum, P. R., & Rubin, D. B. (1984). Reducing bias in observational studies using subclassification on the propensity score. *Journal of the American Statistical Association, 79*, 516–524.

Rosenbaum, P. R., & Rubin, D. B. (1985a). The bias due to incomplete matching. *Biometrics, 41*, 103–116.

Rosenbaum, P. R., & Rubin, D. B. (1985b). Constructing a control group using multivariate matched sampling methods that incorporate the propensity score. *Journal of the American Statistical Association, 39*, 33–38.

Rosenbaum, P. R., & Silber, J. H. (2001). Matching and thick description in an observational study of mortality after surgery. *Biostatistics, 2*, 217–232.

Rossi, P. H. (1980). The presidential address: The challenge and opportunities of applied social research. *American Sociologic Review, 45,* 889–904.

Rubin, D. B. (1977). Assignment to treatment group on the basis of a covariate. *Journal of Educational Statistics, 2,* 1–26.

Rubin, D. B. (1978). Bayesian inference for causal effects: The role of randomization. *Annals of Statistics, 6,* 34–58.

Rubin, D. B. (1980). Randomization analysis of experimental data: The Fisher randomization test comment. *Journal of the American Statistical Association, 75,* 591–593.

Smith, J. A., & Todd, P. E. (2001). Reconciling conflicting evidence on the performance of propensity-score matching methods. *American Economic Review, 91,* 112–118.

Smith, J. A., & Todd, P. E. (2005). Does matching overcome LaLonde's critique of nonexperimental estimators. *Journal of Econometrics, 125,* 305–353.

StataCorp (2003). *Stata statistical software* (Vol. Release 8.0.). College Station, TX: StataCorp.

Tiebout, C. M. (1956). A pure theory of local expenditures. *Journal of Political Economy, 64,* 416–424.

Winship, C., & Morgan, S. L. (1999). The estimation of causal effects from observational data. *Annual Review of Sociology, 25,* 659–706.

CHAPTER SIXTEEN

USING CAUSAL DIAGRAMS TO UNDERSTAND COMMON PROBLEMS IN SOCIAL EPIDEMIOLOGY

M. Maria Glymour

Epidemiologists typically seek to answer causal questions using statistical data: We observe a statistical association between poverty and early mortality and seek to determine whether poverty causes early death. An essential component of epidemiologic training is therefore learning what statistical relations imply, or do not imply, about causal relations. This is why the cliché "correlation does not imply causation" is the mantra of introductory epidemiology classes. But correlations, and other forms of statistical association, do give us information about causal relations, and this is why—despite the oft-repeated warnings— quantitative statistical analyses are the mainstay of epidemiology.

Diagrams are routinely used informally to express beliefs and hypotheses about relations among variables. These informal uses can be greatly expanded by adopting formal rules for drawing the diagrams so that they meet the criteria for causal Directed Acyclic Graphs (DAGs). Causal DAGs are a simple, flexible device for demonstrating the statistical associations implied by a given set of assumptions about the causal structure relating variables. Knowing this, we can also move in the other direction: Given a set of statistical associations observed in the data, we can identify all of the causal structures that could have given rise to these associations. Learning the rules for reading off statistical associations from the causal assumptions represented in a DAG can take a little time and practice. Once mastered, though, these rules turn out to be extremely practical for a number of tasks (for example, choosing regression covariates, understanding selection bias, interpreting tests of "direct" effects, or assessing natural experiments). Using DAGs makes it easier to recognize and avoid mistakes in these and a number of other analytic decisions. The rules linking causal relations to statistical associations are grounded in mathematics, and one way to think of the usefulness of causal diagrams is that they allow non-mathematicians to draw rigorous, mathematically based conclusions about certain types of statistical relations.

In this chapter, some language and background assumptions are first introduced; then the rules for drawing causal DAGs and the associated rules linking the causal assumptions encoded in a DAG to the statistical relations implied by these structural assumptions are described; and finally, a few applications of DAGs within social epidemiology are discussed. Some readers may prefer to begin with the examples and refer back to the definitions and rules for DAGs as needed; however, the material described in the section on the *d*-separation rules is essential for following the examples. A number of excellent and more comprehensive introductions to DAGs, many written by the researchers who developed the ideas, are available elsewhere (Greenland et al. 1999; Pearl 2000; Robins 2001; Spirtes et al. 2000). The goal of this chapter is to provide a basic introduction to demonstrate the utility of DAGs for applied social epidemiology researchers.

Some Background Definitions

Causal inference is an important problem in many applied disciplines, and much of the work written on the topic has been addressed to readers in fields other than epidemiology. The writing on causal inference can sometimes be dense or technical. The chapter begins by explaining how key terms are used. Note that some of these uses (for example, the definition of *cause*) are controversial, and the reader is encouraged to see others who disagree. Debating the definitions is beyond the scope of this chapter, and little of the discussion of DAGs would be affected by adopting such alternative definitions.

Define X and Y as random variables. We say X **causes** Y if, had X taken a different value than it actually did—*and* nothing else temporally prior to or simultaneous with X differed—then Y would have taken a different value. To accommodate the possibility that causation is not deterministic, we can say that had X taken a different value, this would have resulted in a different probability distribution for Y.

It is invaluable to frame our research question in terms of a hypothetical intervention on X. For example, instead of asking, "Does income affect diabetes risk among Cherokee tribal members?" we ask, "Would sending each tribal member an annual check for $4,000 from the Cherokee Nation government change their diabetes risk?" The effect of such a check might differ from other ways of changing income—for example, increasing wages or providing in-kind donations or changing tax rates—even if these approaches had identical net monetary value. Most important, referring to a hypothetical intervention distinguishes the causal question from related statistical questions, such as "Do high-income individuals have lower diabetes risk compared with low-income individuals?" The hypothetical intervention must directly affect only the exposure X, although other things might also change if they are consequences of exposure (Pearl 2000; Spirtes et al. 2000). For example, an intervention such as sending a check may affect diet as well as income, but only because recipients use the extra income to buy different foods. It need not be possible for the researcher to conduct the intervention; there must merely be some conceivable way that X could take a different value, even if by random assortment. The definition of "cause" is the topic of heated and extensive debate; see for example (Dawid 2000; Glymour 1986; Hernán 2004; Holland 1986a, 1986b; Kaufman and Cooper 1999, 2001; Parascandola and Weed 2001; Pearl 2000; Woodward 2003).

We say X and Y are **statistically independent** if knowing the value of X does not provide any information about the value of Y (if X is independent of Y, Y is also independent of X). Conversely, we say X and Y are **statistically dependent** if knowing the value of X gives us some information about the likely value of Y, even if this information is very limited and amounts to a modest change in the probability distribution of Y. If there is some value X of X that is informative about the probability distribution of Y, we say that X and Y are statistically dependent. Note that statistical dependency may be assessed with various statistical parameters, some of which depend on additional assumptions (for example, regression coefficients, odds ratios, t tests, chi-square tests, or correlation coefficients).

It is very helpful to distinguish between words that denote causal relations and words that denote statistical relations (Pearl 2001). "Cause," "influence," "change," "increase," "decrease," and "promote" are all examples of **causal language.** Association, prediction, and any specific measures of statistical association such as regression coefficients and so forth are examples of **statistical language.** When a statistical association is reported in an epidemiology article, it is generally with the hope (sometimes unstated) of using this to give insight into a causal relation. Surveillance reports and predictive (as opposed to etiologic) models are exceptions; in these cases, causal inference is not of primary interest.

If we examine the distribution of one variable, Y, *within* levels of a second variable X, we say that we are examining the distribution of Y **conditional** on X. Conditional relations are often denoted in equations with the symbol " $|$ ". For example, if $p(Y)$ denotes the probability distribution of Y, a formal definition of statistical independence is:

$$p(Y \mid X) = p(Y) \tag{1}$$

which would be read "the probability distribution of Y conditional on X equals the marginal (or unconditional) probability distribution of Y." In other words, knowing the value of X does not give us information about the distribution of Y (for any value x of X).

Similarly, if we examine the relations between two variables within levels of a third variable—for example, the relation between income and mortality within levels of education—we say we are examining the conditional relation. Stratification, restriction, matching, and covariate adjustment in regression models are all statistical techniques that are special types of conditioning. If two variables X and Y are statistically independent without conditioning on any other variables, we say X and Y are **marginally independent.** If X and Y are independent, conditional on Z, then:

$$p(Y \mid X, Z) = p(Y \mid Z) \tag{2}$$

Although causal dependence and statistical dependence are not the same, they are related phenomena. To understand how causal and statistical relations are linked, note that statistical dependency between two variables X and Y could reflect any of five situations (or combinations of these):

1. Random fluctuation.
2. X caused Y.
3. Y caused X.
4. X and Y share a common cause[1]
5. The statistical association was induced by conditioning on a common effect of X and Y (as in selection bias).

The task epidemiologists typically face is to decide which of these explanations is consistent with our data and background knowledge and rule out all others. Often we are especially interested in demonstrating that X likely caused Y (perhaps because this may offer the best prospects for publication). Confidence intervals and p-values are used to assess the plausibility of the first explanation for a statistical association. Temporal order can rule out explanation three, and this is why longitudinal studies are advantageous for demonstrating causation. Ruling out common prior causes, explanation four, is the goal of most covariate

[1]Note that a variation on this situation is the possibility that the sample is composed of two subsamples, each of which has a different marginal probability distribution of X and of Y. In the combined population, X and Y may be statistically dependent even if they were independent in each of the subsamples. This is sometimes considered a sixth possibility to explain a statistical dependency between X and Y. In this chapter, we treat this as a special case of situation four, however. To frame it this way, consider subsample membership to be a variable that is a common cause of X and Y.

adjustment in regression models. Covariate stratification is also frequently, though not universally, motivated by the desire to eliminate the possibility of common prior causes. Explanation five—the association was induced by conditioning on a common effect—is confusing for many people, and it is perhaps for this reason that this possibility is often ignored. This phenomenon is crucial in many settings, though, so we will try to give an intuitive explanation here (it will come up again in the examples section of the chapter).

Why does conditioning on a common effect of two variables induce a statistical association between those variables? The easiest way to hold onto this idea is to find a simple anecdote that describes the phenomenon. For example, suppose you believe that two factors determine basketball prowess: height and speed. Exceptional players must be either extremely tall or extremely fast. If you examined everyone in the world, height and speed might be statistically independent. Short people are not necessarily fast, nor are tall people; however, if you look only at professional basketball players, you would confidently guess that the short ones are *very* fast. People without the advantage of height must compensate with lightening speed in order to become great ball players. By restricting to pro basketball players, you have conditioned on a common effect of height and speed, and within this stratum of pro ball players, height and speed are (inversely) associated. This is not a perfect association, because some of the tall players may also be fast. And it is also possible that speed and height are correlated in the general population. The point is merely that, whatever the association between speed and height in the general population, it is quite different among professional basketball players.

This phenomenon—the change in association between two variables when conditioning on their common effect—is sometimes called **collider bias** because the two causes "collide" at the common effect. It can be induced by sample selection, stratification, or covariate adjustment if some of the covariates are effects of the other independent variables (Hernán et al. 2004).

We say the association between X and Y is **confounded** if the statistical association between X and Y does not equal the causal relation between the two variables. For example, if X and Y are both influenced by Z, the crude (marginal) relation between X and Y is likely confounded, although the relation between X and Y conditional on Z may be unconfounded. If conditioning upon a set of covariates **Z** will render the association between X and Y unconfounded, then we say **Z** is a **sufficient** set of covariates for estimating the relation between X and Y. A sufficient set may be empty (if the crude relation between X and Y is unconfounded), or it may contain one or many variables. Furthermore, there may be several alternative sufficient sets for any pair of variables X and Y (Greenland and Robins 1986; Greenland et al. 1999).

Graphical Models

With this background and common language, we now turn to causal DAGs. First, the rules for expressing causal assumptions in a DAG are outlined. Next, the d-separation rules, which describe how to read from the DAG the set of statistical associations implied by the causal assumptions encoded in that DAG, are explained. Formal introductions to graphical models, explanations of how DAGs relate to conventional structural equation models, and proof of the mathematical equivalence between the rules we apply to DAGs and Robins' g-computation formula can be found elsewhere (Greenland et al. 1999; Pearl 2000; Robins 1987, 1995; Spirtes et al. 2000).

Drawing a Causal DAG[2]

Causal DAGs visually encode an investigator's a priori assumptions about causal relations among the exposure, outcomes, and covariates. In a causal DAG, we say that a variable X causes a variable Y *directly* (relative to the other variables in the DAG) if there is an arrow from X to Y or *indirectly* if there is a sequence of directed arrows that can be followed from X to Y via one or more intermediate variables. In Figure 16.1, X causes Y directly and Z indirectly. The **descendants** of a variable are the other variables in the DAG affected either directly or indirectly by that variable. If two variables shown in a DAG share a common cause, that common cause must also be included in the DAG or else the DAG is not considered "causal." It is not necessary to include all causes of individual variables in the DAG; only causes of two or more variables in the DAG must be included. If unknown or unmeasured common causes are assumed to exist, these should be represented in the diagram as unknown common causes with arrows to the variables that they are thought to affect. The absence of a sequence of directed arrows linking two variables in a DAG represents the assumption that there is no causal relation between the two variables. If a prior value of Y affects X, which affects a subsequent value of Y, these must each be shown as separate variables (for example, $Y_0 \rightarrow X_1 \rightarrow Y_2$). Directed acyclic graphs must not have any cycles between variables, consistent with the general intuition that if X causes Y, Y cannot also cause X at the same moment.

---

[2]This section, the following section on d-separation rules, and Figure 16.1 are taken substantially from Appendix Two in Glymour et al. (2005). "When is baseline adjustment useful in analyses of change? An example with education and cognitive change." *American Journal of Epidemiology,* 162(3) 267–278, by permission of Oxford University Press.

FIGURE 16.1.   AN EXAMPLE CAUSAL DAG.

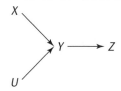

Causal assumptions represented in DAG 1:

- X and U are each direct causes of Y (direct with respect to other variables in the DAG).
- Y is a direct cause of Z.
- X is not a direct cause of Z, but X is an indirect cause of Z via Y.
- X is not a cause of U and U is not a cause of X.
- U is not a direct cause of Z, but U is an indirect cause of Z via Y.
- No two variables in the DAG (X, U, Y, or Z) share a prior cause not shown in the DAG, e.g., no variable causes both X and Y, or both X and U.

Statistical relations implied by the assumptions in the example causal DAG (note that this is not a comprehensive list of all the conditional relations and that the statistical dependencies listed here assume faithfulness):

- X and Y are statistically dependent.
- U and Y are statistically dependent.
- Y and Z are statistically dependent.
- X and Z are statistically dependent.
- U and Z are statistically dependent.
- X and U are statistically independent (the only path between them is blocked by the collider Y).
- X and U are statistically dependent, conditional on Y (conditioning on a collider unblocks the path).
- X and U are statistically dependent, conditional on Z (Z is a descendant of the collider Y).
- X and Z are statistically independent, conditional on Y (conditioning on Y blocks the path between X and Z).
- U and Z are statistically independent, conditional on Y.

The d-Separation Rules Linking Causal Assumptions to Statistical Independencies

After drawing a DAG to represent our causal assumptions, we can apply the d-separation rules to find the statistical relations implied by these assumptions. Before introducing the d-separation rules, three assumptions adopted throughout the rest of the chapter are mentioned. These assumptions are discussed in more detail at the conclusion of this section.

1. The Causal Markov Assumption (CMA): Any variable X is independent of any other variable Y conditional on the direct causes of X, unless Y is an effect of X. The CMA is consistent with most accounts of causation and, although rarely stated in these words, is often implicitly invoked in applied research.

2. Faithfulness: Positive and negative causal effects never *perfectly* offset one another; that is, if X affects Y through two pathways, one positive and one negative, the net statistical relation between X and Y will be either positive or negative. If the two paths perfectly offset one another, the net statistical association would be zero, in which case we say the statistical associations are **unfaithful** to the causal relations. Under faithfulness, we assume this situation never occurs.

3. Negligible randomness: Statistical associations or lack of associations are not attributable to random variation or chance (that is, we assume a large sample size).

The DAG expresses a set of assumptions about the causal relations or absence of causal relations among the variables. If the assumptions of a causal DAG are correct, then two variables in the DAG will be statistically independent conditional on a set of covariates if every **path** between the two variables is **blocked.** What is a path and what does it mean to block it? A path is any sequence of lines (also called edges) connecting two variables *regardless of the direction of the arrowheads*. The direction of arrowheads is important to identify variables on a path that are **colliders.** If arrowheads from A and B both point to a variable C (as in: $A \rightarrow C \leftarrow B$), then C is referred to as a collider on that path between A and B: the causes collide at C. In other words, a collider is a common effect of two variables on the path (the collider itself must also be on the path). All other variables on a path are non-colliders. A path is blocked by conditioning on a proposed set of variables $\mathbf{Z}$ if either of two conditions holds:

1. One of the non-colliders on the path is in the set of variables $\mathbf{Z}$, or;
2. There is a collider on the path, and neither the collider nor any of the collider's descendants is in $\mathbf{Z}$.

These rules fit with the intuition that two variables will be correlated if one causes the other or there is an uncontrolled common prior cause of the two variables. The rules also reflect the fact that a statistical association between two variables can be induced by conditioning on a common effect of the two variables (Greenland et al. 1999; Hernán et al. 2002), as described in the pro basketball example. Note that if a collider on a path is in the proposed covariate set, this collider does not block the path. If a DAG contains no unblocked paths between A and B, the two variables will be marginally independent; that is, without conditioning on any other variables, A and B will be independent. If we assume faithfulness, two variables in a DAG will be statistically dependent if there is an unblocked path between them. Rule (2) implies that conditioning on a variable may unblock a path between A and B and induce a correlation if that variable is a collider or a descendant of a collider on a path between A and B.

To make these ideas more concrete, consider the example DAG in Figure 16.1. This figure shows a causal DAG and lists the causal assumptions represented by that DAG and the statistical associations implied, under the d-separation rules, by those causal assumptions. For example, the assumptions encoded in the DAG imply that X and U are marginally independent but become statistically associated after conditioning on either Y or Z. In contrast, X and Z are marginally dependent but become statistically independent after conditioning on Y.

The Assumptions for Using Causal DAGs

Now we return to the assumptions we stated earlier: Causal Markov, faithfulness, and negligible randomness. Why do we need these assumptions and should we accept them? The Causal Markov Assumption (CMA) is consistent with intuition: if we hold constant the factors that are direct causes of a variable X, then other factors will be independent of fluctuations in X, unless these other variables are themselves influenced by X. Imagine a string of dominos with letters from A to Z lined up in order. Flipping domino A will cause all of the downstream dominos to fall as well. You can interrupt the sequence of falling dominos by removing one in the middle (or holding it up so it doesn't fall). If you hold F up, then flipping E will not affect G or any subsequent domino; however, holding F will not interrupt the effect of flipping G on H or I (see Glymour 2001, pp. 21–27, for a more extensive but accessible discussion of the CMA). Standard epidemiologic reasoning often appeals to the CMA. For example, the injunction against conditioning on mediators if you wish to estimate the total effect of an exposure on the outcome implicitly relies on CMA.

The faithfulness assumption, that positive and negative effects never perfectly offset one another, is valuable because, formally, the d-separation rules define the statistical *independencies* implied by the assumptions in the DAG. Although the statistical independencies are interesting, we would often like to know about the statistical *dependencies*. These do not automatically follow from the d-separation rules, because two variables in a DAG might be statistically independent even though this independence is not implied by the causal structure. If two pathways with equal and opposite counterbalancing effects link two variables in a DAG, these two variables will be statistically independent despite their causal connection. To extend the d-separation rules to define the statistical dependences implied by a DAG, we must assume faithfulness. Some researchers contend that faithfulness is commonly violated in the real world. Nonetheless, the major implications from the examples in the rest of the chapter would stand if we did not assume faithfulness.

We assume negligible randomness, because DAGs give no information on whether statistical relations are likely to have arisen by chance due to random variation. To focus on DAGs we will assume that effects due to random variation can be ignored (for example, because you are looking at statistical associations in a very large sample). Without this assumption, the examples in the rest of the chapter would hold asymptotically.

These three assumptions should be clearly distinguished from the content-specific causal assumptions encoded in DAGs, which relate specifically to the substantive question at hand. By assuming CMA, faithfulness, and negligible randomness, we can link the causal assumptions in the DAG to probability statements about the variables. The CMA is fundamental for the d-separation rules. Faithfulness allows us to predict statistical associations instead of just statistical independencies. Negligible randomness lets us ignore random variations that would appear in small samples.

Applying DAGs to Answer Questions in Social Epidemiology

Why are DAGs useful? In general, we wish to test a hypothesis about how the world works within the context of our prior beliefs. This is linked, sometimes implicitly, to a desire to know what would happen if we intervened to change the value of some treatment or exposure. Directed acyclic graphs help us answer the question: under my prior assumptions, would the statistical analysis proposed here provide a valid test of this causal hypothesis? Consider Figure 16.2 and imagine you are interested in testing whether X has a causal effect on Y (that is, you are unsure if there should be an arrow from X to Y). Other than this question, you believe the causal structure is as drawn in Figure 16.2. It is immediately evident from the DAG that the analysis must condition on U; U confounds the effect of X on Y. But suppose that you are interested in estimating the effect of Z on Y. In this case, you need not condition on U. The relation between Z and Y is unconfounded (as is the relation

FIGURE 16.2. A DAG DEPICTING CONFOUNDING.

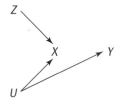

between Z and X). Directed acyclic graphs provide a way to state explicitly one's prior beliefs about causal relations or alternative sets of plausible prior assumptions. We base decisions such as selection of covariates on these priors, although the way in which priors shape these decisions is not always explicit.

We now turn to a number of examples in which DAGs can be used to clarify epidemiologic ideas. In some cases, the DAGs simply provide a convenient way to express well-understood concepts. In other examples, the DAGs illuminate a point of common confusion regarding the biases introduced by proposed analyses or study designs. In all these cases, the findings can be demonstrated mathematically or by using any number of informal arguments. The advantage of DAGs is that they provide a simple, common tool for understanding an array of different problems.

Why Conventional Rules for Confounding Are Not Reliable

Earlier, confounding in terms of contrasting statistical and causal associations were defined. A statistical association between two variables is confounded if it differs from the causal relation between the two variables. This definition implies graphical criteria for choosing a **sufficient set** of covariates, which is a set such that within strata of the covariates the statistical relation between exposure and outcome is unconfounded. That is, after specifying background causal assumptions using a DAG, we can identify from the DAG a sufficient set of covariates Z for estimating or testing for an effect of X on Y; Z is such a sufficient set if (1) no variable in Z is a descendant of X and (2) every path between X and Y that contains an arrow into X is blocked by Z.

These rules are often called the "back-door" criteria, tapping the idea that paths with arrows into X are "back-doors" through which a spurious (non-causal) statistical association between X and Y might arise. When the back-door criteria are fulfilled by a set of measured covariates, it is possible to estimate the total average causal effect of X on Y. Under the graphical criteria, it is clear that there may be several alternative sufficient sets to control confounding. Thus, it is possible that a given variable is included in one sufficient set but not in another. A related point is that these rules do not define a "confounder" but instead describe when a conditional statistical association between two variables will be confounded (see Maldonado 2002 for a helpful discussion of this distinction). Detailed discussion of the graphical criteria can be found in Greenland et al. (1999) and Pearl (2000, p. 79).

How do the graphical criteria relate to conventional criteria for identifying confounders? In both intuition and application, the graphical and conventional criteria overlap substantially. For example, Hennekens and Buring explain that confounding occurs when "an observed association . . . is in fact due to a mixing of effects between the exposure, the disease, and a third factor . . ." (1987, p. 35). Rothman and Greenland describe confounding as "a distortion in the estimated exposure effect that results from differences in risk between the exposed and unexposed that are not due to exposure" (1998, p. 255). The intuitions are similar.

Variations on the following specific criteria for identifying confounders are frequently suggested, although it is often noted that these criteria do not "define" a confounder:

1. A confounder must be associated with the exposure under study in the source population.[3]
2. A confounder must be a risk factor for the outcome, though it need not actually cause the outcome.
3. The confounding factor must not be affected by the exposure or the outcome.

These rules are based on statistical associations, and we will refer to them as the conventional statistical criteria for confounding (a slight misnomer because criterion [3] refers to a causal relation). As it turns out, these statistical criteria often agree perfectly with the back-door criteria—that is, you would choose the same set of covariates using either criteria. For example, in Figure 16.2, both the graphical and statistical criteria indicate that one should condition on U to derive an unbiased estimate of the effect of X on Y. It fulfills the graphical criteria because U is not an effect of X, and the only path between X and Y that contains an arrow into X is blocked by U. It fulfills the statistical criteria because U and X will be statistically associated, U will also predict Y, and U is not affected by X or Y. There are cases when the statistical and graphical criteria disagree, however, and when they diverge, it is the statistical criteria that fail.

The DAG in Figure 16.3 gives one example. We are interested in whether having low education increases risk of type II diabetes; the DAG in Figure 16.3 depicts the causal null that education has no effect on diabetes. We have measured mother's diabetes status, but we do not have measures of the family's income when

---

[3]Sometimes this criterion states, instead, that the confounder must affect the outcome under study. Under this alternative statement of the statistical criteria, the basic argument still follows, in that there are situations in which the statistical and graphical criteria differ, and when this occurs the graphical criteria are correct. The DAGs under which such a discrepancy emerges are slightly more complicated than that in Figure 16.3, but an example is discussed in detail in Greenland et al. (1999).

FIGURE 16.3. A DAG UNDER WHICH CONVENTIONAL CONFOUNDING RULES FAIL.

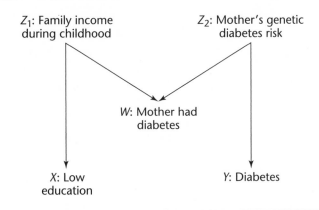

the individual was growing up or if the individual's mother had any genes that would increase risk of diabetes. Under the assumptions in the DAG in Figure 16.3, should we adjust our analysis for mother's diabetes status? First we consider how we would answer this question with the statistical criteria for a confounder, and then we address it with the graphical criteria. The DAG in Figure 16.3 reflects the assumption that family income during childhood affects both educational attainment and mother's diabetes status. The reasoning is that if an individual was poor as a child, his or her mother was poor as an adult, and this poverty increased the mother's risk of developing diabetes (Robbins et al. 2001, 2005). Mother's diabetes status will be statistically related to the respondent's education, because under these assumptions they share a common prior cause. It will also be related to the risk that the respondent has diabetes, because the mother's genetic risk profile affects both her own and her offspring's diabetes risk. Mother's diabetes is not affected by the respondent's own education level or the respondent's own diabetes status. Thus, mother's diabetes meets all three statistical criteria for a confounder. With the statistical criteria, you would choose to adjust the analysis for mother's diabetic status.

What about the graphical criteria? Would conditioning on mother's diabetes block the back-door path between low education and diabetes? First, note that there is one path between low education and diabetes, and mother's diabetes is a collider on that path. If we do *not* adjust for mother's diabetes, it blocks the path between our exposure and outcome. Adjusting for mother's diabetes *unblocks* this path and induces a spurious statistical association between low education and diabetes. Under the graphical criteria, one should not include mother's diabetic status as a covariate.[4]

The intuition here is very similar to the reasoning that pro basketball players who are short will tend to be very fast. Assume that mothers developed diabetes owing either to a genetic predisposition or to experiencing poverty as adults (while raising their children). There may be other reasons as well, but assume these are two non-trivial determinants of a mother's diabetic status. Consider respondents whose mothers had diabetes but no genetic risk factors. These people's mothers likely developed diabetes owing to poverty, implying that the respondents themselves grew up in poverty. Conversely, among respondents with diabetic mothers who did not grow up in poverty, there is probably a genetic risk factor. Conditional on mother's diabetic status (for example, examining only those whose mothers were diabetic), childhood poverty and genetic risk factors will tend to be inversely related; individuals whose mothers did not carry a genetic risk factor will tend to have grown up in poverty. Because of this association, among people with diabetic mothers, low education will be inversely associated with diabetes risk. If low education increases diabetes risk, adjusting for mother's diabetic status (under the assumptions in Figure 16.3) will underestimate this effect. Appendix 16.1 provides some example Stata code to generate data consistent with the causal assumptions in DAG 3 in order to demonstrate this phenomenon.

---

[4]A variation on the statistical criteria can be used to determine whether, given a sufficient set of covariates $\mathbf{Z}$, it is possible to drop any variables from $\mathbf{Z}$ and still have a sufficient set for identifying the effect of X on Y. Assume that the sufficient set $\mathbf{Z}$ consists of two subsets $\mathbf{A}$ and $\mathbf{B}$, and no variable in set $\mathbf{A}$ or set $\mathbf{B}$ is affected by either X or Y. It is unnecessary to adjust for the variables in $\mathbf{B}$, given the variables in $\mathbf{A}$, if $\mathbf{B}$ can be broken into two disjoint subsets $\mathbf{B_1}$ and $\mathbf{B_2}$ (no variable in $\mathbf{B_1}$ can also be in $\mathbf{B_2}$ and all variables in $\mathbf{B}$ must be in either $\mathbf{B_1}$ or $\mathbf{B_2}$) such that 1) $\mathbf{B_1}$ is independent of X within strata defined by $\mathbf{A}$ *and* 2) $\mathbf{B_2}$ is independent of Y within strata defined by X, $\mathbf{A}$, and $\mathbf{B_1}$. The implications of these criteria are consistent with the graphical criteria (Greenland et al. 1999). To apply this to the situation in Figure 16.3, imagine that we know conditioning on W, Z_1, and Z_2 is sufficient to identify the effect of X on Y. We would like to know whether conditioning on the empty set (call this set $\mathbf{A}$; note that a set of variables can be broken down into two sets—one empty and the other the same as the original set) is sufficient. Now break set $\mathbf{B}$ (W, Z_1, and Z_2) into $\mathbf{B_1}$ (Z_2) and $\mathbf{B_2}$ (W and Z_1). Z_2 is marginally independent of X, meeting the first criteria above. Z_1 and W are both independent of Y within strata defined by X and Z_2, meeting the second criteria. Thus, if we know that conditioning on all three variables is sufficient, we can use these statistical criteria to establish that conditioning on none of the three variables would also be sufficient. The result might be more easily established using the graphical criteria, however.

Why Sample Selection Threatens Internal Validity as well as Generalizability

Samples for observational epidemiologic studies are drawn using a variety of criteria. For example, the sample may be drawn from members of a certain occupation (for example, nurses, doctors, or nuns) or residents of a certain community (for example, Framingham or Leisure World Laguna Woods). The possibility that such selection criteria might compromise generalizability is widely recognized. What is sometimes overlooked, however, are the circumstances under which selection criteria can affect internal validity. The sample selection process may sometimes result in spurious statistical associations (that is, associations that do not reflect causal relations between variables measured on the sample population). This potential for bias is of special interest to social epidemiologists, because some of the sample population selection rules use socially relevant characteristics.

On a DAG, we represent selection into the sample as a variable and say that all analyses of a sample are conditioned on selection into that sample. That is, we conceptualize selection as a variable with two values, zero = not selected and one = selected; analyses are restricted to observations where selection = one. The value of this selection variable may be influenced by any number of other variables, including the exposure, the outcome, or other factors that influence the exposure or the outcome (or both). Selection bias may occur if the likelihood of being admitted to the sample depends on both the exposure and the outcome or their respective causes.

To take an extreme example, imagine a study of education's effect on Alzheimer's dementia (AD). Suppose the eligibility criteria for the study are (1) college education or higher, *or* (2) memory impairment. Within the sample, you find a strong inverse correlation between education and AD. In fact, everyone with less than a college education has memory impairment (strongly associated with AD), because otherwise they would not have been eligible for the study. All the sample members with good memory turn out to have high education. Thus, in this sample, higher education is associated with lower risk of AD. Obviously, this is a completely spurious statistical relationship, induced by conditioning sample membership on education and memory impairment. All analyses of the sample are conditional on sample membership, and sample membership is a common effect of the exposure and outcome of interest. No matter what the causal relation between education and Alzheimer's, the statistical associations in the selected sample will differ substantially.

Note that the bias in this example was not a result of drawing a nonrepresentative sample from the "target population" and was not simply a problem

FIGURE 16.4.   A DAG FOR SELECTION BIAS.

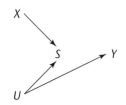

of generalizability. Instead, this bias arises from how the target population is defined, regardless of whether a representative sample is drawn from that target population. One may well define the target population to be college graduates or those with memory impairment and ask whether, for these people, education protected against AD. Within this population, however, the statistical associations between education and AD will not equal the causal relations.

This example is obvious because the selection criteria were direct measures of the exposure and outcome. Selection may be more subtly related to factors that influence exposure and outcome, however. Imagine that you choose to test the hypothesis that education affects AD risk in a sample with selection based on membership in a high-prestige occupation. Achievement of a high-prestige occupation is likely to be influenced by education, but many people with limited education obtain prestigious jobs by virtue of native talent or intellect (or any number of other explanations, but we will focus only on the intelligence factor). Some evidence indicates that intelligence protects against diagnosis of AD (Schmand et al. 1997). Consider the DAG in Figure 16.4. In this DAG, S represents selection into the sample (based on occupation), and it is influenced by X (representing education) and U (intellect), which is itself a cause of Y (AD). Among the high-prestige job holders, people with limited education are likely to have high intellect, whereas those with low intellect are likely to have quite a lot of education. This is not to say that everyone in the sample with extensive schooling will be dim or that all the smart people will be high-school dropouts. The selection process will merely bias the education–intellect association away from the association in the population as a whole. The strength of the spurious association will depend on the details of the selection process, that is, how strongly education and intellect each affect occupation and whether they interact in any way to determine occupation. Note, however, that if high-education sample members are slightly less likely to have high intellect than low-education sample members, this will increase the AD risk of high-education sample members relative to the low-education sample members commensurately. Whatever the true causal relation between education and AD, in a study of high-prestige job holders, that relation will tend to be underestimated, *unless it is possible to also condition on intellect.* Alternatively, if the effect of intellect on AD is mediated entirely by some measured covariate, adjusting for that covariate will eliminate the selection bias. This problem is not resolved by using a longitudinal study design unless the effect of intellect on AD is mediated entirely by some measured baseline variable.

Telling the story as in the preceding paragraphs is complicated and prone to generating confusion, but analyzing the DAG is quite straightforward. Given the DAG in Figure 16.4, we can see that S is a collider between X and U; X and U are statistically associated conditional on S. Thus, conditional on S, X and Y are also statistically associated, even under the assumption shown in this DAG that X has no causal effect on Y (the null hypothesis). Note that whether selection exacerbates or reduces bias in estimating a specific causal effect depends crucially on the causal relations among variables determining selection. If we added an arrow from U to X to the DAG in Figure 16.4, selection on S might reduce bias in estimating the effect of X on Y. The relation between collider bias and selection bias is described by Spirtes et al. (1993) and Pearl (1995) and explicated within the framework of epidemiologic study designs by Hernán et al. (2004).

Survivor bias can be thought of as a special case of selection bias. In life-course research on early life exposures and health in old age, a large fraction of the exposed are likely to die before reaching old age, so survivor bias could be influential. Effect estimates for many exposures–outcome combinations are larger among the young and middle-aged than among the old (Elo and Preston 1996; Tate et al. 1998). An especially striking example of this phenomenon is the black–white mortality crossover: Mortality is greater for blacks and other disadvantaged groups relative to whites at younger ages, but the pattern reverses at the oldest ages (Corti et al. 1999; Thornton 2004). Does the diminishing magnitude of effect estimates among the elderly indicate that the early life exposures become less important causes of the outcome among the old? Not necessarily. Selective survival models show that attenuated estimates among aged cohorts need not imply diminished effects (Howard and Goff 1998; Mohtashemi and Levins 2002). In a selected group of survivors to old age, observed coefficients for early life exposures may differ from the causal coefficients in the following situations: (1) probability of survival is influenced by early life exposure and some other unmeasured factor, (2) the combined effect of the unmeasured factor and early life exposure on *survival* is not perfectly multiplicative, and (3) the unmeasured factor influences the outcome of interest. This can occur even if the unmeasured factor is statistically independent of exposure at birth (as in the numerical example) and thus would not be considered a confounder.

Consider a simple numerical example of this phenomenon (illustrated in Figure 16.5). If interest is in how mother's socioeconomic status (SES) affects one's stroke risk, and we enroll surviving members of the 1920 birth cohort when they are age sixty, roughly 40 percent of the birth cohort will have died prior to enrollment (Arias 2004). Suppose that those whose mothers had low SES were twice as likely to die as those whose mothers had high SES. Furthermore, suppose there is a "bad" gene, carriers of which have twice the chance of dying before age sixty as non-carriers and also have twice the chance of incident stroke after age sixty. Suppose that at birth, these two risk factors are independent and exactly one-half the population are carriers of each (thus 25 percent of the population are high-SES non-carriers, 25 percent are high-SES carriers, 25 percent are low-SES non-carriers, and 25 percent are low-SES carriers). These factors are perfectly multiplicative for death; that is, risk of death before age sixty for high-SES non-carriers is 18 percent, risk of death for low-SES non-carriers is 36 percent, risk of death for high-SES carriers is 36 percent, and risk of death for low-SES carriers is 72 percent. Given this pattern of death, what are the associations among the survivors? The population, which was 25 percent of each risk combination at birth, at age sixty is 34 percent high-SES non-carrier, 27 percent low-SES non-carrier, 27 percent high-SES carrier, and 12 percent low-SES carrier. Thus, 44 percent of the high-SES group are carriers, whereas only 31 percent of the low-SES group are carriers. Suppose high SES actually had no effect on stroke risk after age sixty (that is, if, for everybody in the sample, had we intervened to flip their mother's SES, they would nonetheless have had the same stroke outcome). Even under this assumption of no causal effect, we would observe that high-SES survivors had an elevated risk of stroke compared with low-SES survivors. Although the spurious statistical association between SES and stroke would vanish within strata of the gene, if the gene is unmeasured, the crude association is biased. Whatever protection (or risk) having a high-SES mother might have conferred against having a stroke after age sixty, it will be biased toward looking harmful among the survivors (in this case, the bias is not very large).

This reasoning follows immediately from a causal DAG such as that in Figure 16.4, showing survival (S) affected by mother's SES (X) and an unmeasured risk factor (U) that also affects stroke (Y). Although the numerical example here makes high SES seem spuriously harmful, survivor bias can operate in either direction, depending on how mother's SES and the unmeasured risk factor combine to affect survival (that is, whether there is interaction). The direction and magnitude of the bias can be estimated under various assumptions about the causal structure, although the assumptions needed are more detailed than those shown in DAGs. In some cases, the plausible range of the bias may be too small to be of concern, but this is not always the case.

FIGURE 16.5. A SIMPLE NUMERICAL EXAMPLE OF SURVIVOR BIAS.

This example assumes that high-SES carriers of the "bad" gene have a relative risk of 2 for death before age sixty compared to high-SES non-carriers; low-SES non-carriers have a relative risk of death of 2 compared to high-SES non-carriers; and low-SES carriers have a relative risk of death of 4 compared to high-SES non-carriers. Forty percent of the birth cohort is assumed to die before age sixty. The gene is assumed to double risk of stroke after age sixty, while SES has no effect on stroke after age sixty. Very few low-SES carriers will survive to age sixty. If the RR for stroke of high vs low-SES individuals is calculated among survivors at age sixty without conditioning on the carrier status, high-SES will be associated with increased risk of stroke. The numbers do not total exactly due to rounding.

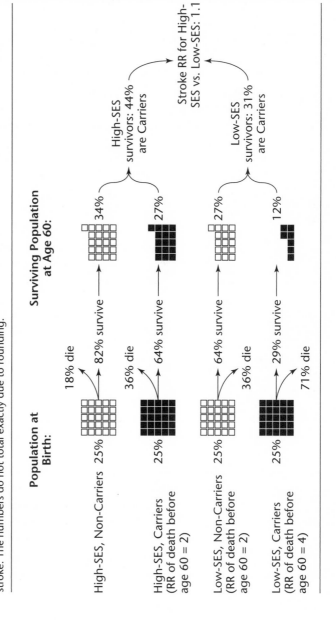

Why Handling Missing Data with Indicator Variables Is Biased Even If the Data Are Missing Completely at Random

Even the best of studies are usually compromised by missing data. Often, the missingness comes here and there, scattered across a large percentage of the observations in the data set. Earl didn't want to reveal his income, Esther was happy to report her income but refused questions on sexual behaviors, Viola broke into tears when asked about participation in community activities such as bridge, and the medical record forms for twelve other sample members were lost. Several methods for handling missing data are available, many of which are unbiased under some assumptions but biased under alternative scenarios (Greenland and Finkle 1995; Little and Rubin 1987). To many researchers, two goals are of preeminent importance: (1) retain everybody in the study so there is still a good chance of getting a statistically significant result, and (2) avoid a lot of extra work. A popular approach to handling missing data that fulfills both goals is to create indicator variables for missingness on each variable (0 = observed, 1 = missing). The variable in question is centered at its mean and all missing values are set to zero. In this way, we can retain everybody in a regression analysis, even if they skipped one or more items. As many a tired researcher has discovered, this approach is also pretty easy to implement. But, we might well ask, does it produce the right answer? Suppose we optimistically assume that the data are missing completely at random. In other words, Viola's shyness regarding social relations had nothing to do with her actual social isolation or any other observed or unobserved characteristic of Viola. The missing data are completely random with respect to exposure and outcome. In this case, would using the missing indicator method to adjust for a putative confounder provide an unbiased effect estimate?

Examine the DAG in Figure 16.6. We are interested in estimating the effect of X on Y, and we recognize that it is important to adjust for Z, a common prior cause of X and Y. Unfortunately, we do not have measures of Z for everyone in our sample. When Z is missing, the variable Z_{ms} takes the value of 1; otherwise it is 0. Because the data are missing completely at random, there are no arrows pointing into Z_{ms} in the DAG. We define a new variable, Z^*, that equals Z whenever Z is observed and equals c (the mean value of observed Z) everywhere else; Z^* is thus determined by both Z and Z_{ms}, and Z^* is thus influenced by both Z_{ms} and Z. Using the missing indicator method, we examine the statistical association between X and Y conditional on Z^* and Z_{ms}.

We can see from this DAG that conditioning on Z^* does not block the backdoor path from X to Y via Z; Z^* is correlated with Z, and that correlation is proportional to the fraction of the sample with observed values of Z. If Z does in fact

FIGURE 16.6. CONDITIONING ON A MISSING VARIABLE INDICATOR.

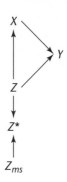

confound the association between X and Y, there will be residual confounding when adjusting for Z^*, and this residual confounding will be proportional to the fraction of missing. A similar issue will arise in general when confounders are mismeasured. The limitations of this approach to handling missing data are well-demonstrated in the literature (Greenland and Finkle 1995; Little and Rubin 1987); the DAG here is merely a device for clarifying the concepts. It is also clear from the DAG that a complete case analysis, in which we condition on Z and consider only observations where $Z_{ms} = 0$, is unbiased under these assumptions (that is, missing completely at random). The DAG can be extended to consider alternative assumptions about the determinants of missingness.

Why Adjusting for a Mediator Does Not Necessarily Estimate the Indirect Effect

Heated arguments in social epidemiology often focus on questions of mediation. Is the effect of sex on depression mediated by hormonal differences between men and women or differences in social conditions? Are education effects on health in old age mediated by credentials, cognitive differences, or behaviors? Is the association between occupational status and heart disease attributable to psychological consequences of low occupational status or material consequences of low-paying low-status jobs? Mediation tests are crucial for identifying the paths between social factors and health differences. We are often at somewhat of a loss as to how to change the "fundamental" cause of the outcome, but have more optimism that we could change a putative mediator, and the preferred policy response would obviously depend on the primary mediators. Implicitly, the question of what mediates observed social effects informs our view of which types of inequalities are socially acceptable and which types require remediation by social policies. For example, a conclusion that women are "biologically programmed" to be depressed more than men may ameliorate the social obligation to try to reduce gender inequalities in depression. Yet if people get depressed whenever they are, say, sexually harassed—and women are more frequently sexually harassed than men—this suggests a very strong social obligation to reduce the depression disparity by reducing the sexual harassment disparity.

One definition of the direct effect of exposure X on outcome Y *not mediated by Z* is the effect of X on Y when everyone in the population is forced to receive the same level of Z. A slightly different definition of direct effects, which I adopt here, is the effect of X on Y when everyone in the population is forced to receive the level of Z they would have received for a specific, constant level of X (for example, if X were 0). The distinction between these definitions is important when discussing the decomposition of a total effect into direct and indirect effects. For a discussion of alternative definitions and issues that arise when the exposure interacts with the mediator, see (Kaufman et al. 2004; Robins and Greenland 1992). Although it is possible that the direct effect of X on Y differs depending on the value of Z, assume for the remainder of this discussion that it does not.

When Z is believed to partially mediate the effect of X on Y, a common approach to quantifying the direct effect is to compare the regression coefficients for X predicting Y in a model simultaneously adjusted for Z to the regression coefficients for X in a model not adjusted for Z (Baron and Kenny 1986; Judd and Kenny 1981). That is:

$$E(Y) = \beta_0 + \beta_1 X + \beta_2 Z \qquad (3)$$

Assuming that it is known that X affects Z, rather than that Z affects X, the coefficient β_1 is interpreted as the direct effect of X on Y. To calculate the mediated effect, a second regression, unadjusted for Z, is estimated:

$$E(Y) = \gamma_0 + \gamma_1 X \qquad (4)$$

The contrast between γ_1 and β_1 is interpreted as the portion of the effect of X on Y that is mediated by Z. Clearly, this interpretation is not correct if Z is a common prior cause of X and Y or to the extent that Z is measured with error. A more subtle problem occurs if X affects Z but there are unmeasured common causes of Z and Y. In this case, the approach described above does not generally give correct estimates of either the direct or indirect effects of X on Y. These

FIGURE 16.7. TESTS FOR DIRECT VERSUS MEDIATED EFFECTS.

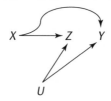

unmeasured common causes may be completely unassociated with X; if they affect both Z and Y they will nonetheless bias the estimate of the direct effect of X on Y. This may be surprising because we are not used to considering carefully whether our mediator covariates might have unidentified confounders with the outcome.

The reason the standard approach to testing for mediation fails whenever the putative mediator is confounded is immediately evident from the DAG in Figure 16.7. The variable Z is a common effect of X and U. Within levels of Z, X and U become statistically associated, even if they were marginally statistically independent, and this introduces a spurious statistical association between X and Y within levels of Z. Whatever the causal relation between X and Y, when Z is held constant the statistical association will reflect this causal relation plus the spurious association via U.

We can describe this same phenomenon with an example. Suppose we are interested in knowing whether the relation between education and systolic blood pressure (SBP) is mediated by adult wealth (say, at age sixty). Unfortunately, we do not have any measure of occupational characteristics, and it turns out that having a high-autonomy job promotes the accumulation of wealth and also lowers SBP (perhaps owing to diminished stress). Returning to Figure 16.7, now X represents education, Y represents SBP, Z represents wealth at age sixty, and U represents job autonomy. To estimate the effect of education on SBP not mediated by wealth, we need to compare the SBP in people with high and low education if the value of wealth were not allowed to change in response to education. For example, if we gave someone high education but intervened to hold their wealth to the wealth they would have accumulated had they had low education (but changed no other characteristics of the situation), how would SBP change compared with giving the person less education? Unfortunately, we cannot conduct such an intervention. The mediation analysis described previously instead compares the SBP of people with high versus low education but who happened to have the same level of adult wealth. Overall, someone with high education will also tend to be wealthier than someone with low education. A high-education person with the same wealth as a low-education person is likely to have accumulated less wealth than expected for some other reason, such as a low autonomy job. Thus, the mediation analysis will be comparing people with high education but low job autonomy to people with low education and average job autonomy. If job autonomy affects SBP, the high-education people will seem to be worse off than they would have been if they had average job autonomy. This will in effect underestimate the direct effect of education on SBP. Under the traditional analysis plan, if we underestimate the direct effect, we will automatically overestimate the mediated effect. This same phenomenon can be explained more formally using counterfactual language. The point here is to note that with a causal DAG, one can see quickly that adjusting for a confounded mediator will induce a spurious association (which may be in either direction) between the primary exposure and outcome.

This observation can be frustrating, because estimating mediation is so important in social epidemiology. In fact, it is so frustrating that researchers sometimes prefer to ignore the problem because, if honestly confronted, it seems to render progress impossible. This is a mistake. First, the injunction that hypothesized mediators be unconfounded in order to draw causal inferences is not any more severe than the demand that primary exposures be unconfounded in order to draw causal inferences. We accept the latter injunction without irritation. Second, if the hypothesized mediators are confounded, we can conduct sensitivity analyses to understand our true uncertainty about the magnitude of the direct or mediated effects. Cole and Hernán (2002) wrote an accessible discussion of this problem walking through a numerical example. Blakely (2002), in a response to Cole and Hernán, called for careful sensitivity analyses to determine whether substantial bias is introduced under realistic assumptions about the strengths of the causal relations.

When Is an Alleged Natural Experiment Valid?

Observational epidemiologists are (or at least should be) constantly concerned that they have not adequately measured and controlled for all common prior causes of their exposure and outcome. For this reason, randomized experiments are strongly preferred to observational studies for demonstrating causality (despite the many other limitations of randomized trials). A randomized trial is represented in the DAG in Figure 16.8. Here Z represents random assignment to treatment group. We will ignore the variable W on this DAG for the moment. Random assignment

FIGURE 16.8. IDENTIFYING A VALID NATURAL EXPERIMENT.

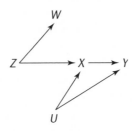

affects treatment received (X), although it does not perfectly determine X because some participants do not adhere to their assigned treatment. There are no causal connections between Z and Y except via X. In the DAG, we show an unmeasured variable U that confounds the association between X and Y, thus forcing us to use the experimental design to test whether X affects Y. The crucial assumption here is that, if we find that average Y differs by treatment assignment Z, this implies that Z affects Y. If Z covaries with Y, this implies that X affects Y, because there is no other possible pathway which would lead to an association between Z and Y except the one via X.

Note that the causal assumptions for a valid trial may be met even if the researcher did not assign the values of Z: the crucial assumption is simply that Z was assigned in a manner otherwise unrelated to the outcome, and its association with X is the only plausible reason it might predict Y. Various natural experiments may fulfill this assumption. We may think that the day of the week one falls ill determines the quality of hospital care received, but there is no other reason for day of illness to influence ultimate health outcomes. In this case, day of symptom onset provides a natural experiment for the effect of quality of hospital care on outcome. A similar idea using hour of birth as an instrument for postpartum length of stay is developed in the study by Malkin et al. (2000). We may think that the weather in the summer before a subsistence farmer's child is born determines the calories that child receives in his first year of life, but weather during that period should have no other effect on the child's health at age ten. Weather then provides a natural experiment for the effect of early caloric intake on later health. We may believe that infants born in hospitals that provide lactation counseling to postpartum mothers are more likely to be breastfed but that being born in such a hospital has no other effect on child health. In this case, being born in a hospital with lactation counseling provides a natural experiment for the effect of breastfeeding on child health. We may believe that women whose mothers or sisters had breast cancer are unlikely to take hormone therapy at menopause but that having relatives with breast cancer has no other causal link to cardiovascular disease risk. If so, having female relatives with breast cancer is a natural experiment for the effect of hormone therapy on cardiovascular disease.

These examples highlight the core criteria upon which putative natural experiments must be assessed: is there any other reason for the treatment assignment (that is, day of symptom onset, weather in the summer before birth, birth in a hospital with lactation counseling) to influence the outcome besides via the exposure of interest? For example, if we believe that hospitals with lactation counselors also tend to provide better care in other respects, then we cannot attribute a difference in health between children born at lactation-counseling or non-counseling hospitals strictly to breastfeeding. The natural experiment is not valid. Data from natural experiments are often analyzed with an Instrumental Variables (IV) analysis, in which treatment assignment is referred to as an **instrument** for the effect of X on Y. Specifically, given a causal DAG, we say Z is a valid instrument for the effect of X on Y if Z and X are statistically dependent and if every unblocked path connecting Z and Y contains an arrow pointing into X. An IV effect estimate can be calculated as the ratio of the relation between the instrument and the outcome (the intent-to-treat effect estimate) and the relation between the instrument and the treatment. To interpret this parameter, we assume that some people would have been treated regardless of the value of the instrument, other people would *not* have been treated no matter what value the instrument took, whereas still a third group, sometimes called the cooperators, would receive the treatment if and only if assigned to receive it by the instrument. We assume nobody in the population is a contrarian (that is, receives treatment only if assigned *not* to receive treatment and avoids treatment only if assigned to receive it). Under these assumptions, the IV estimate provides a consistent estimate of the average effect of receiving treatment on those who received the treatment owing to the value of the instrument.

One interesting and somewhat surprising observation from the DAGs is that an instrument need not directly affect exposure. In Figure 16.8, the relation between W and Y may provide a valid test of the hypothesis that X affects Y even though W does not itself directly affect X but rather shares a common prior cause with X. Here Z affects both W and X, and they are thus statistically associated. Neither W nor Z has any other pathways linking them to Y. If W and Y are statistically associated, under these assumptions it implies that X affects Y. Natural experiments and IV analyses are discussed in more detail in Chapter 17 of this book. For accessible discussions of the use of IV analyses to estimate causal effects see (Angrist and Krueger 2001; Currie 1995; Greenland 2000).

Why It Is a Mistake to Condition on the Dependent Variable

For various reasons, it may be appealing to examine relations between X and Y within a certain range of values of Y. For example, one might want to know whether the effect of education on mental status among individuals with below average mental status is the same as the effect of education among individuals with above average mental status. Alternatively, one might suspect that the outcome measurement available becomes increasingly unreliable at high levels and therefore wish to exclude any high-scoring respondents from the analysis.

These decisions can introduce important bias into an analysis, and this can be seen with a DAG such as that in Figure 16.9. In this DAG, we are interested in the effect of X on Y; Y is also influenced by U, but U is statistically independent of X. Under these assumptions, a simple analysis of the statistical relation between X and Y (without statistical adjustment for any other covariates) gives an unbiased estimate of the causal effect. Suppose however, that we condition on some values of Y. Let us define a variable Y^* that is one if Y is above a threshold value and zero if it is below. Now we examine the relation between X and Y only among those with $Y^* = 1$. This turns out to have an undesirable consequence: X and U are likely to be statistically associated among respondents with $Y^* = 1$. As a result, the statistical relation between X and Y will now be confounded by the effect of U on Y (although the direction of confounding will not necessarily be the same as the direction of the effect of U on Y).

Let us consider the question of education's effect on mental status, using the mini-mental status exam (MMSE) as a measure of mental status. The MMSE ranges from zero to thirty, and an MMSE score below twenty-four is considered a clinically important threshold for impairment (Folstein et al. 1975). Suppose we ask whether the effect of education on MMSE is the same for respondents with MMSE equal to or above twenty-four as for respondents with MMSE below twenty-four. We assume that MMSE score is influenced by education and also influenced by intelligence (IQ), although IQ is unrelated to

FIGURE 16.9. CONDITIONING ON THE DEPENDENT VARIABLE.

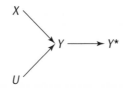

education (if IQ itself affects education, the analysis is obviously confounded, but we make the optimistic assumption here that IQ does not affect education). Thus, in the DAG in Figure 16.9, U represents IQ, X represents education, Y represents MMSE, and Y^* is an indicator for whether MMSE is above twenty-four. In general, under this setup, we will underestimate the association between education and MMSE in both strata of Y^* unless we are able to simultaneously adjust for IQ. Among the high-functioning individuals (those with high MMSE scores), those with low education are more likely to have unusually high IQ. Among the low-functioning individuals, those with high education are more likely to have unusually low IQ. Even though IQ and schooling are statistically independent in the population, they are inversely correlated within strata of their common effect, MMSE. Note that the rules for drawing causal DAGs described earlier in the chapter would not require that U in Figure 16.9 be shown, because U is not a direct cause of more than one other variable in the DAG. The rules for drawing causal DAGs specify what is required for the d-separation rules to be applicable, but this phenomenon is not addressed by the d-separation rules.

This phenomenon is also relevant when considering how to respond to an artificial ceiling on the measurement of Y. One tempting but erroneous approach is to drop all of the observations with ceiling values of Y. This is effectively conditioning the analysis on the value of Y and will bias the statistical association between X and Y. An important caveat is that the preceding discussion only applies if X actually does affect Y. If X has no effect on Y, then Y is not a common effect of X and U. In this situation, conditioning on Y should not influence the estimated relation between X and Y—it should be zero in every strata. This finding is discussed in introductory econometrics texts, including Kennedy (1998) and Wooldridge (2002), although it is not generally demonstrated with DAGs.

Why Adjusting for Baseline Values Can Bias Analyses of Change

Our final example of how DAGs can clarify otherwise confusing analysis decisions relates to analyses of change. When the substantive question is whether an exposure X, measured at baseline, affects changes in the value of Y over a follow-up time period, an important analytic decision is whether to condition on the value of Y as measured at baseline. This conditioning may take the form of restriction or stratification, but most frequently the decision is whether to include Y at baseline as an independent variable in a regression model. Let us take as a substantive example the effect of exposure to violence (ETV) in early childhood on changes in depressive symptoms in adulthood. Suppose that adults at average age thirty are enrolled, and depressive symptoms are assessed with the Centers for Epidemiologic Studies Depression scale at baseline ($CESD_1$) and again after five years of follow-up ($CESD_2$). The CESD is a continuous scale ranging from zero to sixty, in which higher scores indicate worse depressive symptoms (Radloff 1977). Our (hypothetical) ETV measure is dichotomous and based on exposures before age fifteen. At baseline, when respondents are average age thirty, ETV is associated with higher average CESD scores. We would like to know if ETV also causes increases in depressive symptoms over the five-year follow-up of adults. That is, for any given person who was not exposed to violence in childhood, would her change over the five-year follow-up period have differed had she in fact been exposed to violence?

One possible analysis would be to estimate a baseline-adjusted change score model using regression, where the CESD change score is the difference between CESD at follow-up and CESD at baseline:

$$CESD_2 - CESD_1 = \gamma_0 + \gamma_1 ETV + \gamma_2 CESD_1 + \varepsilon_i \qquad (5)$$

It has been shown elsewhere (Laird 1983) that the previous model provides the same coefficient for $ETV(\gamma_1)$ as does a lagged-effects model such as:

$$CESD_2 = \gamma_0 + \gamma_1 ETV + \gamma_2^* CESD_1 + \varepsilon_i \qquad (6)$$

We will focus on whether the statistical analysis in equation (5) answers our causal question, but keep in mind that if the analysis in equation (5) fails to answer this question, estimation of equation (6) will also fail. Alternatively, we could estimate a change score model without baseline adjustment:

$$CESD_2 - CESD_1 = \beta_0 + \beta_1 ETV + \varepsilon_i \qquad (7)$$

In either regression model a number of other covariates believed to directly affect ETV and change in depressive symptoms might also be included. It turns out that β_1 and γ_1 are frequently quite different numbers, so they both cannot represent the "right" answer to a specific causal question. Figure 16.10 is a causal DAG under which a baseline adjusted analysis (as in equation [5]) would give a positively biased estimate of the effect of ETV on change in depression, but an unadjusted analysis, as in equation (7), would give an unbiased estimate under the null. The major conceptual point in this DAG is that CESD is an imperfect measure of a latent construct: depressive symptoms. The CESD score is influenced both by true underlying depression and by some error in measuring that depression. This reflects the well-documented finding that the CESD scale has imperfect reliability (McDowell and Newell 1996). The phenomenon in the following description could also occur because of instability in the construct of depression, but that is outside

FIGURE 16.10. AN EXAMPLE WHEN BASELINE ADJUSTMENT BIASES ANALYSES OF CHANGE.

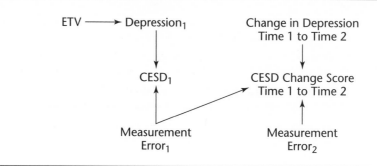

the scope of this discussion. Because ETV and $CESD_1$ are correlated and ETV is temporally prior to $CESD_1$, we assume that ETV affects baseline depressive symptoms. Over the five-year follow-up, some true change in depressive symptoms will occur. We are not privy to the true change, but we will observe the change in CESD scores, which is strongly influenced by true change. Unfortunately, the change in CESD scores is *also* influenced by the error in measuring CESD at baseline. If the baseline error was positive, the CESD change score will tend to be negative, purely due to regression to the mean. If the baseline error was negative, regression to the mean will tend to push the change score in a positive direction. The error in measuring $CESD_2$ will also influence the change score, and if the two errors are perfectly correlated, there will be no regression to the mean; however, psychometric assessments of the CESD scale indicate substantial measurement error that is uncorrelated across time periods. This is the reasoning for drawing the DAG as we did in Figure 16.10. Under these assumptions, if ETV has no effect on change in depression during the follow-up period, ETV and change in CESD score will be statistically independent: the β_1 estimated in equation (7) is unbiased. The only path in the diagram connecting ETV and change score (ETV—Depression$_1$—$CESD_1$—error$_1$—CESD change score) is blocked by $CESD_1$ (a collider). Thus, analyses not adjusted for $CESD_1$ provide unbiased estimates of the overall (that is, total) effect of ETV on change.

Conditional on $CESD_1$, however, ETV and CESD change score are spuriously correlated, because conditioning on $CESD_1$ "unblocks" the previously described path. The intuition is just as with the previous examples of conditioning on common effects. Anyone with a high $CESD_1$ has either severe baseline depression symptoms (high depression$_1$) or large positive measurement error$_1$ (or both). A person without depression who has a high $CESD_1$ must have a positive error$_1$. If a person with severe depressive symptoms scores a low CESD$_1$, error is negative. Thus, *within levels of CESD$_1$*, depression$_1$ and error$_1$ are inversely correlated, and ETV and error$_1$ are inversely correlated. Because error$_1$ contributes negatively to change score, change score and error$_1$ are negatively correlated, an example of the regression to the mean phenomenon. Hence, conditional on CESD$_1$, ETV and CESD change score are positively correlated. Therefore baseline-adjusted ETV coefficients are positive, even when ETV does not affect change in depressive symptoms. The spurious correlation is proportional to the error in the CESD measure and the strength of the ETV-CESD$_1$ relationship. This finding has been demonstrated mathematically (Yanez et al. 1998) and with an applied example (Yanez et al. 2002). The issue is discussed in more detail using DAGs in Glymour et al. (2005).

Caveats and Conclusion

Directed acyclic graphs do not convey information about important aspects of the causal relations, such as the magnitude or functional form of the relations (for example, linearity, interactions, or effect modification). This can be frustrating because not all biases are created equal, and it would be nice to establish which ones can safely be ignored. For example, Greenland (2003) compares the likely bias introduced by adjusting for a collider with the bias that would result from failing to adjust for a common prior cause. His findings suggest that if the collider is not a direct effect of the exposure and the outcome, one might prefer to adjust on the grounds that the bias potentially introduced by *failing* to adjust for the variable is likely to be larger than the bias potentially introduced by mistakenly adjusting for it. Exploring the magnitude of potential biases under a range of assumptions is invaluable, and there are many approaches to doing this. One option is to generate simulated data sets based on DAGs, for example as in the simple code in Appendix 16.1. More sophisticated simulations can be conducted in many statistical packages, including freeware available online (TETRAD, 2005)[5].

Drawing a DAG that adequately describes our prior beliefs or assumptions is sometimes difficult. To the extent that using DAGs forces greater clarity about

---

[5]TETRAD is a project on statistical data and causal inference. The causal discovery algorithms used by the accompanying software package have been controversial (see for example, Robins and Wasserman, 1999 and rejoinders). Apart from this debate regarding the reliability of the causal inference algorithms, the software includes a convenient routine to simulate data sets based on assumptions in structural equation models without specifying programming code.

assumptions, this seems advantageous. Though it may seem an impossible task to draw a "true" DAG, to the extent that we are uncertain about how to specify the DAG, we should also be uncertain about the causal interpretation of our statistical tests.

Directed acyclic graphs are a convenient device for expressing ideas explicitly and understanding how causal relations translate into statistical relations. Causal DAGs provide a simple, flexible tool for thinking about many epidemiological problems. The goal of this chapter was to demonstrate how an array of apparently disparate problems in epidemiologic reasoning can be expressed and resolved with causal DAGs. This is part of the remarkable convenience of learning the d-separation rules. Rather than considering each case of a potential bias as a separate problem and struggling for the "right" answer, DAGs help provide a unified way of evaluating a potential analysis plan for any specific question of interest and set of causal assumptions. Although in some cases the issues raised are especially pertinent in research on social determinants of health, these problems are by no means limited to social epidemiology. The last two decades of progress on causal inference, of which the use of causal DAGs is only a part, has the potential to substantially enhance applied epidemiologic work, and these improvements may be especially beneficial in social and life-course epidemiology.

APPENDIX 16.1

The following Stata commands create a data set with five normally distributed variables: W, X, Y, $Z1$, and $Z2$. Variable $Z1$ affects X and W; $Z2$ affects W and Y. There are no other causal relations between variables (for example, we assume the null hypothesis that X has no effect on Y). This is the same causal structure as shown in Figure 16.3, although all variables are assumed to be continuous. Under these assumptions, W meets conventional statistical criteria for a confounder but not the graphical criteria. As shown in the two regressions, conditioning on W induces a negative statistical association between X and Y.

Manipulating the path coefficients can illustrate how the size of the bias induced by adjustment for W depends on the strength of these relations. Please note that several assumptions about the causal structure are implicit in the following code but *not* encoded in the corresponding DAG. For example, the code specifies linear and additive causal effects. The DAG encodes no such assumptions and would thus be consistent with other specifications. The magnitude of the bias induced by conditioning on W is sensitive to these assumptions about functional form.

```
set obs 10000
* Generate constants that determine the magnitude of
the causal effects (that is, path coefficients).
gen Z1toX = 1
gen Z1toW = 1
gen Z2toW = 1
gen Z2toY = 1
* Generate Z1 and Z2 as normally distributed random
variables.
gen Z1 = invnorm(uniform())
gen Z2 = invnorm(uniform())
* Generate random components for all other variables:
W, X, and Y
gen W_random = invnorm(uniform())
gen X_random = invnorm(uniform())
gen Y_random = invnorm(uniform())
* Generate W as a function of Z1, Z2, and a random
component
gen W = Z1toW*Z1 + Z2toW*Z2 + W_random
* Generate X as a function of Z1 and a random component
gen X = Z1toX*Z1 + X_random
* Generate Y as a function of Z2 and a random component
gen Y = Z2toY*Z2 + Y_random
* Describe the data generated means
corr W X Y Z1 Z2
* Run regressions with and without adjustment for W to
estimate the effect of X on Y.
reg Y X
reg Y X W
```

Acknowledgments

I wish to thank the following people for helpful comments and suggestions on earlier drafts of this chapter: Jennifer Weuve, Katherine Hoggatt, Clark Glymour, James Robins, David Rehkopf, and Sander Greenland. All remaining errors and confusions are my own.

References

The asterisks indicate especially accessible or influential references.

Angrist, J. D., & Krueger, A. B. (2001). Instrumental variables and the search for identification: From supply and demand to natural experiments. *Journal of Economic Perspectives, 15,* 69–85.

Arias, E. (2004). United States life tables, 2001. *National Vital Statistics Report, 52.*

Baron, R. M., & Kenny, D. A. (1986). The moderator mediator variable distinction in social psychological-research—conceptual, strategic, and statistical considerations. *Journal of Personality and Social Psychology, 51,* 1173–1182.

Blakely, T. A. (2002). Commentary: Estimating direct and indirect effects—fallible in theory, but in the real world? *International Journal of Epidemiology, 31,* 166–167.

*Cole, S. R., & Hernán, M. A. (2002). Fallibility in estimating direct effects. *International Journal of Epidemiology, 31,* 163–165.

Corti, M. C., Guralnik, J. M., Ferrucci, L., et al. (1999). Evidence for a Black-White crossover in all-cause and coronary heart disease mortality in an older population: The North Carolina EPESE. *American Journal of Public Health, 89,* 308–314.

Currie, J. (1995). Welfare and the well-being of children. In F. Welch (Ed.), *Fundamentals of pure and applied economics* (p. 165). Chur, Switzerland: Harwood Academic Publishers.

Dawid, A. P. (2000). Causal inference without counterfactuals. *Journal of the American Statistical Association, 95,* 407–424.

Elo, I. T., & Preston, S. H. (1996). Educational differentials in mortality: United States, 1979–85. *Soc Sci Med, 42,* 47–57.

Folstein, M. F., Folstein, S. E., & McHugh, P. R. (1975). "Mini-mental state." A practical method for grading the cognitive state of patients for the clinician. *Journal Psychiatric Research, 12,* 189–198.

Glymour, C. (1986). Statistics and causal inference—statistics and metaphysics. *Journal of the American Statistical Association, 81,* 964–966.

Glymour, C., Spirtes, P., & Richardson, T. (1999). On the possibility of inferring causation from association without background knowledge. In C. Glymour, & G. Cooper (Eds.), *Computation, causation, and discovery* (p. 323–331), Menlo Park, CA, and Cambridge, MA: AAAI Press/The MIT Press.

Glymour, C., (2001). *The mind's arrows: Bayes nets and graphical causal models in psychology.* Cambridge, MA: MIT Press.

Glymour, M. M., Weuve, J., Berkman, L. F., Kawachi, I., & Robins, J. M. (2005). When is baseline adjustment useful in analyses of change? An example with education and cognitive change. *American Journal of Epidemiology, 162,* 267–278.

Greenland, S. (2003). Quantifying biases in causal models: Classical confounding vs. collider-stratification bias. *Epidemiology, 14,* 300–306.

Greenland, S. (2000). An introduction to instrumental variables for epidemiologists. *International Journal of Epidemiology, 29,* 722–729.

Greenland, S., & Finkle, W. D. (1995). A critical look at methods for handling missing covariates in epidemiologic regression analyses. *American Journal of Epidemiology, 142,* 1255–1264.

Greenland, S., & Robins, J. M. (1986). Identifiability, exchangeability, and epidemiological confounding. *International Journal of Epidemiology, 15,* 413–419.

*Greenland, S., Pearl, J., & Robins, J. M. (1999). Causal diagrams for epidemiologic research. *Epidemiology, 10*, p. 37–48.

Hennekens, C. H., & Buring, J. E. (1987). *Epidemiology in medicine* (1st ed., p. 383). Boston/Toronto: Little, Brown and Company.

*Hernán, M. A. (2004). A definition of causal effect for epidemiological research. *Journal of Epidemiology and Community Health, 58*, 265–271.

*Hernán, M. A., Hernandez-Diaz, S. & Robins, J. M. (2004). A structural approach to selection bias. *Epidemiology, 15*, 615–625.

Hernán, M. A., Hernandez-Diaz, S. Werler, M. M. & Mitchell, A. A. (2002). Causal knowledge as a prerequisite for confounding evaluation: An application to birth defects epidemiology. *American Journal of Epidemiology, 155*, 176–184.

Holland, P. W. (1986a). Statistics and Causal Inference. *Journal of the American Statistical Association, 81*, 945–960.

Holland, P. W. (1986b). Statistics and causal inference—rejoinder. *Journal of the American Statistical Association, 81*, 968–970.

Howard, G., & Goff, D. C. (1998). A call for caution in the interpretation of the observed smaller relative importance of risk factors in the elderly. *Annals of Epidemiology, 8*, 411–414.

Judd, C. M., & Kenny, D. A. (1981). Process analysis—estimating mediation in treatment evaluations. *Evaluation Review, 5*, 602–619.

Kaufman, J. S., & Cooper, R. S. (1999). Seeking causal explanations in social epidemiology. *American Journal of Epidemiology, 150*, 113–120.

Kaufman, J., Maclehose, R., & Kaufman, S. (2004). A further critique of the analytic strategy of adjusting for covariates to identify biologic mediation. *Epidemiologic Perspectives and Innovations, 1*, 4.

Kaufman, J. S., & Cooper, R. S. (2001). Commentary: Considerations for use of racial/ethnic classification in etiologic research [see comment]. *American Journal of Epidemiology, 154*, 291–298.

Kennedy, P., (1998). *A guide to econometrics* (4th ed., p. 468). Cambridge, MA: The MIT Press.

Laird, N. (1983). Further comparative analyses of pretest-posttest research designs. *The American Statistician, 37*, 329–330.

Little, R., & Rubin, D. B. (1987). *Statistical analysis with missing data. Wiley series in probability and mathematical statistics applied probability and statistics.* New York: Wiley.

Maldonado, G., & Greenland, S. (2002). Estimating causal effects. *International Journal of Epidemiology; 31*, 422–429.

Malkin, J. D., Broder, M. S., & Keeler, E. (2000). Do longer postpartum stays reduce newborn readmissions? Analysis using instrumental variables. *Health Services Research, 35*, 1071–1091.

McDowell, I., & Newell, C. (1996). *Measuring health: A guide to rating scales and questionnaires* (2nd ed.). New York: Oxford University Press.

Mohtashemi, M., & Levins, R. (2002). Qualitative analysis of the all-cause Black-White mortality crossover. *Bull Math Biol, 64*, 147–173.

Parascandola, M., & Weed, D. L. (2001). Causation in epidemiology. *Journal of Epidemiology and Community Health, 55*, 905–912.

Pearl, J. (1995). Causal diagrams for empirical research. *Biometrika, 82*, 669–688.

*Pearl, J. (2000). *Causality* (p. 384). Cambridge, UK: Cambridge University Press.

*Pearl, J. (2001). Causal inference in the health sciences: A conceptual introduction. *Health Services & Outcomes Research Methodology, 2*, 189–220.

Radloff, L. S. (1977). The CES-D scale: A self-report depression scale for research in the general population. *Applied Psychological Measurement, 1,* 384–401.

Robbins, J. M., Vaccarino, V., Zhang, H. P., & Kasl, S. V. (2001). Socioeconomic status and type 2 diabetes in African American and non-Hispanic white women and men: Evidence from the Third National Health and Nutrition Examination Survey. *American Journal of Public Health, 91,* 76–83.

Robbins, J. M., Vaccarino, V., Zhang, H. P., & Kasl, S. V. (2005). Socioeconomic status and diagnosed diabetes incidence. *Diabetes Research and Clinical Practice, 68,* 230–236.

Robins, J. (1987). A graphical approach to the identification and estimation of causal parameters in mortality studies with sustained exposure periods. *Journal of Chronic Diseases, 40,* 139S–161S.

Robins, J. M. (1995). Comment on Judea Pearl's paper, "Causal diagrams for empirical research." *Biometrika, 82,* 695–698.

Robins, J., & Wasserman, L. (1999). On the impossibility of inferring causation from association without background knowledge. In C. Glymour, & G. Cooper (Eds.), *Computation, causation, and discovery* (p. 305–321). Menlo Park, CA, and Cambridge, MA: AAAI Press/The MIT Press.

*Robins, J. M. (2001). Data, design, and background knowledge in etiologic inference. *Epidemiology, 12,* 313–320.

*Robins, J. M., & Greenland, S. (1992). Identifiability and exchangeability for direct and indirect effects. *Epidemiology, 3,* 143–155.

Rothman, K. J., & Greenland, S. (1998). *Modern epidemiology* (2nd ed.). Philadelphia, PA: Lippincott-Raven.

Schmand, B., Smit, J. H., Geerlings, M. I., & Lindeboom, J. (1997). The effects of intelligence and education on the development of dementia. A test of the brain reserve hypothesis. *Psychological Medicine, 27,* 1337–1344.

Spirtes, P., Glymour, C., & Scheines, R. (1993). *Causation, prediction, and search. Lecture Notes in Statistics* (Vol. 81). New York: Springer-Verlag.

*Spirtes, P., Glymour, C. & Scheines, R. (2000). *Causation, prediction, and search* (2nd ed.). Cambridge, MA: MIT Press.

Tate, R. B., Manfreda, J., & Cuddy, T. E. (1998). The effect of age on risk factors for ischemic heart disease: The Manitoba Follow-Up Study, 1948–1993. *Annals of Epidemiology, 8,* 415–421.

TETRAD (2005). *The Tetrad project.* Retrieved on January 16, 2006, from www.phil.cmu.edu/projects/tetrad.

Thornton, R. (2004). The Navajo-US population mortality crossover since the mid-20th century. *Population Research and Policy Review, 23,* 291–308.

Woodward, J. (2003). *Making things happen: A theory of causal explanation* (p. 410). New York: Oxford University Press.

Wooldridge, J. M. (2002). *Econometric analysis of cross section and panel data* (p. 752). Cambridge, MA: Massachusetts Institute of Technology.

Yanez, N. D., Kronmal, R. A., & Shemanski, L. R. (1998). The effects of measurement error in response variables and tests of association of explanatory variables in change models. *Statistics in Medicine,* 17, 2597–2606.

Yanez, N. D., Kronmal, R. A., Shemanski, L. R., & Psaty, B. M. (2002). A regression model for longitudinal change in the presence of measurement error. *Annals of Epidemiology,* 12, 34–38.

CHAPTER SEVENTEEN

NATURAL EXPERIMENTS AND INSTRUMENTAL VARIABLE ANALYSES IN SOCIAL EPIDEMIOLOGY

M. Maria Glymour

Motivation for Using Instrumental Variables in Social Epidemiology Research

Demonstrating the existence of causal relations between social exposures and health and quantifying the magnitude of those relationships are central tasks in social epidemiology research. Unfortunately, the core analytic tools of the discipline frequently fail to accomplish one or both of these tasks. Unmeasured confounding is a persistent threat in analyses of observational data, ameliorated only imperfectly by stratification or statistical adjustment for common prior causes of exposure and outcome. Even with data from randomized experiments, the intent-to-treat (ITT) estimate of the exposure effect is biased if subjects in the trial sometimes fail to adhere to their randomly assigned treatment regimens. Instrumental variables (IV) analyses are useful to address both of these problems. Given randomized trial data, IV analyses can provide an estimate of how those who received treatment were affected by it. In observational data, if a valid instrument is available, IV analyses can potentially circumvent the problem of unmeasured confounders. The validity and interpretation of IV effect estimates are premised on strong assumptions, however. The usefulness of IV depends on the plausibility of the assumptions for the specific instrument and causal relation in question.

429

Randomized trials are considered the "gold standard" for establishing the existence of a causal relation between a treatment and an outcome (Abel and Koch 1999; Byar et al. 1976; DeMets 2002). Intent-to-treat analyses, in which the outcomes of those assigned to treatment are contrasted with the outcomes of those assigned to control, are a standard analytical method. Because of non-compliance, the ITT parameter does not estimate the effect of *receiving* the treatment on the outcome. Instead, ITT analysis estimates the effect of *being assigned to receive the treatment* on the subjects' health. If the ITT effect estimate in a valid randomized controlled trial (RCT) is significantly different from zero, this indicates the existence of a causal relation between treatment and outcome but not the magnitude of that relationship. Often, the primary research question relates to the magnitude of the effect of receiving the treatment. Directly comparing compliers with non-compliers or the treated with the untreated are well-known and long-rejected options (Hennekens and Buring 1987; Weiss 1998). Instrumental variables analyses, however, provide a substantively meaningful estimate of the effect of treatment on those who received the treatment even if non-compliers differ considerably from compliers with respect to the outcome.

In the absence of randomized trial data, epidemiologists attempt to draw causal inferences from observational data by conditioning on common prior causes (confounders) of the exposure and the outcome. Such conditioning may take the form of covariate adjustment, stratification, restriction, or propensity score matching, for example, and can be applied in almost any sort of statistical analysis from chi-square tests to multi-level regression models. These approaches have a common goal: find a set of covariates such that within strata of those covariates, the statistical association between treatment and outcome is entirely due to the causal effect of one upon the other (Greenland et al. 1999). The limitation of all of these conditional analyses, and a leading reason epidemiologists lose sleep, is that it is difficult to find such a set of covariates. Even if all the common prior causes of the exposure and the outcome are known at a conceptual level, have they been well-measured? Does the regression model specify the correct functional form? Residual confounding threatens the internal validity of the analysis if the crucial covariates are badly measured or if the functional form for those confounders is mis-specified. With a valid instrument, IV can be used to estimate the effect of the treatment even if important confounders of the treatment-outcome relation are unmeasured or even unknown.

In short, IV analyses use data from either researcher-randomized or natural experiments to estimate the effect of an exposure on those who were exposed as a result of the experiment. Instrumental variables analyses depend strongly on the assumption that the data were generated by a "valid" experiment (that is, that subjects were effectively randomized), even if the randomization was not by the intent of the researcher and adherence to random assignment was low. For many of the exposures of interest in social epidemiology, opportunities to intentionally randomize are few and far between. Social phenomena such as schooling, poverty, employment, and even features of personal relationships are influenced by administrative policies, state and local laws, and other forces external to the individual (Angrist and Krueger 2001; Currie 1995). These policies sometimes create natural or quasi-experiments in which an individual's probability of exposure to adverse social conditions is influenced by a policy that is uncorrelated with personal characteristics. Such natural experiments—in which a random factor influences the probability of exposure but is not under the control of the investigator—provide a powerful approach to test causal claims.

This chapter begins by providing an intuition for IV analyses and then develops greater detail in subsequent sections. The first section gives a brief introduction to the assumptions required to interpret IV estimates as causal parameters and then explains how the IV estimate is calculated. The next section frames natural experiments and IV estimates in terms of the general problem of causal inference and walks through a simple numerical example comparing the IV estimate with other parameters. We then discuss a few examples of specific instruments that seem especially clever or potentially relevant to social epidemiology. The concluding sections address common points of confusion regarding IV analyses, link the discussion to a typical econometrics account, and reiterate the limitations of IV.

Much of the description in this chapter focuses on the motivating ideas. More formal introductions to IV are available in several excellent articles published elsewhere (Angrist and Krueger 2001; Angrist et al. 1996; Greenland 2000; Pearl 2000). Instrumental variables analysis is also discussed in standard econometrics textbooks (Greene 2000; Kennedy 1998; Wooldridge 2002), although the language and treatment adopted by economists may be unfamiliar to epidemiologists.[1]

---

[1]Although the basic idea of instrumental variables is intuitive and fairly consistent across disciplines and presentations, there are several topics related to IVs that are still active areas of research. These areas include the causal interpretation of the IV estimate under various sets of assumptions and the properties of IV estimators. This chapter focuses on the Angrist Imbens Rubin "local average treatment effect" interpretation, but much can be learned from instruments that do not fit the Angrist et al. example.

The Core Idea in IV Analyses

The IV estimate can be interpreted as the average effect that receiving treatment had on those individuals who received the treatment as a result of the value of the instrument. This interpretation rests on the assumption that the instrument is valid and monotonically related to the treatment.[2] Understanding these assumptions helps clarify the rationale for IV estimates.

Assumptions

The motivation and assumptions for a valid instrument can be concisely expressed using a causal directed acyclic graph (DAG). Figure 17.1a shows the basic causal structure under which we would be interested in calculating an IV effect estimate. Because this is a causal DAG, all common prior causes of two or more variables in the DAG are also shown in the DAG (that is, there are no confounders that do not appear in the DAG). We are interested in the effect of X on Y, but the relation is confounded by an unmeasured common prior cause U. The measured variable Z affects X, but has no direct effect on Y and no prior causes in common with Y. We can imagine the scenario in Figure 17.1a as an RCT, in which Z is random assignment to treatment, X represents receiving the treatment, and Y is the outcome of interest. If Z and Y are statistically related, it must be because Z affects X and X affects Y (setting aside the possibility of chance). The traditional instrument is a variable that directly affects exposure, and this is the structure we will focus on for much of the chapter. Note, however, that for the purpose of testing whether X affects Y, the causal structure in Figure 17.1b also depicts a valid instrument. In this causal structure, the instrument and exposure share a common prior cause, as in Figure 17.1b, which is acceptable provided this common cause does not itself directly affect the outcome.

---

[2]We also assume throughout that the effect of the treatment on one individual does not depend on the treatment that others in the population receive (that is, the Stable Unit Treatment Value Assumption, SUTVA). Without this assumption, the number of possible causal effects for each individual in the population increases exponentially with the number of other people in the population. Violations of this assumption could be represented on a DAG by showing the relevant feature of the distribution of treatment as a separate variable with a path into the outcome (Y). This new variable would in general have an unblocked path linking it to Z. Regardless, SUTVA may be questionable for some social exposures, but the issues raised are not unique to instrumental variables analyses. For further discussion of this assumption in general, see Little and Rubin (2000) or Winship and Morgan (1999) or, related to social exposures, Kaufman et al. (2003) or Oakes (2004).

FIGURE 17.1A AND B. CAUSAL DIAGRAMS DEPICTING A VALID INSTRUMENT.

A valid instrument must be associated with the predictor of interest and all unblocked paths between the instrument and the outcome must pass through the predictor.

1a. The instrument directly affects exposure but has no other effect on the outcome.

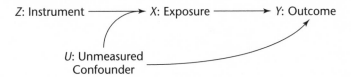

1b. The instrument is statistically associated with the exposure, and all of the common causes of the instrument and the outcome operate via the exposure.

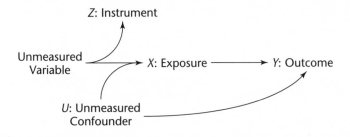

Given a causal DAG, we say Z is a valid instrument for the effect of X on Y if Z and X are statistically dependent (associated) and if every unblocked path connecting Z and Y contains an arrow pointing into X[3]. If there were a path directly from Z to Y, then Z would not be a valid instrument (Figure 17.2a). If there were a path directly from Z to U, then Z would not be a valid instrument (Figure 17.2b).

---

[3]Please see Chapter Sixteen for a more complete discussion of DAG terminology. A path is a sequence of lines connecting two variables regardless of the direction of the arrowheads. A path is blocked if two arrows on the path point to the same variable (as in: $A{\rightarrow}C{\leftarrow}B$; that is, if there is a collider on that path). It is also possible to block (or unblock) a path by conditioning on variables along that path. Formally, a path is blocked by conditioning on a proposed set of variables Z if either of two conditions holds: (1) one of the non-colliders on the path is in the set of variables Z, or (2) there is a collider on the path and neither the collider nor any of the collider's descendants is in Z. This is described in more detail in Chapter Sixteen and Pearl (2000).

FIGURE 17.2A, B, AND C. CAUSAL DIAGRAMS DEPICTING INVALID INSTRUMENTS.

2a. If there is a direct path from Z to Y that does not pass through X, Z is not a valid instrument for the effect of X on Y.

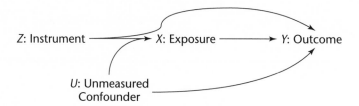

2b. If there is a path from Z to a common prior cause of X and Y, Z is not a valid instrument for the effect of X on Y.

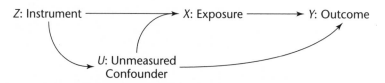

2c. If there is a prior cause of Z that directly affects Y (not exclusively mediated by X), then Z is not a valid instrument for the effect of X on Y.

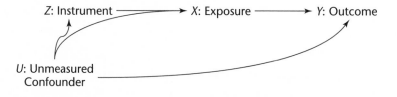

If there were a path from U to Z, then Z would not be a valid instrument (Figure 17.2c). Each of these scenarios would invalidate the instrument because the statistical relation between Z and Y would not arise exclusively owing to the causal effect of X on Y. Note that a valid instrument for the effect of X on Y is *not* a confounder of the relation between X and Y. If Z confounds the relation between X and Y, for example because it is a common prior cause of X and Y as in Figure 17.2a, then Z is not a valid instrument.

To interpret IV effect estimates as causal parameters, we need additional assumptions beyond those encoded in the causal structures presented in Figure 17.1a and b. We focus on the interpretation of the IV estimate possible under the monotonicity assumption. Under monotonicity, we assume that the direction of the effect of Z on X is the same for everyone in the sample. That is, if Z increases X for one person, it must either increase or not affect X for all other people as well. It cannot increase X for some people and decrease it for others. For example, in an RCT, the monotonicity assumption implies that there is nobody who would have refused the treatment if assigned to treatment but would have (perversely) sought out the treatment if assigned to control.

Obtaining IV Estimates

There are several ways to calculate IV estimates. The intuition is best exemplified with what is sometimes called the Wald estimator. To calculate the Wald IV estimate, first calculate the relationship between the instrument and the outcome (Z and Y). If Z is treatment assignment in an RCT, this is the ITT estimate. The relationship between Z and Y provides a test of the claim that X affects Y: if X has no effect on Y then Z and Y should be independent. Conversely, if X affects Y, then Z and Y will *not* be independent, although the association between Z and Y will not be of the same magnitude as the association between X and Y. To estimate the effect of X on Y, we must take into account the fact that Z does not perfectly determine X. This is the second step in calculating the Wald IV estimate: we *scale up* the effect of Z on Y by a factor proportional to the effect of Z on X. The IV estimate of the effect is simply the ratio of the difference in Y across different values of Z to the difference in X across different values of Z. Define $E(Y = 1 | Z = 1)$ as the mean value of Y among subjects for whom $Z = 1$, (that is, those people randomized to receive treatment). Then the IV estimate of the effect of X on Y is

$$\frac{E(Y = 1 | Z = 1) - E(Y = 1 | Z = 0)}{E(X = 1 | Z = 1) - E(X = 1 | Z = 0)} \tag{1}$$

Note that if everyone followed their assigned treatment, the denominator would be one and the IV effect estimate would equal the ITT effect estimate. As adherence declines, the denominator drops from one to zero, inflating the ITT estimate in proportion to the severity of non-adherence in the trial.

The two-stage-least-squares estimator (2SLS) can be applied more generally for instruments with multiple values or to simultaneously adjust for other covariates. A 2SLS analysis consists of regressing X on Z, calculating predicted values of X based on this regression (as in equation [2]), and using these predicted values of X as independent variables in a regression model of Y (as in equation [3]). The coefficient on the predicted value of X (β_1 below) is then interpreted as the 2SLS IV estimate of the effect of X on Y. The estimated effect of the instrument on treatment, α_1 in equation (2), is sometimes called the first-stage coefficient.

$$\hat{X} = \alpha_0 + \alpha_1 Z + \alpha_k \text{ Other Predictors} \tag{2}$$

$$Y = \beta_0 + \beta_1 \hat{X} + \beta_k \text{ Other Predictors } + \varepsilon \tag{3}$$

The 2SLS estimators provide the intuition for IV analyses, but IV estimates based on 2SLS are potentially biased toward the ordinary least squares estimates when there are multiple instrumental variables with weak effects on the treatment (Bound et al. 1995). This bias occurs because the first stage of the 2SLS models (the effect of the instrument on treatment) is not known with certainty; it must be estimated from the observed data. The estimated coefficients for each term may be unbiased estimates of the "true" causal effects, but they are based on a finite sample and will not be identical to the population causal coefficients. These deviations between the true and maximum likelihood estimated first stage coefficients will be in the direction that most improves the prediction of treatment. As a result, the predicted values of treatment from the estimated first stage coefficients will be slightly correlated with the other, unmeasured, causes of treatment. Typically this correlation is very weak, but it increases with the number of instruments per observation. Because of this, when there are multiple instruments, an alternative to the 2SLS IV estimator is preferred. The properties of alternative IV estimators, such as limited information maximum likelihood (LIML), jackknife instrumental variables (JIVE) models, or two-sample or split-sample IV estimators (Angrist and Krueger 2001; Greene 2000; Kennedy 1998; Wooldridge 2002) is a topic of much econometrics research. Limited information maximum likelihood estimates the first-stage coefficients while constraining the structural parameters to avoid the finite sample bias. Jackknife instrumental variables models jackknife the estimated first stage coefficients, so that for each observation, the predicted value of the endogenous variable is estimated with coefficients calculated excluding that observation. Split-sample methods estimate the first stage on a different sample than the second stage. As of this writing, LIML has the substantial practical advantage of being automated in SAS and Stata.

Framing Natural Experiments and IVs Causally

We now turn to a discussion of the general problem of causal inference, and frame IVs as an approach to overcoming this problem. Framing IVs in terms of counterfactuals helps clarify why they work and how they relate to other methods of drawing causal inferences from observational data (Winship and Morgan 1999).

The Fundamental Challenge of Drawing Causal Inferences

A fundamental challenge in epidemiology is to draw causal inferences when, by definition, we cannot directly observe a causal contrast. For each individual, to directly estimate the causal effect of one treatment compared with another, we would need to observe the individual's outcome under the treatment she received (the actual outcome) and also her outcome under the treatment she did not receive (the counterfactual outcome). Of course, we can only observe her outcome under the actual treatment and are left to infer the counterfactual response. That is, we cannot know what her outcome would have been had we intervened to "set" or force her to receive a treatment other than the one she actually received (for a more formal definition of causal effects, see Pearl 2000, p. 70, and his discussion of the "do" operator). This is the case even if we have data from a randomized experiment. Define $Y_{X=1}$ as the value that Y would take if X were set to 1 and $Y_{X=0}$ as the value that Y would take if X were set to 0. We can only observe $E(Y_{X=1} | X = 1)$, that is, the value Y takes if X is set to 1 among those for whom X in fact equals 1; we can never observe $E(Y_{X=1} | X = 0)$.

Why Randomization Overcomes This

Usually, we draw an inference about the average value of the counterfactual outcomes for a group of people who received one treatment based on the average actual outcomes of a comparison group of people who received the other treatment. In other words, we observe the difference in average value of the outcome between those exposed to X and those not exposed and use this difference as an estimate of the average difference in counterfactual outcome values.

Observed difference in Y between exposed and unexposed:

$$E(Y | X = 1) - E(Y | X = 0) \qquad (4)$$

Causal effect of X on Y:

$$E(Y_{X=1} - Y_{X=0}) \qquad (5)$$

A core assumption for drawing causal inferences from observational data is that the average outcome of the group exposed to one treatment regimen represents the average outcome the other group would have had *if* they had been exposed to the same treatment regimen; that is, the groups are exchangeable (Hernán 2004). For example, if we are examining the effect of high-school completion on health, we typically assume that the health of high-school dropouts represents the health the high-school graduates would have experienced *had they left school before graduation*. Randomization helps ensure that each person's expected outcome with or without treatment is independent of which treatment that person actually receives. Treatment group assignment in a perfectly conducted RCT is independent of both the known and unknown confounders, thus ensuring exchangeability (with a large enough sample).

If treatment is not randomly assigned, the assumption of exchangeability may not be plausible. We may suspect, for example, that individuals who completed high school are somehow different from those who left school early, and thus the graduates would have had better health even if they had left school early. Treatment received (more education or less education) is not independent of the outcomes the individual would have had under either treatment regime. For example, the amount of education received and subsequent health may have a common prior cause that confounds the relationship.[4] Covariate adjustment is a standard response to this problem in epidemiology research: we attempt to measure and adjust for a set of covariates such that within strata of these covariates, the treated and untreated are exchangeable. Although we have reason to believe (based on comparisons of observational and randomized studies) that covariate adjustment is frequently successful, in many other circumstances it is not plausible that we have adequately measured all confounding pathways.

How Natural Experiments Mimic Randomized Trials

Natural experiments mimic RCTs in that the mechanism determining each person's exposure is independent of the outcome that individual would experience under either exposure value. The factor that determines the chance that an individual is exposed is an instrument for the effect of the exposure on the outcome (Angrist et al. 1996; Pearl 2000), in exactly the sense shown in Figure 17.1a. Treatment group assignment in an RCT is an example of an ideal instrument. Let us assume that adherence to assigned treatment is imperfect because some people do not take the treatment to which they are assigned, as is typical in RCTs. The experiment can still be used to assess whether the treatment affects the outcome, provided we assume that nobody perversely seeks the treatment contrary to their assigned treatment (that is, assuming monotonicity). Natural experiments created by circumstances outside of researchers' control (for example, policy changes, weather events, or natural disasters) are another approach to avoiding confounding. The natural experiment provides an instrument. This leads to the counterfactual definition of a valid instrument: Z is not independent of X, but Z is independent of Y_X (the counterfactual value of Y for any value of X) (Pearl 2000).

---

[4]Confounding may also occur if the association arose by chance rather than because of a common cause.

For example, recent work exploits changes in state compulsory schooling laws (CSLs) as a natural experiment for the effect of schooling. Although all states had CSLs in place by 1918, states differed substantially with respect to the number of years required (that is, the age of mandatory primary school enrollment and the age of permitted drop out). Over the course of the century, many states changed their schooling requirements, some more than once. As a result, some elderly U.S. residents were born in states that required only a few years of school before a child could drop out, whereas others were born in places that required up to twelve years. Lleras-Muney (2002) demonstrated that CSLs influenced completed schooling for children born in each state; individuals born in states with long CSL requirements completed more years of schooling, on average, than individuals born in states with short CSL requirements. She used this approach to estimate the effect of years of completed schooling on all-cause mortality (Lleras-Muney 2005). The analysis treated year of birth and state of birth as "treatment assignments" that influenced but did not perfectly determine the amount of schooling children complete.

In terms of hypothesized causal structure, natural experiments and RCTs ideally both follow the structure shown in Figure 17.1a, where Z represents treatment assignment. In a natural experiment, this might be an indicator for whether the observation was before or after a policy change; X represents the treatment received, (for example, how much education the individual actually completed). This structure may be incorrect for either an RCT or for a natural experiment. The important difference between RCTs and natural experiments, however, is the extent to which we might put faith in the hypothesized causal structure.

The common threats to validity in RCTs can be described as modifications to the causal structures in Figure 17.1. Clinical trial participants or treating physicians are typically blinded with respect to treatment assignment on the grounds that knowing treatment status could affect how symptoms are perceived or the outcome assessment (Friedman et al. 1996; Weiss 1998, pp. 4, 23). This would be represented by drawing an arrow directly from Z to Y, as in Figure 17.2a. With such an arrow, Z is no longer a valid instrument for the effect of X on Y. This same diagram would explain why the phenomenon termed "compensatory behavior"—in which trial participants aware that they were assigned to placebo compensate by taking other efforts to improve their outcomes—is a threat to validity in trials (Friedman et al. 1996; Neuman 1997). Many of the internal validity threats listed in Cook and Campbell's classic text (1979), such as resentful demoralization or compensatory rivalry, could be summarized as alterations to the causal structure presented in Figure 17.1a. Despite these concerns, natural experiments often appear to meet the assumptions for a valid instrument; that is, we may consider Figure 17.1a a plausible causal structure to describe the data generated by a natural experiment.

In this case, natural experiments provide valid tests for the existence of causal relations and can further be used to estimate the magnitude of the causal effect for people whose treatment was influenced by the exposure.

The ITT Estimate Versus the IV Estimate

The extent of non-adherence is a second important difference between RCTs and natural experiments. Imperfect adherence is the norm in RCTs, leading to extensive work on analyses of "broken experiments" (Barnard et al. 1998), but the level of adherence in natural experiments is often much lower than in RCTs. A crucial insight for using IVs is to understand that, although high adherence is preferable for many reasons, with a valid instrument it is possible to derive consistent estimates of the causal effect even if adherence is low. The ITT estimate can be calculated with data generated by either RCTs or natural experiments. In either case, the ITT estimate provides a consistent test of the null hypothesis that treatment has no effect on the outcome (although this does not hold for trials comparing two alternative treatments, when the null is that the two alternatives have equivalent effects (Robins and Greenland 1996). As adherence declines, however, the magnitude of the ITT estimate will be increasingly distant from the magnitude of the true causal effect of receiving the treatment (assuming this effect is non-zero). Thus, when analyzing natural experiments in which the instrument had only a modest effect on probability of treatment, it is crucial to adjust for non-adherence in order to estimate the effect of receiving the treatment. The same point can be made for RCTs; it is just a matter of degree.

How can we derive an effect estimate that accounts for non-adherence? First, we will discuss the problems with either an as-treated analysis, in which the treated are compared with the non-treated, or a per-protocol analysis, in which compliers in the treated group are compared with compliers in the control group (that is, compliers in the $Z = 1$ group with compliers in the $Z = 0$ group). We will then explain why the IV estimate does not have the same problems as the other approaches.

Consider the example data shown in Figure 17.3. These data were generated according to rules consistent with the causal diagram shown in Figure 17.3a. There are three exogenous variables: Z (a dichotomous instrument or treatment assignment), U_1 (a three-level variable that affects both the treatment received, X, and the outcome, Y), and U_2. Note that the causal diagram in Figure 17.3a is nearly structurally identical to the diagram for a valid instrument shown in Figure 17.1a, except that the variable U_2 is omitted from Figure 17.1a (because U_2 affects only one other variable in the diagram, namely Y).

To make this more concrete, imagine that this represents an experiment in which participants are randomly assigned to receive a scholarship for college tuition (Z, with the goal of estimating the effect of completing college (X) on later health (Y). Let U_1 represent the education of the participant's mother, classed into three levels, which affects both likelihood of completing college and the participant's later health. Let U_2 represent a genetic determinant of health, which is independent of college completion and mother's education. The diagram in Figure 17.3a specifies

FIGURE 17.3A, B, AND C.   EXAMPLE CONTRASTING ITT, IV, AND POPULATION AVERAGE CAUSAL EFFECT IN TWO POPULATIONS.

3a. Causal DAG consistent with the data for population 1.

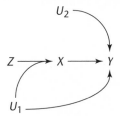

3b. Table showing the distribution of observed and counterfactual variables in populations 1 and 2.

Exogenous Variables

	Z	U_1	(Type)	U_2	$X_{z=0}$	$X_{z=1}$	X	$Y_{x=0}$	$Y_{x=1}$	Y	*n* (Popln 1)	*n* (Popln 2)
Control	0	0	(never)	0	0	0	0	0	0	0	200	100
	0	1	(cooperator)	0	0	1	0	0	1	0	200	200
	0	2	(always)	0	1	1	1	0	1	1	200	300
	0	0	(never)	1	0	0	0	0	1	0	200	200
	0	1	(cooperator)	1	0	1	0	1	1	1	200	200
	0	2	(always)	1	1	1	1	1	1	1	200	200
Treatment	1	0	(never)	0	0	0	0	0	0	0	200	100
	1	1	(cooperator)	0	0	1	1	0	1	1	200	200
	1	2	(always)	0	1	1	1	0	1	1	200	300
	1	0	(never)	1	0	0	0	0	1	0	200	200
	1	1	(cooperator)	1	0	1	1	1	1	1	200	200
	1	2	(always)	1	1	1	1	1	1	1	200	200

Individuals whose mothers had low education ($U_1 = 0$) are never treated, that is $X = 0$ regardless of the value of Z. Individuals whose mothers had high education ($U_1 = 2$) are always treated, that is, $X = 1$ regardless of the value of Z. Individuals whose mothers had middle levels of education, ($U_1 = 1$) are called "cooperators", because in these people $X = Z$. Y is determined by X, U_1, and U_2. $Y = 0$ unless either a) X and U_2 are both equal to 1, or b) $U_1 > 0$ and $X = 1$, or c) $U_1 > 0$ and $U_2 = 1$.

FIGURE 17.3A, B, AND C.   EXAMPLE CONTRASTING ITT, IV, AND POPULATION AVERAGE CAUSAL EFFECT IN TWO POPULATIONS. *(Continued)*

3c. Table of parameter estimates calculated from populations 1 and 2.

	Popln 1	Popln 2
$Pr(Y=1|Z=1)$	0.67	0.75
$Pr(Y=1|Z=0)$	0.50	0.58
ITT Risk Difference	**0.17**	**0.17**
$Pr(X=1|Z=1)$	0.67	0.75
$Pr(X=1|Z=0)$	0.33	0.42
Randomization Effect on Treatment	**0.33**	**0.33**
IV Risk Difference	**0.50**	**0.50**
$Pr(Y_{x=0}=1)$	0.33	0.33
$Pr(Y_{x=1}=1)$	0.83	0.92
Population Average Causal Risk Difference	**0.50**	**0.58**
$Pr(Y_{x=0}=1|cooperators)$	0.50	0.50
$Pr(Y_{x=1}=1|cooperators)$	1.00	1.00
Risk Difference Among Cooperators	**0.50**	**0.50**
$Pr(Y_{x=0}=1|never)$	0.00	0.00
$Pr(Y_{x=1}=1|never)$	0.50	0.67
Risk Difference Among Never-Takers	**0.50**	**0.67**
$Pr(Y_{x=0}=1|always)$	0.50	0.40
$Pr(Y_{x=1}=1|always)$	1.00	1.00
Risk Difference Among Always-Takers	**0.50**	**0.60**

the existence of causal relations but not the details of these relationships. The data in Figure 17.3b were generated by assuming a population distribution (shown in column "n (Popln 1)") for the three exogenous variables (Z, U_1, and U_2) and using the following two rules to determine the values of X and Y. The first rule specifies the value of college completion (X), given scholarship (Z) and mother's education (U_1). The three values of U_1 (0, 1, or 2) correspond to three "types" of people: those with the lowest value of mother's education will not receive treatment X (complete college) regardless of their random assignment to scholarship (they are never-takers); individuals with the middle level of mother's education ($U_1 = 1$) will receive treatment X if and only if assigned to $Z = 1$ (they are cooperators); and those with the highest values of mother's education will receive treatment X regardless of their assignment (always-takers). This is summarized in the following rule.

Rule 1) $X = 0$ if $Z + U_1 < = 1$; $X = 1$ if $Z + U_1 > 1$.

Consistent with monotonicity, this rule assumes that there are no "contrarians" in the population who receive treatment X if and only if assigned to $Z = 0$. That is, there is nobody in the population who would complete college without a scholarship but would fail to complete college if he received a scholarship. The second rule used to generate the population distribution 1, shown in Figure 17.3b specifies the value Y will take, given the values of X, U_1, and U_2.

Rule 2) $Y = 0$ unless either:

$-X$ and U_2 are both equal to 1, or

$-U_1 > 0$ and $X + U_2 \geqslant 1$.

In other words, the person is healthy if he (1) both completes college and has a good genetic endowment or (2) his mother has one of the two higher values of education and he either completes college or has a good genetic endowment.

These two rules specify all counterfactual values of X and Y under all possible combinations of values for the exogenous variables, Z, U_1, and U_2. Figure 17.3b shows the counterfactual values of X, for alternative values of Z, and the counterfactual values of Y, given alternative values of X. The counterfactual values in the two randomized groups are identical; the goal of randomization has been achieved. The *actual* values differ because randomized assignment affects the values of X (for people who follow their assigned treatment), which affects the value of Y. The causal risk difference (cRD) for the effect of X on Y can be calculated as the weighted average of the difference in the counterfactuals:

$$\text{Causal RD} = \text{cRD} = [\Pr(Y_{X=1} = 1) - \Pr(Y_{X=0} = 1)]$$
$$= [(1000/1200) - (400/1200)] = 0.5 \tag{6}$$

What is the risk difference (RD) calculated with an intent-to-treat analysis?

$$\text{ITT RD} = [\Pr(Y = 1 \mid Z = 1) - \Pr(Y = 1 \mid Z = 0)]$$
$$= [(800/1200) - (600/1200)] = 0.17 \tag{7}$$

The ITT RD is much smaller than the causal RD because the randomized assignment only affected treatment in one-third of the population (the cooperators).

We might also calculate the as-treated RD, comparing people who received treatment with those who did not:

$$\text{As Treated RD} = \Pr(Y = 1 \mid X = 1) - \Pr(Y = 1 \mid X = 0)$$
$$= (1200/1200) - (200/1200) = 0.83 \tag{8}$$

Finally, we could compare cooperators in the treatment group with cooperators in the control group—that is, subjects in the scholarship group ($Z = 1$) who completed college ($X = 1$) versus subjects in the control group ($Z = 0$) who did not complete college ($X = 0$). We will call this the per-protocol RD.

$$\text{Per-Protocol RD} = \Pr(Y = 1 \mid Z = 1, X = 1) - \Pr(Y = 1 \mid Z = 0, X = 0)$$
$$= (800/800) - (200/800) = 0.75 \tag{9}$$

The as-treated RD and the per-protocol RD are both larger than the causal RD. This is because the relationship between the treatment received (X) and health is confounded by U_1. By using treatment *received* instead of treatment *assigned*, we are throwing away the advantage of the randomized trial and are again vulnerable to all the validity threats in any observational study.

Under our assumptions, the ITT underestimates and the adherent RD overestimates the causal RD. The IV estimate uses the ITT RD and scales it up in inverse proportion to the level of adherence in the study. In this population, one-third of the people in the control group received the treatment, and two-thirds of the people in the treatment group received the treatment. Thus, adherence can be estimated as $\Pr(X = 1) \mid Z = 1) - \Pr(X = 1 \mid Z = 0) = 0.33$. The ITT RD reflects the causal effect of X on Y in the third of the population whose treatment *changed* as a result of their randomized assignment. The ITT RD is thus diluted by a factor of three compared with the causal RD, but the IV estimate reflects a correction for this:

$$\text{IV RD} = (\Pr(Y = 1 \mid Z = 1) - \Pr(Y = 1 \mid Z = 0))/(\Pr(X = 1 \mid Z = 1)$$
$$- \Pr(X = 1 \mid Z = 0)) = 0.17/0.3 = 0.5 \tag{10}$$

The IV RD equals the causal RD in this example, but it obscures an important caveat in IV analyses. The example data were created assuming the effect of X on Y did not differ between never-takers, cooperators, and always-takers. This need not be the case, however. In general, the IV estimate is consistent for the causal effect of exposure among cooperators, that is, those subjects who would have taken the treatment if and only if assigned to the treatment. In our causal structure, these are people with $U_1 = 1$. The effect of treatment on the outcome among cooperators may or may not be the same as the effect among never-takers or always-takers. To see this substantively, consider the example of college scholarships. Suppose that individuals whose mothers have the lowest education would benefit the *most* from a college degree. There are many reasons that college completion may have heterogenous treatment effects: for example, the degree might afford improved access to medical care, which is especially beneficial to people who had limited resources in childhood, or perhaps mother's education (U_1) happens to be associated with genetic risk (U_2). We can demonstrate this in our numerical example by changing the sample size for each type of person (for example, for each row in Figure 17.3). Imagine that the sample sizes were as described for population 2 in Figure 17.3, with fewer than 200 people in rows one and seven, and more in rows three and nine. This change does not violate the assumption of randomization (the distribution is still identical between those with $Z = 0$ and those with $Z = 1$). Note, however, that this causal structure is not consistent with the diagram shown in Figure 17.3a, because it implies that the variables U_1 and U_2, which were statistically independent in population 1, are statistically associated in population 2.

In this new population, the causal RD among cooperators is 0.50, the causal RD among the always-takers is 0.60, and the causal RD among the never-takers is 0.67. The IV RD is 0.50, which is identical to the causal RD for cooperators.

The preceding discussion is premised on the assumption that there is nobody in the population who will complete college if and only if assigned *not to receive the scholarship.* That is, although some respondents' behavior may not be affected by the treatment assignment, nobody will perversely pursue the opposite of his or her assigned treatment. If there are any such people in the population, sometimes called contrarians or defiers, the IV effect estimate does not converge to the causal effect among the cooperators. As discussed previously, the interpretation of the IV estimator depends on this monotonicity assumption (Angrist et al. 1996). This assumption is often considered a major limitation of IV analyses, but note that if we believe the population includes defiers, the ITT estimate is similarly uninterpretable.

In summary, the IV estimate can be used to derive causal effect estimates for that part of the sample whose exposure was affected by the instrument. This is sometimes termed the local average treatment effect or LATE. The IV estimate may or may not differ from other causal parameters of interest, such as the average causal effect for the entire sample or the effect of treatment on the treated (TOT). These other causal parameters may be estimated under additional assumptions. For example, if we assume either that there are no "always-takers" in the population, or that the effect of the treatment on the always-takers is the same as the effect on the cooperators, the IV estimate is equal to the TOT. This assumption may be plausible if the treatment is very difficult to obtain except by participating in the experiment. Without these assumptions, it may be possible to at least estimate the bounds of possible values of these causal parameters (Balke and Pearl 1997). Unlike effect estimates derived by contrasting outcomes in trial participants who adhered to their assigned treatment, the IV estimate is consistent even if there is an unmeasured factor that affects both adherence and the outcome.

The relevance and interest of the IV versus the ITT or other causal parameters depend on the substantive question (Robins and Greenland 1996). In many cases, it seems plausible that the treatment has a similar effect on everyone or, at least, that the average causal effect of treatment on those whose treatment was affected by the instrument would be identical to the average causal effect of treatment on those unaffected by the instrument. For example, one might argue that, when considering asbestos exposure in an occupational setting, the effect of exposure on the exposed and the unexposed is likely to be similar. On the other hand, social phenomena may have different effects on population subgroups, and these subgroups may be more or less likely to respond to an instrument in a natural experiment. For example, a long-standing debate in social science research concerns the differential financial returns to education for blacks and whites (Link et al. 1976; Welch 1973), and recent findings suggest similar interaction between education and race in affecting health (Farmer and Ferraro 2005). Similarly, some evidence suggests that social connections and psychosocial interventions have different effects on women than on men (Unger et al. 1999). Different effects on subgroups who take up the treatment may occur even when treatment is explicitly randomized. Evidence from the Moving to Opportunity trial (Kaufman et al. 2003; Liebman et al. 2004) suggests that uptake of a randomized treatment offer (a voucher to move to housing in low-poverty communities) was complex and possibly influenced by the perceived benefit of the treatment (for further discussion of this issue in relation to this trial, see Kaufman et al. 2003). In some cases, it seems plausible that the "marginal" person who would be treated if and only if assigned to treatment by the instrument will have less to gain from the treatment than others. If an individual stands to gain a great deal from a specific treatment, he or she would probably have pursued it regardless of the instrument. Consider a medical treatment known to be beneficial to patients with extreme values of a clinical indicator but of uncertain value for patients with less extreme values of the clinical indicator (for example, hypertension medication). Patients with extremely high blood pressure probably stand the most to gain from medication, and they are thus the most likely to be treated. It is patients with borderline hypertension who may or may not receive treatment, and it is the effect of medication on these "gray area" patients that would be the most useful for informing future medical practice. An appropriate instrument might influence whether or not these marginal patients received medication and thus could identify exactly the effect of interest. Clearly, this reasoning only makes sense for some types of treatment and some instruments. Research on the effects of changes in the Swedish compulsory schooling laws (CSLs) on earnings suggests that increases in compulsory schooling had the largest influence on education of high-ability children from disadvantaged socioeconomic backgrounds and the additional schooling benefited these children more than others (Meghir and Palme 2005).

The potential discrepancy between the IV estimate and the average causal effect does not invalidate the IV effect estimate; it merely indicates that the effect of forcing the entire population to receive the treatment would not be accurately estimated by the IV estimate. It may be considered an advantage that the IV estimate corresponds to the effect of treatment for the "marginal" person, that is, the person who would not receive the treatment except for the instrument. If the IV estimate is not of interest, another option is to attempt to derive bounds for the population average causal effect, as discussed in detail by Pearl (2000).

A Good Instrument Is Hard to Find

Thinking of good natural experiments for the exposure at hand requires a depth of understanding of the processes that lead individuals to be exposed:

> ... the natural experiments approach to instrumental variables is fundamentally grounded in theory, in the sense that there is usually a well-developed story or model motivating the choice of instruments. Importantly, these stories have implications that can be used to support or refute a behavioral interpretation of the resulting instrumental variable estimates (Angrist and Krueger 2001, p. 76).

Recognizing potential instruments requires substantive knowledge about the exposure of interest combined with a mental knack: a backwards leap of imagination from the exposure to the factors that determined that exposure. Finding testable implications of a particular story about why an instrument influences the exposure can substantially buttress one's confidence in the instrument, and this also requires substantive knowledge about the exposure and the instrument. Countless IV analyses have been published in the social science literature, some more compelling than others. Instrumental variables methods are also gaining acceptance in health services research (McClellan and Newhouse 2000; Newhouse and McClellan 1998). A few specific examples and some critiques of these examples are reviewed in the following paragraphs.

In an influential but controversial paper, Angrist and Krueger (1991) took advantage of a quirk in CSLs to estimate the effect of education on earnings. Many states' CSLs effectively require less schooling for children born in January than for children born in December. An example of such a law would require that children enter school in the fall of the calendar year in which they turn six but may quit school on their sixteenth birthday. The result of this difference is that there is a seasonal effect on completed education. On average, U.S. children born in the fourth quarter of the year complete slightly more school than children born in the first quarter of the year. Arguing that month of birth should not have any other reason to affect earnings, Angrist and Krueger therefore used quarter of birth as an instrument to estimate the effect of years of completed schooling on earnings. They found that first-quarter-born children had slightly lower earnings than children born later in the year. Others (Bound and Jaeger 1996) have criticized this instrument on the grounds that season of birth is associated with personality characteristics (Chotai et al. 2001), shyness (Gortmaker et al. 1997), height (Weber et al. 1998), mortality (Gavrilov and Gavrilova 1999), and schizophrenia risk (Mortensen et al. 1999). Any of these factors might affect health through mechanisms other than completed education. It is difficult to directly eliminate these alternative explanations. Angrist and Krueger bolstered their claim by pointing out that the alternatives tend to emphasize *season* of birth rather than the administrative concept of quarter of birth. Seasons do not have abrupt thresholds. Angrist and Krueger show abrupt differences in education and income between December births and January births, suggesting that season-based explanations are not adequate. They also provided evidence that the differences in schooling emerge in middle and high school, as would be expected if they were due to CSLs.

A popular approach to finding instruments exploits state-level policies, such as the state and temporal variation in CSLs as mentioned earlier. For example, Evans and Ringel used state cigarette taxes as an instrument for smoking during pregnancy, because cigarette prices tend to affect smoking rates but would have no other obvious mechanism to influence birth outcomes. They found IV estimates of the causal effect of smoking on birth weight very similar to effect estimates derived from a randomized trial of a prenatal smoking cessation program (Evans and Ringel 1999; Permutt and Hebel 1989). Because state policies or characteristics are ecological variables, using them as instruments invites criticism. Any one state policy likely correlates with numerous other state-level characteristics, potentially rendering the instrument invalid. Instrumenting based on changes in state policies over time may help alleviate this problem, especially if it is possible to combine geographic differences with temporal differences to define the instrument.

Other notable IV applications in health research have included estimating the impact of intensive treatment on outcome of acute myocardial infarction, using differential distance to alternative types of hospitals as an instrument (McClellan et al. 1994); the effect of length of postpartum hospital stay, instrumented with hour-of-delivery, on risk of newborn readmission (Malkin et al. 2000); the influence of prenatal care visits, instrumented with a bus drivers' strike, on birth outcomes (Evans and Lien 2005); and waiting time on liver transplant outcomes, instrumented with blood type (Howard 2000). Hoxby (2000) used the number of streams in a metropolitan area as an instrument for school choice, on the grounds that streams would have influenced the boundaries of school districts when they were defined in the eighteenth and nineteenth centuries. Cutler uses the same variable as an instrument for residential racial segregation (Cutler and Glaeser 1997). This work is fascinating because of the substantive relevance of residential segregation to social epidemiology research, but the exact exposure influenced by the instruments is somewhat ambiguous.

Epidemiology has a long history of using natural experiments to test causal effects (Costello et al. 2003; Dow and Schmeer 2003; Susser and Stein 1994). Unfortunately, these experiments are occasionally analyzed in ways that ignore the instrument and focus on differences in the exposure or treatment actually received.

Such analyses throw away the advantages of the natural experiment and are fraught with the same potential biases as any observational study.

Some natural experiments may not be amenable to calculating a classic two-stage IV estimate, for example because a direct measure of the treatment is not available. The number of days in the school term seems a promising instrument for estimating the effect of time in a school classroom on health: term length varied substantially between states in 1900 and increased in most states between 1900 and 1950. An IV effect estimate cannot be directly calculated, however, because in most epidemiologic studies, years of schooling is the only available measure of the time an individual spent in a classroom. Years of schooling will have the same value for someone who completed ten years of school in a 180-day term length school as for someone who completed ten years of school in a 120-day term length school, although the former student would have spent 50 percent more time in the classroom. Assuming that longer term lengths increase the average amount of time a student spends in the classroom, even if actual classroom time is unknown, we can still use the reduced form coefficient (ITT estimate) to test the hypothesis that classroom time affects health. We cannot directly calculate the IV estimate without additional assumptions about the unobserved number of days in a classroom.

In a study on the effects of psychological stress on mortality, Phillips et al. (2001) hypothesized that anticipating bad events increased mortality risk. To test this, they took advantage of the observation that the number four is considered unlucky by many ethnic Japanese and Chinese Americans and that many ethnic Chinese consider the fourth day of the month to be bad luck. They hypothesized that mortality rates for Chinese- and Japanese-American elderly would show a spike on the fourth day of the month. With twenty-six years of mortality records, they found exactly this spike, due primarily to an increase in deaths from chronic heart disease. Furthermore, they demonstrated that it was not observed among whites (for whom the number four does not have negative connotations). This analysis was not amenable to calculation of an IV effect estimate, because the psychological stress associated with the unlucky day was not measured. Nonetheless, the association between the instrument (day of the month) and the outcome (death) supports the hypothesis that stress exacerbates mortality risk. The controversy surrounding this study highlights a disadvantage of using a natural experiment when the exposure of interest is not directly measured. Subsequent work failed to replicate this finding in other samples (see Smith 2002 and review in Skala 2004), but without a measure of stress, we cannot tell whether this is because stress does not affect mortality or because the fourth day of the month does not induce much anxiety.

In some cases, the instrument is a policy change, and the ITT estimate itself may be of primary substantive interest. The ITT estimate in this case gives the estimated effect of changing the policy. This is especially common in social epidemiology, for which the desired outcome of a successful research finding is not that individuals take a certain pill but rather that an institution such as the government changes a policy or an administrative standard.

Although natural experiments without measures of the primary exposure can be informative, a good natural experiment combined with solid measurement of the exposure variable is invaluable. During the Dutch Famine Winter of 1944, the Netherlands was occupied by Nazis who limited food access for urban residents in retaliation for resistance activities. The calorie restrictions were very severe, and the timing is fairly well documented. As a result, a host of studies have been generated focusing on infants conceived and born during the Famine Winter and showing how calorie restriction at specific sensitive time points affects various health outcomes (Susser and Stein 1994; Susser et al. 1999).

Mendelian randomization—the idea of exploiting genetic variations to draw inferences regarding environmental causes of diseases (Smith 2004)—can also be considered in the framework of IV analyses (Thomas and Conti 2004). Under some circumstances, genotype can be a valid instrument for estimating the causal effect of a phenotype (the physical manifestations of the gene) on a disease. Knowledge of the causal link between the phenotype and disease may highlight many potentially manipulable environmental determinants of that phenotype. For example, Katan (2004) originally proposed using allelic variations of the apoE gene as instruments to estimate the effect of cholesterol level on cancer, with an eye to informing dietary choices. The primary challenges of Mendelian randomization studies—pleiotropy, developmental compensation, and confounding due to population stratification (Smith and Ebrahim 2003)—each correspond to violations of the assumptions for a valid instrument. For example, the apoE gene may affect several phenotypes in addition to lipid metabolism; because not all of the paths linking the apoE gene to cancer are mediated by cholesterol level, it is a questionable instrument to estimate the effect of cholesterol on cancer.

A final note on examples of instruments is that randomized studies with encouragement designs and regression discontinuity models often exploit the idea of an IV analysis, although this is not always explicit.

A Few Other Points

An instrument may be valid for estimating the effect of X on Y but invalid for estimating the effect of X on some other outcome W. There may be no common prior causes of X and Y but several common prior causes of X and W. In many cases, however, the substantive argument for the instrument validity in one case extends to other outcomes.

We have focused on a simple example with a dichotomous instrument and a dichotomous exposure. Instrumental variables estimates can be calculated when either or both the instrument and the exposure of interest take multiple values. When the exposure is not binary, the IV estimate is a weighted average of the causal effect of each level of exposure among the subpopulation of individuals whose exposure was affected by the instrument (Angrist and Imbens 1995). It is often desirable to have multiple instruments. Multiple instruments can be useful both to improve the statistical power of an IV analysis and, if power is adequate, to test the validity of instruments against one another. Finally, some instruments may be valid only after conditioning on a measured covariate. A common prior cause of the instrument and the outcome renders the instrument invalid, unless that confounder can be measured and statistically controlled. Of course, instruments with no such common prior cause are far more appealing than instruments that can be "fixed" by statistical adjustment. A valid instrument need not directly affect the exposure of interest. It merely needs to be statistically associated with this exposure, and this association may arise from sharing a prior cause (Pearl 2000, p. 248), although in this case a modified set of assumptions is required to define the causal interpretation of the IV estimate.

The two-stage-least-squares (2SLS) technique is sometimes confused with propensity score models, because the first step in both methods is to model the predicted value of the exposure of interest. The approaches should not be confused; they are aimed at accomplishing different goals and are technically distinct. The goal of propensity score modeling is to improve adjustment for measured confounders. The goal of IV analysis is to derive an unbiased effect estimate even when we have not measured all of the important confounders. The second stage of a propensity score model might include either adjusting for both observed X and the propensity score or matching on the propensity score. The second stage of a 2SLS IV model regresses the outcome variable on all the covariates and the predicted value of the exposure (X) but *excludes* the actual value of X.

Instrumental Variables in Economics Research

The conduct of scientific research is extensively influenced by disciplinary cultures. Although the problem of unmeasured common prior causes is a fundamental challenge in both economics and epidemiology, the typical response to this problem differs between the two disciplines. Epidemiologists tend to rely on statistical adjustment for ever-longer lists of covariates, whereas natural experiments and IV analyses have traditionally been considered more compelling in the economics literature. Many of the most interesting IV analyses have been conducted to address research questions in economics. Typically, skepticism about either approach can be justified, given the limitations of our knowledge. One can nearly always imagine an unmeasured confounder that might influence both exposure and outcome. Similarly, it is extremely difficult to think of instruments that are beyond reproach. Beyond the obvious implication that one should never give a talk that will be attended by both epidemiologists and economists, the take-home lesson is the importance of humility about all of our methods. Familiarity breeds acquiescence, and the scientific literature is littered with bandwagon moments, in which everyone starts agreeing with a false claim simply because it's been made so often. Testing hypotheses with multiple approaches, especially if the alternative methods depend on different assumptions, can be invaluable.

Economists rarely use causal diagrams or even causal language to discuss IVs. It may therefore be helpful to review the standard economic account of IV analyses and explain why it coincides with the explanation we give. An introductory econometrics textbook authored by Kennedy states, "The IV procedure produces a consistent estimator in a situation in which a regressor is contemporaneously correlated with the error" (1998, p. 139).

Instrumental variables here are described as a solution when the data violate one of the assumptions of the classical linear regression model: the residuals must be independent of the independent variables. To translate this to causal language, consider the classical regression model:

$$Y = \beta_0 + \beta_1 X + \varepsilon \qquad (11)$$

The errors (ε) in this model represent both inherent randomness in Y and factors other than X that influence Y. When the unmeasured variables that affect Y also affect X, it implies that the errors will be correlated with the regressor X: exactly the problem described by Kennedy (other situations can also lead to this problem, such as measurement error). The econometric phrasing translates more or less directly into the causal language: IVs are useful to find an effect estimate when the outcome variable and the predictor of interest share an unmeasured prior cause. Kennedy continues:

> This [instrument] is a new independent variable which must have two characteristics. First, it must be contemporaneously uncorrelated with the error; and second, it must be correlated (preferably highly so) with the regressor for which it is to serve as an instrument (1998, p. 139).

This definition of a valid instrument can be given a causal interpretation. The requirement that the instrument be uncorrelated with the error translates to the claim that the instrument does not itself directly affect the outcome and it shares no common prior causes with the outcome, as shown in Figure 17.1. Adding a common prior cause of Z and Y creates an unblocked path from Z to Y that does not pass through X (as in Figure 17.2c) and violates the graphical criterion for a valid instrument. A helpful discussion of the alternative definitions can be found in Pearl (2000, pp. 247–248), where the graphical, counterfactual, and error-based definitions of IVs are considered.

One point of caution: econometrics textbooks frequently suggest using a lagged value of the exposure of interest as an instrument. This approach may be credible for some substantive questions, but it seems unlikely to provide valid instruments for the effects of various social exposures on health. Economists employ IV analyses to overcome two sorts of problems other than omitted variables bias (unmeasured confounding): simultaneous equations and error in measurements of the independent variable. The original application of IV, published in 1928 by Phillip Wright but possibly attributable to his son Sewall, addressed a simultaneous equations problem regarding the supply and demand equations for flaxseed oil (Stock and Trebbi 2003). In recent years, however, interest in using IVs to address omitted variables problems has increased (Angrist and Krueger 2001).

Limitations of IV Analyses

The most devastating critique of an IV analysis is that the instrument is not valid because it either directly affects the outcome or it has a common prior cause with the outcome. If the instrument derives from an ecological variable, these concerns are especially pertinent. The weaker the instrument (that is, the worse the non-adherence), the greater is the dependence of the IV estimate on the assumption of a valid instrument. The adjustment for compliance in the IV estimator simultaneously inflates any bias in the ITT estimate. Even a small association between the instrument and the outcome that is not mediated by the exposure of interest can produce serious biases in IV effect estimates for the exposure. For this reason, criticisms of the validity of the instrument must be taken seriously, even if they hypothesize fairly small relationships.

Comparing IV estimates with estimates from models without instruments, such as ordinary least squares (OLS) models, can provide a validity test. Often, the researcher has a pre-existing view about the direction of bias in the OLS estimates. In the case of education and health, we might expect OLS analyses to overestimate the true causal effect, because personal characteristics such as intelligence that prompt someone to attend school longer also affect health through various other pathways. On these grounds, we anticipate the IV effect estimate for a year of education will be smaller than the OLS effect estimate. In fact,

Lleras-Muney (2005) found that using an instrument for education produced larger effect estimates compared with models estimated without an instrument (for example, weighted least squares). This is not unusual with IV analyses: several important IV analyses have unexpectedly found effect estimates as large as or larger than the comparable OLS effect estimates. Results such as this do not necessarily indicate an invalid instrument, although that is an obvious concern. One possible explanation is that OLS underestimates the causal effect due to measurement error in the independent variable. As previously discussed, the IV effect may also differ from the population average effect because the cooperators either benefit more or less from the treatment than others in the population. A related concern about IVs based on natural experiments is that natural experiments may be more vulnerable to the presence of defiers than typical randomized controlled trials (RCTs).

A general criticism of IV estimates is that it is impossible to identify the particular subpopulation to which the causal effect estimate applies—those whose exposure was affected by the instrument. For any one person, we observe the level of exposure they received given the value the instrument actually took, but not the level of exposure they would have received had the instrument taken on a different value. Although we know the IV effect estimate is the causal effect among cooperators, we generally have no way to identify who is a cooperator. This is even more complicated with an exposure with multiple levels or intensities (for example, schooling may range from zero to sixteen or more years).

Sample size poses an additional challenge in applying IV methods in epidemiology. Because IV analyses identify causal effects based on changes in the subgroup of the population whose exposure was affected by the instrument, the effective sample size for the analysis is much smaller than the actual sample size. For example, only a small fraction of students are constrained by CSLs (that is, drop out of school as soon as it is legal for them to do so). Angrist and Krueger (1991) estimated that only 4 percent of sixteen-year-olds in a 1944 birth cohort were constrained to stay in school by state CSLs (which equated to keeping roughly one-third of the likely drop outs in school). As a result of the small effective sample size, the confidence intervals for IV effect estimates are often very wide. Confidence intervals can be tightened by using instruments with a greater effect on the exposure or increasing the sample size. Because of the potential for bias in weak instruments, finding "better" natural experiments (that is, instruments that have a large effect on the exposure of interest or are unequivocally valid) is generally preferable to increasing the sample size.

A more prosaic challenge in interpreting IV estimates from natural experiments is truly understanding what the instrument represents, that is, what the relevant X variable is. For example, CSLs affect the age children begin school, the age children leave school (and enter the labor market), the amount of time children spend in a classroom, the schooling credentials children receive, and whether or not they are exposed to occupational hazards at very young ages. It is possible to tell a story focusing on any of these phenomena as the crucial mediator between CSLs and health. This is one reason it is extremely appealing to use multiple instruments. For example, we may be able to find an instrument that affects time in the classroom but does not affect schooling credentials.

Multiple instruments are also appealing as validity checks (Chu et al. 2001). If the instruments truly affect the same mediating variables, then we would expect the IV estimates from the two instruments to be identical. Formal tests for instrument validity rely on this assumption. The caveat here, though, is that instruments may not affect the same mediator. Two IV estimates based on different instruments may each accurately estimate the causal effect of a slightly different exposure. For example, extending compulsory school by lowering the age for first enrollment may have different effects than extending compulsory school lengths by increasing the age for school drop out. The cognitive effect of a year of school in early childhood may differ from the effect of completing an additional year of schooling in adolescence (Gorey 2001; Mayer and Knutson 1999).

IVs in Social Epidemiology

Distinguishing between causal and non-causal explanations for the association between social conditions (interpreted broadly) and health is crucial in order to identify potential interventions. Epidemiology, and social epidemiology in particular, is troubled by a fundamental dilemma. The RCT is often considered the "gold standard" for estimating causal effects (Abel and Koch 1999; Byar et al. 1976; DeMets 2002), but observational designs are essential for exposures that, for practical or ethical reasons, cannot be randomly assigned in a trial. Social gradients in health are extremely well-documented, but the extent to which these gradients are "causal" is still hotly debated (Smith 1999), in part because of the difficulties of explicitly randomizing the exposure. Insisting on RCTs as the only valid source of evidence rules out the pursuit of many critically important lines of research. If we suspect that social factors are among the most important determinants of health, it is incumbent upon us to aggressively seek rigorous scientific approaches to test these determinants and estimate their effects.

In the absence of RCTs, epidemiologists typically rely on covariate adjustment or stratification to estimate causal parameters from observational data. Researchers often reason that if several studies find similar results in various populations, this provides compelling evidence that the relationship is causal. Frequently, however, each study adjusts for a similar set of covariates and is thus subject to a similar set of biases. Repeated analyses of the correlation between education and old age cognition can do little to test causal claims, because the validity of each study depends on essentially identical assumptions. These assumptions are never directly tested, and repeating similar study designs provides very little new information. Although some investigators have reported remarkable consistency between effect estimates from well-designed observational studies and RCTs (Benson and Hartz 2000; Concato et al. 2000), troubling inconsistencies have also been documented in the past decade (Omenn et al. 1996; Rossouw et al. 2002). Discrepancies between RCT results and observational studies of high-profile epidemiologic questions have reinvigorated the debate about the reliability of causal inferences in the absence of trial data.

Despite the difficulty of conducting full scale randomized trials of social exposures, natural experiments occur with regularity. Instrumental variables analyses, when applied to data from these natural experiments, offer useful causal tests because they are based on different, albeit strong, assumptions. Although much of the prior work using IVs has been conducted in the context of economic or other social science research questions, many of the exposures are extremely relevant to social epidemiology.

Although IV analyses can substantially strengthen claims about the causal effects of social factors, the method also has important limitations. The assumptions for a valid instrument are very strong, and small violations can lead to large biases (Bound et al. 1995). The core critique of any IV analysis is that the instrument influences the outcome in question through some pathway other than the exposure of interest. The major strength of the IV approach is that the assumptions for valid estimation are generally quite different than the assumptions for valid causal estimates from ordinary regressions. When regression models have repeatedly demonstrated an association, an additional regression estimate adds little new information because the analysis depends on the same assumptions. Instrumental variables analyses, however, are generally premised on a different set of assumptions, which may (or may not) be more palatable. At a minimum, natural experiments and IV analyses provide a valuable complement to other analytic tools for examining causal relations in social epidemiology.

Acknowledgments

I wish to thank the following people for helpful comments and suggestions on earlier drafts of this chapter: Joanna Asia Maselko, James Robins, and Manoj Mohanan. All remaining errors and confusions are my own.

References

The asterisks indicate especially accessible or influential references.

Abel, U., & Koch, A. (1999). The role of randomization in clinical studies: Myths and beliefs. *Journal of Clinical Epidemiology, 52,* 487–497.

Angrist, J. D., & Imbens, G. W. (1995). 2-stage least-squares estimation of average causal effects in models with variable treatment intensity. *Journal of the American Statistical Association, 90,* 431–442.

*Angrist, J. D., & Krueger, A. B. (1991). Does compulsory school attendance affect schooling and earnings? *The Quarterly Journal of Economics, 106,* 979–1014.

*Angrist, J. D., & Krueger, A. B. (2001). Instrumental variables and the search for identification: From supply and demand to natural experiments. *Journal of Economic Perspectives, 15,* 69–85.

*Angrist, J. D., Imbens, G. W., & Rubin, D. B. (1996). Identification of causal effects using instrumental variables. *Journal of the American Statistical Association, 91,* 444–455.

Balke, A., & Pearl, J. (1997). Bounds on treatment effects from studies with imperfect compliance. *Journal of the American Statistical Association, 92,* 1171–1176.

Barnard, J., Du, J. T., Hill, J. L., & Rubin, D. B. (1998). A broader template for analyzing broken randomized experiments. *Sociological Methods Research, 27,* 285–317.

Benson, K., & Hartz, A. J. (2000). A comparison of observational studies and randomized, controlled trials. *New England Journal of Medicine, 342,* 1878–1886.

Bound, J., & Jaeger, D. A. (1996). *On the validity of season of birth as an instrument in wage equations: A comment on Angrist and Krueger's "Does compulsory school attendance affect schooling and earnings?"* (p. 27). Cambridge, MA: National Bureau of Economic Research.

Bound, J., Jaeger, D. A., & Baker, R. M. (1995). Problems with instrumental variables estimation when the correlation between the instruments and the endogenous explanatory variable is weak. *Journal of the American Statistical Association, 90,* 443–450.

Byar, D. P., Simon, R. M., Friedewald, W. T., et al. (1976). Randomized clinical trials. Perspectives on some recent ideas. *New England Journal of Medicine, 295,* 74–80.

Chotai, J., Forsgren, T., Nilsson, L. G., & Adolfsson, R. (2001). Season of birth variations in the temperament and character inventory of personality in a general population. *Neuropsychobiology, 44,* 19–26.

Chu, T., Scheines, R., & Spirtes, P. (2001). Semi-instrumental variables: A test for instrument admissibility. In: *Uncertainty in artificial intelligence* (p. 83–90). Seattle: Morgan Kaufmann Publishers.

Concato, J., Shah, N., & Horwitz, R. I. (2000). Randomized, controlled trials, observational studies, and the hierarchy of research designs. *New England Journal of Medicine, 342,* 1887–1892.

Cook, T. D., & Campbell, D. T. (1979). *Quasi-experimentation: Design & analysis issues for field settings.* Boston: Houghton Mifflin Company.

Costello, E. J., Compton, S. N., Keeler, G., & Angold, A. (2003). Relationships between poverty and psychopathology: A natural experiment. *Journal of the American Medical Association, 290,* 2023–2029.

*Currie, J. (1995). Welfare and the well-being of children. In F. Welch (Ed.), *Fundamentals of pure and applied economics* (p. 165). Chur, Switzerland: Harwood Academic Publishers.

Cutler, D. M., & Glaeser, E. L. (1997). Are ghettos good or bad? *Quarterly Journal of Economics, 112,* 827–872.

DeMets, D. L. (2002). Clinical trials in the new millennium. *Statistics in Medicine, 21,* 2779–2787.

Dow, W. H., & Schmeer, K. K. (2003). Health insurance and child mortality in Costa Rica. *Social Science & Medicine, 57,* 975–986.

Evans, W. N., & Lien, D. S. (2005). The benefits of prenatal care: Evidence from the PAT bus strike. *Journal of Econometrics, 125,* 207–239.

Evans, W. N., & Ringel, J. S. (1999). Can higher cigarette taxes improve birth outcomes? *Journal of Public Economics, 72,* 135–154.

Farmer, M. M., & Ferraro, K. F. (2005). Are racial disparities in health conditional on socio-economic status? *Social Science & Med, 60,* 191–204.

Friedman, L. M., Furberg, C. D., & DeMets, D. L. (1996). *Fundamentals of clinical trials* (3rd ed.). St. Louis, MO: Mosby.

Gavrilov, L. A., & Gavrilova, N. S. (1999). Season of birth and human longevity. *Journal of Anti-Aging Medicine, 2,* 365–366.

Gorey, K. M. (2001). Early childhood education: A meta-analytic affirmation of the short- and long-term benefits of educational opportunity. *School Psychology Quarterly, 16,* 9–30.

Gortmaker, S. L., Kagan, J., Caspi, A., & Silva, P. A. (1997). Day length during pregnancy and shyness in children: Results from northern and southern hemispheres. *Developmental Psychobiology, 31,* 107–114.

Greene, W. H. (2000). *Econometric analysis* (4th ed.). Upper Saddle River, NJ: Prentice-Hall.

*Greenland, S. (2000). An introduction to instrumental variables for epidemiologists. *International Journal of Epidemiology, 29,* 722–729.

*Greenland, S., Pearl, J., & Robins, J. M. (1999). Causal diagrams for epidemiologic research. *Epidemiology, 10,* 37–48.

Hennekens, C. H., & Buring, J. E. (1987). *Epidemiology in medicine* (1st ed., p. 383). Boston/Toronto: Little, Brown and Company.

*Hernán, M. A. (2004). A definition of causal effect for epidemiological research. *Journal of Epidemiology and Community Health, 58,* 265–271.

Howard, D. (2000). The impact of waiting time on liver transplant outcomes. *Health Services Research, 35,* 1117–1134.

Hoxby, C. M. (2000). Does competition among public schools benefit students and taxpayers? *American Economic Review, 90,* 1209–1238.

Katan, M. B. (2004). Commentary: Mendelian randomization, 18 years on. *International Journal of Epidemiology, 33,* 10–11.

Kaufman, J. S., Kaufman, S., & Poole, C. (2003). Causal inference from randomized trials in social epidemiology. *Social Science & Medicine, 57,* 2397–2409.

Kennedy, P. (1998). *A guide to econometrics* (4th ed., p. 468). Cambridge, MA: Massachusetts Institute of Technology Press.

Liebman, J. B., Katz, L. F., & Kling, J. R. (2004). *Beyond treatment effects: Estimating the relationship between neighborhood poverty and individual outcomes in the MTO experiment* (p. 1–42). Princeton, NJ: Princeton Industrial Relations Section.

Link, C., Ratledge, E., & Lewis, K. (1976). Black-white differences in returns to schooling— some new evidence. *American Economic Review, 66,* 221–223.

Little, R. J., & Rubin, D. B. (2000). Causal effects in clinical and epidemiological studies via potential outcomes: Concepts and analytical approaches. *Annual Review of Public Health, 21,* 121–145.

Lleras-Muney, A. (2002). Were compulsory attendance and child labor laws effective? An analysis from 1915 to 1939. *Journal of Law & Economics, 45,* 401–435.

Lleras-Muney, A. (2005). The relationship between education and adult mortality in the U.S. *Review of Economic Studies, 72,* 189–221.

Malkin, J. D., Broder, M. S., & Keeler, E. (2000). Do longer postpartum stays reduce newborn readmissions? Analysis using instrumental variables. *Health Services Research, 35,* 1071–1091.

Mayer, S. E., & Knutson, D. (1999). Does the timing of school affect learning? In S. E. Mayer, & P. E. Petterson (Eds.), *Earning and learning: How schools matter* (p. 79–102). Washington, DC: Brookings Institution Press.

*McClellan, M., McNeil, B. J., & Newhouse, J. P. (1994). Does more intensive treatment of acute myocardial infarction in the elderly reduce mortality? Analysis using instrumental variables. *Journal of the American Medical Association, 272,* 859–866.

McClellan, M. B., & Newhouse, J. P. (2000). Overview of the special supplement issue. *Health Services Research, 35,* 1061–1069.

Meghir, C., & Palme, M. (2005). Educational reform, ability, and family background. *American Economic Review, 95,* 414–424.

Mortensen, P. B., Pedersen, C. B., Westergaard, T., et al. (1999). Effects of family history and place and season of birth on the risk of schizophrenia. *New England Journal of Medicine, 340,* 603–608.

Neuman, W. L. (1997). *Social research methods; qualitative and quantitative approaches* (3rd ed.). Needham Heights, MA: Allyn & Bacon.

*Newhouse, J. P., & McClellan, M. (1998). Econometrics in outcomes research: The use of instrumental variables. *Annual Review of Public Health, 19,* 17–34.

Oakes, J. M. (2004). The (mis)estimation of neighborhood effects: Causal inference for a practicable social epidemiology. *Social Science & Medicine, 58,* 1929–1952.

Omenn, G. S., Goodman, G. E., Thornquist, M. D., et al. (1996). Risk factors for lung cancer and for intervention effects in CARET, the Beta-Carotene and Retinol Efficacy Trial. *Journal of the National Cancer Institute, 88,* 1550–1559.

*Pearl, J. (2000). *Causality* (p. 384). Cambridge, UK: Cambridge University Press.

Permutt, T., & Hebel, J. R. (1989). Simultaneous-equation estimation in a clinical trial of the effect of smoking on birth weight. *Biometrics, 45,* 619–22.

Phillips, D. P., Liu, G. C., Kwok, K., Jarvinen, J. R., Zhang, W., & Abramson, I. S. (2001). The Hound of the Baskervilles effect: Natural experiment on the influence of psychological stress on timing of death. *British Medical Journal, 323,* 1443–1446.

Robins, J. M., & Greenland, S. (1996). Identification of causal effects using instrumental variables—Comment. *Journal of the American Statistical Association, 91,* 456–458.

Rossouw, J. E., Anderson, G. L., Prentice, R. L., et al. (2002). Risks and benefits of estrogen plus progestin in healthy postmenopausal women: Principal results from the Women's Health Initiative randomized controlled trial. *Journal of the American Medical Association, 288,* 321–333.

Skala, J. A.,Freedland, K. E. (2004). Death takes a raincheck. *Psychosomatic Medicine, 66,* 382–386.

Smith, G. (2002). Scared to death? *British Medical Journal, 325,* 1442–1443.

Smith, G. D. (2004). Genetic epidemiology: An "enlightened narrative"? *International Journal of Epidemiology, 33,* 923–924.

Smith, G. D., & Ebrahim, S. (2003). 'Mendelian randomization': can genetic epidemiology contribute to understanding environmental determinants of disease? *International Journal of Epidemiology, 32,* 1–22.

Smith, J. P. (1999). Healthy bodies and thick wallets: The dual relation between health and economic status. *Journal of Economic Perspectives, 13,* 145–166.

Stock, J. H., & Trebbi, F. (2003). Retrospectives—Who invented instrumental variable regression? *Journal of Economic Perspectives, 17,* 177–194.

Susser, E. B., Brown, A., & Matte, T. D. (1999). Prenatal factors and adult mental and physical health. *Canadian Journal of Psychiatry-Revue Canadienne De Psychiatrie, 44,* 326–334.

Susser, M., & Stein, Z. (1994). Timing in prenatal nutrition—A reprise of the Dutch Famine Study. *Nutrition Reviews, 52,* 84–94.

Thomas, D. C., & Conti, D. V. (2004). Commentary: The concept of "Mendelian randomization." *International Journal of Epidemiology, 33,* 21–25.

Unger, J. B., McAvay, G., Bruce, M. L., Berkman, L., & Seeman, T. (1999). Variation in the impact of social network characteristics on physical functioning in elderly persons: MacArthur studies of successful aging. *Journals of Gerontology Series B: Psychological Sciences and Social Sciences, 54,* S245–S251.

Weber, G. W., Prossinger, H., & Seidler, H. (1998). Height depends on month of birth. *Nature, 391,* 754–755.

Weiss, N. S. (1998). Clinical epidemiology. In K. J. Rothman & S. Greenland (Eds.), *Modern epidemiology* (pp. 519–528). Philadelphia, PA: Lippincott-Raven.

Welch, F. (1973). Black-white differences in returns to schooling. *American Economic Review, 63,* 893–907.

*Winship, C., & Morgan, S. L. (1999). The estimation of causal effects from observational data. *Annual Review of Sociology, 25,* 659–706.

Wooldridge, J. M. (2002). *Econometric analysis of cross section and panel data* (p. 752). Cambridge, MA: Massachusetts Institute of Technology Press.

NAME INDEX

A

Abel, U., 430, 455
Abramson, J. H., 61
Acevedo-Garcia, D., 171
Acs, G., 121
Adams, P. L., 101
Adelstein, A. M., 87
Aizer, A., 289
Alba, R. D., 101
Alison, S. S., 26
Alison, W. P., 36, 39
Alker, H. R., Jr., 318, 344
Altman, D. G., 243
Angell, K. L., 247
Angrist, J. D., 381, 418, 431,
    436, 438, 445, 447–452,
    451, 453, 454
Arber, S., 65, 66
Arias, E., 410
Armhein, C., 227, 228
Armstead, C., 98
Asada, Y., 137
Asthana, S., 61
Avlund, K., 66

B

Bach, P. B., 142
Backlund, E., 323
Baiocchi, G., 87
Balke, A., 445
Ball, T. J., 249
Banguero, H., 62
Banton, M., 90
Baquet, C., 134
Barker, M., 92
Barnard, J., 440
Barnes, D., 36
Barnett, S., 214
Barnett, V., 381
Baron, R. M., 414
Barry, J., 214
Barth, F., 89
Bartley, M., 48
Bashi, V., 105
Basilevsky, A., 7
Baumann, K. E., 272, 276, 277, 278
Beaglehole, R., 316
Bearman, P. S., 268, 276, 277
Becker, A. B., 245, 249, 254, 256

Beckwith, D., 245
Beebe-Dimmer, J., 56, 57
Beekley, M. D., 14
Bell, D., 216
Bell, W., 178
Bellman, R., 376
Ben-Shlomo, Y., 71, 73
Bénabou, R., 288
Benavides, F. G., 56
Benson, K., 456
Bentham, J., 29
Berger, V. W., 361
Berk, R., 8, 9, 10, 15, 370, 374,
    376, 389
Berkman, L. F., 60, 135, 193, 209,
    217, 229, 267, 268, 269, 271,
    272, 316
Bernstein, I., 9
Bertrand, M., 289
Betson, D. M., 112, 126–127
Bevins, A., 103
Beyers, J. M., 194
Bichat, X., 36
Bingenheimer, J., 317
Bird, C. E., 229

SUBJECT INDEX